S0-AMJ-207

LANGUAGE AND COMMUNICATION IN OLD AGE

ISSUES IN AGING
VOLUME 9
GARLAND REFERENCE LIBRARY OF SOCIAL SCIENCE
VOLUME 1104

Issues in Aging

Diana K. Harris, *Series Editor*

Language and Communication in Old Age

Multidisciplinary Perspectives

Edited by
Heidi E. Hamilton

Garland Publishing, Inc.
A member of the Taylor & Francis Group
New York and London
1999

Copyright © 1999 by Heidi E. Hamilton
All rights reserved

Library of Congress Cataloging-in-Publication Data

Language and communication in old age : multidisciplinary perspectives / edited
  by Heidi E. Hamilton.
    p.   cm. (Garland reference library of social science ; v. 1104. Issues in
aging ; v. 9)
    Includes bibliographical references and index.
    ISBN 0-8153-2356-5 (alk. paper)
    1. Aged—Language. 2. Aged—Communication.   I. Hamilton, Heidi
Ehernberger. II. Series: Garland reference library of social science ; v. 1104.
III. Series: Garland reference library of social science. Issues in aging ; v. 9.
P120.A35L36   1999
408'.2—dc21   98-38853
                                                        CIP

Cover photograph courtesy of AARP (American Association of Retired Persons).

Printed on acid-free, 250-year-life paper
Manufactured in the United States of America

for Siri and Sean
whose courage and joy
are my inspiration

Contents

Series Editor's Foreword

This series attempts to address the topic of aging from a wide variety of perspectives and to make available some of the best gerontological thought and writings to researchers, professional practitioners, and students in the field of aging as well as in other related areas. All the volumes in the series are written and/or edited by outstanding scholars and leading specialists on current issues of considerable interest.

This volume of edited papers covers a wide range of topics dealing with the relationship between old age and language. It offers the reader a diversity of perspectives while at the same time emphasizing their interconnectedness. The three sections in this collection provide an indication of the scope of this book: (1) language and communicative abilities in old age; (2) identity in old age; and (3) social norms, values, and practices in old age. This comprehensive resource on old age and language will be useful to specialists and students alike. It makes a unique and valuable contribution to the literature.

Diana K. Harris
The University of Tennessee

Acknowledgments

First and foremost I would like to thank the contributors to this volume for their enormous patience and trust. Little did they know when they agreed to contribute that, during the early stages of the volume, I would have a baby who would need to undergo bone marrow transplantation. The ensuing roller coaster ride was trying for all concerned, but each and every contributor stayed with the project, frequently voicing both their professional and personal support to me along the way. For that I am eternally thankful.

I am also grateful to Dr. Diana K. Harris, series editor, *Issues in Aging,* for her immediate support of our project. It has been a pleasure working with her as well as with the able editors of Garland Publishing Inc., especially Marie Ellen Larcada, Alexia Meyers, Phyllis Korper, and Chuck Bartelt. Special appreciation goes to Jon Berndt Olsen for generously providing critical technical assistance in the final stages of the manuscript preparation.

My initial guiding lights within the area of language and aging were and continue to be Dr. Loraine K. Obler, Dr. Nikolas Coupland and Dr. Justine Coupland. I will always be grateful to them for showing early interest in my work and supporting me at crucial points in my career. Later, but equally important, influences came from Dr. Mark Luborsky, Dr. Susan Kemper, and Dr. Ellen Ryan.

I cannot imagine a more conducive environment for conceptualizing and carrying out scholarly projects than Georgetown University's Department of Linguistics. Faculty members and students share a love for intellectual challenges while respecting a wide variety of approaches to the study of language. I have especially profited from continuing discussions there with Dr. Deborah Tannen, Dr. Deborah Schiffrin, and Dr. Roger Shuy.

This volume would not have become a reality without the support of my family, especially my husband, Dan, and my parents, Gerald and Claire Ehernberger. Their complete confidence in my abilities and stamina has been vital to my work. And, finally, a thank you as big as the heavens to my children—to Sean, whose joyful courage throughout major health problems has taught me more about life than anyone else could have, and to Siri, who gave her baby brother the most precious gift of life.

Contributors

Martin L. Albert
Boston University School of Medicine
and Boston Veterans Administration Medical Center

Joyce Allman
Texas Christian University

Rhoda Au
Boston University School of Medicine

Barbara A. Barresi
Emerson College and Boston University School of Medicine

Anne R. Bower
Philadelphia Geriatric Center

Maria G. Cattell
Millersville University and
The Field Museum of Natural History

Sandra Bond Chapman
University of Texas at Dallas

Justine Coupland
University of Wales, College of Cardiff

Nikolas Coupland
University of Wales, College of Cardiff

V. Olga B. Emery
Dartmouth Medical School

Heidi E. Hamilton
Georgetown University

Julene Johnson
University of Texas at Dallas

Valerie Cryer McKay
California State University, Long Beach

Chevelle Newsome
California State University, Sacramento

Jon Nussbaum
University of Oklahoma

Lorraine Obermann
Dawnland Center, Montpelier, Vermont

Loraine K. Obler
City University of New York

Shoko Yohena Okazaki
Meiji Gakuin University

Sandra L. Ragan
University of Oklahoma

Elif Tolga Rosenfeld
Georgetown University

Steven R. Sabat
Georgetown University

Ina Samuels
University of Massachusetts, Boston

Pamela A. Saunders
University of Kansas

Lucretia Scoufos
Alabama State University

Hanna K. Ulatowska
University of Texas at Dallas

Introduction

CHAPTER 1

Language and Communication in Old Age

Some Methodological Considerations

Heidi Ehernberger Hamilton

"Inevitably, the lifespan perspective . . . will both inform and challenge established findings in the study of virtually any context of language use."

Coupland, Coupland & Giles (1991:2)

INTRODUCTION

Language and communication in old age is an area of investigation that has been gaining momentum over recent years, although the research generated is small in comparison with that of developmental studies at the other end of the lifespan, i.e., studies of child language. As individuals age, some experience marked mental and/or physical changes; some take on new social roles (due to retirement, for example); some operate within new social networks; and some move to new homes, sometimes in new communities. These changes may be accompanied by changes in the use of language by and with these individuals, changes in their communicative needs, and/or changes in available communicative partners.

Even a quick look at work on the interrelationships between language and old age that has come out over the past twenty years or so produces a dizzying array of topics and approaches. Some scholars (e.g., Obler and Albert, 1980; Bayles and Kaszniak, 1987; and Ulatowska, 1985) describe the language and/or communicative abilities that accompany aging, looking both at healthy individuals and those dealing with health problems that affect language use, such as Alzheimer's disease and aphasia. Others (e.g., Coupland, Coupland, and Giles, 1991; and Giles, Coupland, and Wiemann, 1990) work with the assumption that language choices that people make help to construct their social identities (including an elderly identity) and relate these choices to issues of mental and physical health. Still others (e.g., Hummert, Wiemann, and Nussbaum, 1994; Nussbaum, Thompson, and Robinson, 1989; and Lubinski, 1981) recognize the critical importance of communicative relationships across the lifespan and investigate communication among friends, within the family, and even within nursing homes.

So, one thing seems clear. Like every other age group, elderly individuals use language in a wide variety of contexts—with many different people at different times and places and for different purposes. Where does this leave the scholar interested in exploring issues of language and communication in old age? Which individuals should serve as research subjects? What kind of language should be "tapped"? For what purposes? How? Once the language has been "tapped," how should it best be examined? These and other similar methodological questions will guide the upcoming discussion in this chapter.

In the next section, I discuss disciplinary influences on researchers' choices, ranging from what to study, why that study could be important, and how best to carry out that study. Various conceptualizations of old age in the literature are then explored, leading us to realize the complexity involved when we choose elderly subjects for our study. We then take a look at characteristics of the discourse of four contexts within which language is usually studied as it is related to later life: standardized tests, interviews with the researcher, conversations with the researcher, and real-life situations "listened in on" by the researcher. Relative advantages and disadvantages are discussed for each. Based on the discussion in previous sections, I then argue that multiple perspectives are necessary to reach an understanding of the multifaceted nature of the relationship between old age and language. The final sections provide background information regarding the context within which this volume was conceived, and upcoming chapters are previewed according to their relative focus on issues relating to: 1) language and communicative abilities in old age, 2) identity in old age, and 3) social norms, values, and practices in old age.

QUESTIONS, MOTIVATIONS, AND APPROACHES

A graduate school professor of mine, Dr. Roger Shuy, always expected his students to be able to provide concise answers to two brief questions when proposing paper topics in his courses: "What?" and "So what?" In this way, students were trained to get quickly to the heart of the matter: Could they articulate explicitly *what* the problem was that provided the focus of their proposed work? And, after articulating the problem, could they state clearly why anyone should care about that problem? When using this approach with my own students, I find it useful to have them organize their proposals along the lines of the traditional journalistic questions. In addition, then, to answering the questions "What?" and "Why?" (Shuy's "so what?"), the students must justify the most appropriate approach to the problem (How?), the most appropriate subjects for the study (Who?), and the most appropriate context (Where? When?) in which to study the subjects' language use.

Of course, in practice, the answers to these questions are not fully independent of each other. We would expect two researchers trained in different disciplines to 1) be interested in different problems; 2) choose different contexts for the display of these problems; 3) choose their subjects differently, both in terms of number and characteristics; 4) choose tools from different analytical tool bags; and, finally, 5) justify their interest in the research question in different ways.

Depending on whether one takes a theory-driven or a data-driven approach, the research project will begin by focusing on one of the facets just discussed and letting the others fall subsequently into place. For example, a researcher taking a theory-driven approach would start with a question and motivation that derive from a theory which he or she deems important and relevant; once the motivated question has been posed, the researcher determines which and how many subjects are necessary to carry out the study as well as the context(s) of the subjects' language use. In this approach, the analytical tools necessary to the examination of the language use are usually determined ahead of the actual data collection.

In contrast to the theory-driven approach, the data-driven approach often starts with an interest (which could be understood to be a motivation for the study—albeit a different kind than that emanating from theory) in particular subjects and/or contexts which leads to the collection of language used by these subjects within these contexts. The researcher probably has a general research question in mind, but this question will be allowed to evolve as the investigation proceeds. Interesting patterns and unexpected language use by these subjects within these contexts lead the researcher to decide which analytical tools to try out; the analysis and the research question proceed hand in hand, each informing the other until the reseacher is convinced that he or she has understood the data in an interesting way.

The bottom line is that disciplinary training will often lead researchers to study certain problems and to propose the most effective way of approaching those problems (and, of course, certain problems may indeed be more easily solved by a particular approach); we should take care not to allow this situation, however, to blind us to the possibility of crossing disciplinary boundaries (sometimes they may seem more like barriers) in search of creative solutions to important research questions.[1]

WHO IS OLD? CONCEPTUALIZATIONS OF OLD AGE

Researchers who work with elderly individuals come to the immediate realization that age is much more complex than a simple biological category. A speaker's chronological age tells only a small part of the story. In her research within the Labovian sociolinguistic paradigm of language variation and change, Eckert (1984) began to realize some of the complexity of the notion of age when she found that simple chronological age did not correlate well with the facts of linguistic change; differences in aspirations, roles, and orientation to society needed to be taken into account in order to make sense of the situation. (See Eckert 1997 for a thorough discussion of age as a sociolinguistic variable.)

Counts and Counts (1985), in their work on aging in the Pacific, find the need to differentiate between chronological age, functional age, historical age, and social age. Functional age refers to changes in facility (e.g., senses), in appearance, in activity (both level of interest in community events and level of independence), and in bodily action (physiological and cognitive). Historical age refers to an individual's age as related to a specific event significant to the society in which the individual lives. Social age refers to the rites of passage in a given society.

Boden and Bielby (1986) argue that the perception of one's age is also important to a more complete understanding of age beyond chronological age. The notion of "disjunctive aging" advanced by

Coupland, Coupland, and Giles (1989) seems to extend this idea. By "disjunctive aging," Coupland et al. refer to the phenomenon of individuals feeling older or younger than their actual chronological age.

And, finally, there is the influence of "societal aging," or ageism, where a "generalized other" that does not correspond to their self-image is projected onto individuals (see Copper, 1986:52). Randall (1986:127) elaborates on this influence in the following way: "The dislocation created out of the contradictions between how I feel and look—and WHAT I KNOW—and how society perceives me—physically, socially, economically, emotionally—is a very real element in every day."

Despite the complex situation just discussed, many researchers working in this field still choose to select subjects for their studies based on chronological age, often in conjunction with various measures of health status. Sometimes categories distinguish between the young-old and the old-old or even the oldest-old as a way of taking into account the fact that sixty-five-year-olds are often different in many ways from eighty-five-year-olds or those over one hundred years old. Time constraints frequently do not allow for the kinds of complex evaluations necessary to take into account individuals' *perceived* age, levels of activity and independence, etc. And, of course, in some studies, the researchers are specifically interested in chronological age, not perceived age, as it relates to a variety of other factors.

Feeding into some of the disparities between perceived and chronological age is the extreme heterogeneity that has been found to exist among elderly individuals. Nelson and Dannefer (1992) observed that this increasing diversity over the lifespan does not appear to be specific to any particular domain; i.e., the same general finding emerges across physical, personality, social, and cognitive domains. Elderly individuals may, therefore, differ from each other in terms of memory and/or cognition, attitudes towards self and others, physical health, and communicative needs. Fredrickson and Carstensen (1991), Ulatowska, Cannito, Hayashi, and Fleming (1985), and Wiemann, Gravell, and Wiemann (1990) have all found that elderly individuals judge anticipated positive affect and friendly, social relations to be significantly more important than information-seeking or other task-oriented functions when they are choosing a person to talk with and deciding which contacts to maintain.

Differences may also exist in terms of what kinds of people elderly women and men actually have to talk with as well as where and how often this talk takes place. Issues here include social networks and attitudes of those in the networks both toward the particular individual in question and toward old people in general. Is the individual's lifetime partner (if any) still alive? Does the social network include only persons of the individual's generation or also of younger (and possibly older) generations? Is the individual talking a great deal to persons who hold ageist attitudes?

This extreme variation makes it difficult to talk about normative behavior in terms of language use. Wiemann, Gravell, and Wiemann (1990) discuss the need for standards appropriate to different stages of aging, which are vital to understanding whether a person is aging successfully rather than just comparing them to the communicative, social, and psychological standards of typical middle age, as is usually the case.

Researchers deal with this issue of heterogeneity in different ways. Often researchers argue that the best way of compensating for wide variation is to carry out studies on very large numbers of subjects. The large numbers are seen as means to greater generalization of the findings of the study; i.e., in a large study, it is more likely that researchers will be working with a set of individuals who represent the larger population of elderly individuals in relevant ways. In a case study or one involving very few subjects, it is more likely that the individuals will not represent the larger population in these ways.

On the other hand, proponents of case studies and small-scale studies argue that the extreme variation that exists within the elderly population makes it likely that large-scale studies simply average out these large differences in behavior, and that the averages found, therefore, are actually not representative of large numbers of the elderly population in any meaningful way. Case studies and small-scale studies are seen as being able to investigate in a more in-depth fashion the interrelationships among a variety of communicative behaviors or factors, leading to well-grounded research questions and methodologies that can be used in subsequent large-scale studies (see Caramazza, 1986; McCloskey and Caramazza, 1988; Caramazza and Badecker, 1989; Moody, 1989; and Caramazza, 1991 for further discussion of this issue).

CONTEXTS OF TALK ELICITED/OBSERVED

In this section I characterize four contexts within which language used by elderly individuals has typically been examined. These are (1) standardized tests, (2) interviews, (3) conversations, and (4) real-life interactions "listened in on."

Language within the *standardized test situation* tends to be tightly constrained. The language tasks are very clearly identified so that any deviation from what is expected can be characterized as outside the range of normal. One clear benefit of this context is that the researcher can find out a good deal about a wide range of language/communicative abilities and compare the results with a large number of other individuals who have previously taken the test within a limited amount of time. A disadvantage of this context is that its predetermined tasks limit the display of the test-taker's language/communicative abilities to just those under investigation. Another possible disadvantage of this context is that the test-taker's performance on the test may bear little resemblance to his or her actual linguistic abilities as displayed in everyday situations.

Language used within an *interview with the researcher* tends to be somewhat topically constrained and the participant roles and communicative division of labor are fairly clear-cut. The interviewer is usually understood to be in charge of asking the questions, while the interviewee is expected to answer those questions. Although there may be no "right or wrong" answers to mark the interviewee as being within or outside the range of normal (as is the case with standardized tests), subjects still know that they are not to veer very far off of the proposed topics of discussion. One benefit of this communicative context is that the researcher can find out in a fairly quick and straightforward way what the interviewee has to say about a given set of topics. The use of open-ended questions allows the interviewees to frame their answers in whatever terms they feel are meaningful (in comparison to a questionnaire with predetermined answer options, for example). This freedom gives the researcher not only greater insight into the interviewees' way of thinking but also provides rich discourse for more micro-level analyses of language choices by the interviewee. One disadvantage of the interview (as compared with standardized testing) is that the open-endedness of the questions allows for the possibility that certain linguistic/communicative behavior will not be displayed.[2] Another possible disadvantage of the interview (as compared with conversation) in terms of data collection is the fact that it often plays itself out in an asymmetrical way, the interviewee being at the distinct disadvantage of not knowing "the agenda" of the interview. Depending on the degree to which the interviewee feels uncertain about the purposes of the interview or feels uncomfortable talking with a relative stranger, the answers *about* communicative practice given in the interview may bear little relationship to what the interviewee *actually* does in practice.

The language used in *conversations with the researcher* is usually more free-wheeling than that in the interviews and exam situations discussed above. In conversations, topics come and go relatively freely, being initiated, elaborated upon, and closed by either party. One benefit of undirected conversations is that the researcher can identify issues of importance to the elderly individual that may never have come up in a more topically-constrained discourse. Self-selected and designed conversational contributions can be windows on emotions and reflections that would probably have gone unnoticed within a more constrained context. Additionally, in a conversation that is perceived to be symmetrical, the elderly individual can be expected to display a fuller range of linguistic and communicative abilities than in a context that is seen to contain a power differential. One disadvantage of the conversation (as compared with the testing situation) as well as the interview context is the possibility that not all linguistic abilities judged to be relevant may be displayed. Another disadvantage (as compared with the interview situation) is that it is more difficult for the researcher to maintain any sense of "agenda" when the elderly interlocutor may introduce new topics at any time, choose not to elaborate upon topics introduced by the researcher, etc.

The fourth context in which language of elderly individuals can be examined is in *real life situations "listened in on" by the researcher*. In these situations, the elderly individuals whose language is of interest are going about their business in a usual fashion and "just happen" to be observed, for example, on visits to the doctor (see Coupland and Coupland, this volume) and in support group conversations (see Saunders, this volume). One distinct advantage of this type of interaction, as contrasted with the contexts discussed above, is that there is no direct influence by the researcher on the language used by the elderly individuals. In cases where the researcher is in the immediate vicinity taping the interaction or taking notes, there may be a moderate indirect influence on the interaction due to the observer's paradox (see Labov (1972) for discussion of the fact that it is impossible to observe people who are *not* being observed). Another advantage in situations where the researcher is of a younger generation than his or her subjects (and necessarily is always involved in *intergenerational* encounters with elderly individuals) is that it is possible to gain access to *intra*generational interactions such as conversations held among residents in a nursing home. Additionally, the researcher can examine language used by elderly interlocutors with persons *they* have chosen to talk with in everyday life situations that are meaningful to *them* as contrasted with interactions, such as the tests, interviews, and conversations, which usually take place outside the normal stream of life for these individuals. One possible disadvantage of "listening in on" real-life interactions has to do with the fact that the researcher is not part of the interaction. Because the talk is not constructed with the researcher in mind, it is quite likely that the researcher will not be privy to some of what is being talked about or that the researcher will *think* he or she understands what is going on but actually does not. These problems can be overcome to a certain extent through the use of playback interviews (see Tannen 1984), in which the original participants listen to the taped interaction along with the researcher. During or after the listening session, the researcher can ask questions for clarification, or the original participants can make comments on their own.

EMBRACING MULTIPLE PERSPECTIVES

After reading the preceding discussion, one might feel a sense of anxiety and confusion when faced with the task of addressing the relationships between old age and language. Both Chafe (1994) and Moermann (1996), however, offer us another possibility. Chafe, in an insightful discussion of data and methodologies dealing with linguistics and the mind, argues that no one approach is inherently the correct one. In his opinion (Chafe 1994:12), all types of data "provide important insights, and all have their limitations." Each type of methodology "makes a contribution, but none has an exclusive claim on scientific validity" (Chafe 1994:18). Following Chafe, then, I would argue that all perspectives are potentially valid in the understanding of language as it is related to old age.

In addition, Moerman's (1996:147) recent comparison of the field of conversation analysis to the "swidden" fields of Southeast Asia is helpful in this regard. In contrast to "sessile" farms which are planted with a single crop, these swidden fields support a great variety of mutually sustaining plants. Although they appear untidy in their early stages of growth, these fields are productive and supportive. To carry this analogy over to the study of old age and language, I would argue that we who work in this area are also not yet ready for a single "best" approach. The field is far too complex to be understood in a unidimensional way.

The time is right, it would seem, for a volume that explores a variety of approaches without aiming at true interdisciplinarity. This volume's explicit focus on multidisciplinary perspectives is meant to provide the reader with a look at some of the issues considered to be important by scholars in a variety of disciplines, all embracing the relationship between old age and language.

BACKGROUND TO THE VOLUME

This volume has its roots in a day-long pre-conference session at the 1992 Georgetown University Round Table on Languages and Linguistics (GURT), which brought together researchers from the fields of anthropology, speech and hearing sciences, psychology, and linguistics representing the following institutions: Boston University School of Medicine, Boston Veterans Administration Medical Center, California State University at Long Beach, City University of New York, Dartmouth University Medical School, Dawnland Center (Montpelier, Vermont), Emerson College, the Field Museum of Natural History, Georgetown University, Millersville University, Philadelphia Geriatric Center, the University of Kansas, the University of Massachusetts/Boston, and the University of Texas at Dallas. Additional contributions were later solicited from researchers at the University of Oklahoma, Texas Christian University, the University of Wales College of Cardiff, Meiji Gakuin University (Japan), and Georgetown University in order to balance the original selection of studies.

Given the multidisciplinary nature of the volume, it comes as no surprise that the contributors employ a range of methodologies to language used by and with elderly individuals in a range of contexts, as discussed above. With this in mind, I challenged the contributors to revise their original papers, making them more accessible to readers from a variety of disciplines. This revision included highlighting assumptions made by their disciplines, defining key concepts not necessarily known outside of their disciplines, justifying their choice of methodologies and data bases, and contextualizing their research questions within the scientific literature for their particular approaches. It is my hope that this type of discussion will allow each individual chapter to be understood by readers *generally* interested in issues of language and aging and not only by those experts familiar with a particular research paradigm. If readers proceed through the chapters in the order in which they are presented in the volume, they will suffer no "intellectual whiplash" as they make their way from opening discussions of the relationship of memory to language based on large-scale standardized tests to closing discussions of the ways in which African American grandmothers talk about imparting cultural identity and womanhood to their granddaughters.

PREVIEW OF UPCOMING CHAPTERS

Contributions to this volume fall loosely into three general approaches to the relationship between old age and language as identified by their primary focus on: 1) the relative decline, preservation (often called "sparing" in the literature), or improvement of linguistic and communicative abilities in old age; 2) identity in old age as reflected in and created by language use; and 3) discourse as a carrier of meta-level awareness regarding social norms, values, and practices in old age.

Section I: Language and Communicative Abilities in Old Age

The approach to the relationship between old age and language typically taken by psycholinguists, neurolinguists, and speech-language pathologists looks generally at the relative decline, preservation, or (occasionally) improvement of language and communicative abilities which accompanies human aging. Some researchers look specifically at subgroups of the overall elderly population which are known to have difficulties with communication, such as elderly individuals with clinical depression, aphasia of various types, and Alzheimer's disease. Others attempt to characterize the decline, preservation, or improvement of such abilities within the healthy elderly population. Some of this research is carried out for the primary purpose of learning more about language in general (and only secondarily about how elderly individuals may use it); other such research may be undertaken for the primary purpose of finding out how elderly individuals use language, as a first step towards designing appropriate therapeutic or diagnostic tasks.

In Emery's study comparing the performance of 20 healthy elderly individuals with that of 20 elderly individuals with major depression/unipolar, 12 elderly individuals with depressive dementia, and 20 individuals with Alzheimer's disease on standardized tests for memory (Wechsler Memory Scale and Katzman Test for Delayed Recall) and for language (Western Aphasia Battery and Test for Syntactic Complexity), she provides evidence that the interaction between the cognitive activities of memory and language increases with the severity of deterioration in the brain. Her findings highlight the importance of research on patient populations to inform basic theoretical research on the relationship of memory and language as well as provide important information regarding the ways in which depressive dementia (also called "pseudodementia") may be differentiated from clinical depression and Alzheimer's disease.

Important clinical applications are also proposed by Obler, Oberman, Samuels, and Albert, whose investigation of the language comprehension of nine mid-stage Alzheimer's patients on a standardized language test (Boston Diagnostic Aphasia Examination) suggests that written input may aid the comprehension abilities of these patients. Eight of the nine patients exhibited significantly better comprehension when auditory input was either supplemented with or entirely replaced by written materials.

Barresi, Obler, Au, and Albert sent questionnaires to healthy individuals who had taken part in a longitudinal study of their language and communicative abilities. Correlations of forty subjects' responses regarding a variety of language-related activities with their performance on the Boston Naming Test over a decade provide evidence that naming ability is negatively affected to a significant degree by the amount of television the subjects watched as well as the subjects' age and level of education.

Ulatowska, Chapman, and Johnson tackle the important issue of discourse-level decline related to aging by focusing on tasks which they argue require "deeper" levels of information processing than most of the sentence-level and lexical tasks found in standardized test batteries. These researchers investigated the ability of 15 older middle-aged adults (fifty-seventy years), 15 old-elderly adults (over eighty years), and 15 aphasic adults to provide the gist of six fables and to formulate the moral of each of these fables. Counter to the investigators' expectations, results of the exploratory study indicated that the old-elderly group did not experience more difficulties than the older middle-aged group with these discourse-level processing tasks. As expected, however, the aphasic individuals did exhibit difficulties with these tasks when compared with the other two groups.

Sabat's chapter moves us farther along the naturalness continuum in terms of type of data used, while still maintaining the overall focus on relative decline/preservation/improvement of abilities represented by this first group of papers. Sabat's case study of three conversations he had with one sixty-eight-year-old Alzheimer's patient highlights the influence of the healthy interlocutor in terms of the overall success of these conversations. With assistance from the healthy conversational partner, the Alzheimer's patient in this study was able to participate in meaningful conversations despite his severe linguistic problems as identified on standardized tests. The conversations which form the data base in this study are excerpted at length in this chapter, serving as a useful complement to the more analytical papers in this section. The transcripts provide the reader with an opportunity to "hear" the patient's own voice with regard to the experience of Alzheimer's disease.

Section II: Identity in Old Age

One approach to the relationship between old age and language often taken by social psychologists and sociolinguists looks not at language abilities and disabilities of this group (or, if they do, they are seen as interactional resources individuals can use in identity construction) but attempts to identify patterns and strategies in emergent discourse production by and with (usually healthy) elderly interlocutors. These patterns then enable researchers to compare and contrast communicative behavior of different groups among the healthy elderly, rather than treating the elderly as one homogeneous group to be compared with younger groups of individuals. In her examination of the bereavement stories told by 14 Irish-American widowers between the ages of seventy-five and eighty-four, Bower makes the important point that ethnic group identity accounts for the distinctive profile of the expressive style of these men. In the process, she carefully considers and then rules out three other possible explanations for the narrative differences she identified: cognitive deficit, performance deficit, and inner state. Bower concludes her discussion with a plea that investigations of language produced by both healthy and impaired elderly speakers take into full account "what sociolinguistic parameters and constraints their ethnicity places upon what may be spoken about and how it may be expressed."

Another major group of researchers within this overall approach to identity and old age looks not for systematic differences (such as ethnic or gender identity) among the elderly population *per se* but for the role that "recurring patterns of elderly and intergenerational language use" (Coupland, Coupland, and Giles, 1991:5) play in the construction of elderly identity. Coupland et al. analyze 102 doctor-patient interactions involving 98 patients ages sixty-two to ninety-seven and 8 doctors to determine how doctors and patients negotiate the salience of age. Coupland et al.'s examination links the discourse of the geriatric medical consultation to the construction of health and illness by showing how doctors can work to reconstruct patients' conceptions of their own aging and health.

Rosenfeld's careful investigation of the language used by artist Georgia O'Keeffe in a movie celebrating her ninetieth birthday extends our understanding of the management of the salience of age to variations within single interactions by identifying linguistic features which correspond to various registers, footings, and roles taken by O'Keeffe. Rosenfeld argues that the notion of age is not always relevant to O'Keeffe or to her interlocutors in these interactions. In those cases where old age *was* found to be relevant, the participants may evaluate it either positively or negatively. Rosenfeld's examination of variation in language used within single interactions allows us to see the subtlety with which old age is presented as part of an individual's identity.

Okazaki's investigation of one conversation she had with a sixty-eight-year-old woman, Mary, focuses on one of the discourse strategies identified by the Couplands (Coupland, Coupland, Giles, and Wiemann 1988), that of painful self-disclosure. In this case, the disclosure is of Mary's relatively recent inability to drive a car, which Okazaki argues is understood differently by Japanese and Americans. The differing points of view on this socially significant ability due to cultural difference and to age difference result in what Okazaki identified as cross-talk (Gumperz) in the mutual disclosure discourse.

Section III: Social Norms, Values, and Practices in Old Age

The general approach to the relationship between old age and language typically taken by anthropologists and as initial steps by some communication scientists is to use discourse of elderly individuals to understand their social norms, values, and practices. In contrast to the two approaches described above, this approach does not always involve microanalysis of the language *per se* but often focuses on the *content* of the discourse. The way in which individuals talk about their values and norms does not always correspond to their behavior in real-life situations: ideology and praxis do not always match. On the other hand, listening to individuals talk about issues of significance to them helps to provide the researcher with an insider's (or "emic") perspective on issues critical to an ethnographically-sound analysis.

In the first contribution in this section, Saunders discusses the social norms of elderly women as expressed in weekly support group meetings. Instead of an approach based on answers to questions posed specifically to gain an understanding of these norms, Saunders uses a more indirect approach, analyzing the women's gossip for evidence of social norms regarding femininity and sexual activity, for example. She suggests that, even though the group explicitly discourages the practice of gossiping outside the group, gossip about outsiders during the meetings serves both to convey information between members and to reinforce social norms of the local and greater speech communities. Saunders shows how two specific discourse devices, overlapping speech and interrogative utterances, function to construct gossip as a multi-party interaction involving both active and passive gossipers.

Just as Saunders uses gossip to uncover group members' social norms, Cattell examines complaints of old people in rural Kenya and in urban Philadelphia to reach an understanding of these individuals' perceptions of social and cultural change. Based on a variety of data sets, including conversations, interviews, and responses to written surveys, Cattell argues that being old often entails transformations of the self in terms of personal identity and social roles. Complaining (for example, about loss of control in the neighborhood or problems with family obligations) may then be understood as an attempt by the complainers to defend social norms in the face of unceasing change around them.

Allman, Ragan, Newsome, Scoufos, and Nussbaum present an approach diametrically opposed to that taken in the chapters in section

I. Through the use of unstructured interviews with 20 ambulatory female patients sixty-five years of age and older, Allman et al. offer the reader a window into these women's perceptions of physicians' communicative behaviors and the importance of these behaviors to their overall health care. Allman et al. attempt to give older women a voice in a scientific literature that overwhelmingly focuses on men by allowing them to talk about their own real concerns. This chapter can be seen as an important first step towards the identification of issues for future studies of health care services to older women.

Like Allman et al., McKay is concerned with providing a corrective to what she argues is the reductionist nature of traditional social scientific inquiry by giving voice to women who have traditionally been ignored in such studies. In her interviews with 10 African American grandmother-granddaughter pairs, McKay examines the way that these women understand their relationships with each other. Using the actual words spoken by the participants in response to questions about role models, cultural and family traditions, family stories, the meaning of the African American woman today, and advice, McKay argues that a key function of the relationship between generations of African American women is to convey womanhood and cultural values such as determination, strength, and independence, giving the granddaughters an increased understanding of who they are.

CONCLUDING REMARKS

The goal of understanding how language and old age are related to each other challenges us to understand how language is used by a large number of elderly individuals in many and varied contexts, both experimental and natural. This valuable goal can be achieved with much collaborative research in the future. Despite the fact that the contributors to this volume base their findings and discussions on language produced by *different* elderly individuals in *different* contexts, each study makes some bold strokes in the overall sketch of these interrelationships. As we continue to work towards a comprehensive understanding, it is important to remember that each participant in each study is a more complete human being than is apparent in any given context of language use. Therefore it would be instructive to hear what a seventy-five-year-old woman with a score of, for example, 94 on the Western Aphasia Battery Repetition Test (standardized test context) has to say about her interactions with doctors (in an interview with a researcher), examine how she talks about trying to remain independent (in a conversation with a researcher), and "listen in on" the language she uses with her doctor and the language her doctor uses with her during her annual medical check-up. It is hoped that future research will attempt to provide this larger context for investigations of language in later life.

Language and Communication in Old Age: Multidisciplinary Perspectives offers the interested reader a glimpse into the full range of approaches to the issues of old age and language through a direct and explicit comparison of a variety of disciplinary assumptions, key concepts, methodologies, data bases, and relevant research questions. As such, I hope that it not only provides experienced researchers in the field of language and aging with an increased awareness of different but related perspectives but also serves as a provocative and informative introduction for those new to these issues.

NOTES

1. For example, when I began my investigations of natural conversations with an elderly woman who had been diagnosed with Alzheimer's disease in the early 1980s (as written up in Hamilton 1991, 1994a, 1994b, 1996), most scholars I talked with indicated to me that I should carry out my research within the paradigms recognized by psycholinguistics or neurolinguistics. The existing theoretical frameworks and methodologies in those literatures did not, however, allow me to capture what I sensed was potentially most significant about my subject's communicative abilities and how they were interrelated with my own communicative behavior in our conversations. In the face of these comments and recommendations, I had to continually ask myself what a sociolinguistic approach to this problem would look like and, indeed, whether it was possible. I found as time went on that such a crossing of the boundaries was not only possible but fruitful.

2. It has often been noted, for example, that individuals with early stages of Alzheimer's disease can "mask" the degree of their communicative problems, such as naming difficulties, by cleverly giving answers in such a way as not to point to the problem areas.

REFERENCES

Bayles, Kathryn, and Kaszniak, Alfred. 1987. *Communication and Cognition in Normal Aging and Dementia*. Boston: Little, Brown and Company.

Boden, Deirdre, and Bielby, Denise. 1986. The way it was: topical organization in elderly conversation. *Language and Communication* 6:73–89.

Caramazza, A. 1986. On drawing inferences about the structure of normal cognitive systems from the analysis of impaired performance: the case for single-patient studies. *Brain and Cognition* 5:41–66.

Caramazza, A. 1991. Data, statistics, and theory: a comment on Bates, McDonald, MacWhinney, and Applebaum's "A maximum likelihood procedure for the analysis of group and individual data in aphasia research." *Brain and Language* 41:43–51.

Caramazza, A., and Badecker, William. 1989. Patient classification in neuropsychological research. *Brain and Cognition* 10: 256- 295.

Chafe, Wallace. 1994. *Discourse, Consciousness, and Time*. Chicago: University of Chicago Press.

Copper, Baba. 1986. Voices: On becoming old women. In J. Alexander et al., eds., *Women and Aging*. Corvallis, Oregon: Calyx Books. 47–57.

Counts, Dorothy Ayers, and Counts, David R. 1985. *Aging and Its Transformations: Moving toward Death in Pacific Societies*. Lanham, Maryland: University Press of America.

Coupland, Nikolas, Coupland, Justine, and Giles, Howard. 1989. Telling age in later life: Identity and face implications. *Text* 9:129–151.

Coupland, Nikolas, Coupland, Justine, and Giles, Howard. 1991. *Language, Society and the Elderly*. Oxford: Blackwell.

Coupland, Justine, Coupland, Nikolas, Giles, Howard, and Wiemann, John. 1988. My life in your hands: Processes of self-disclosure in intergenerational talk. In N. Coupland, ed., *Styles of Discourse*. New York: Croom Helm.

Eckert, Penelope. 1984. Age and linguistic change. In David Kertzer and Jennie Keith, eds., *Age and Anthropological Theory*. Ithaca: Cornell University Press.

Eckert, Penelope. 1997. Age as a sociolinguistic variable. In Florian Coulmas, ed., *The Handbook of Sociolinguistics*. Oxford: Blackwell Publishers. 151–167.

Frederickson, B. L., and Carstensen, Laura L. 1991. Social selectivity in old age. Paper presented at the 44th Annual Scientific Meeting of the Gerontological Society of America, November 22–25, 1991. San Francisco, California.

Giles, Howard, Coupland, Nikolas, and Wiemann, John M. 1990. *Communication, Health and the Elderly*. Manchester: Manchester University Press.

Hamilton, Heidi. 1991. Accommodation and mental disability. In H. Giles, J. Coupland, and N. Coupland, eds., *Contexts of Accommodation: Developments in Applied Sociolinguistics*, Cambridge: Cambridge University Press. 157–186.

Hamilton, Heidi. 1994a. *Conversations with an Alzheimer's Patient: An Interactional Sociolinguistic Study.* Cambridge: Cambridge University Press.

Hamilton, Heidi. 1994b. Requests for clarification as evidence of pragmatic comprehension difficulty: The case of Alzheimer's disease. In Ron Bloom, Loraine Obler, Susan De Santi, and Jonathan Ehlich, eds., *Discourse in Adult Clinical Populations*. Hillsdale, New Jersey: Lawrence Erlbaum Associates, Inc. 185–199.

Hamilton, Heidi. 1996. Intratextuality, intertextuality and the construction of identity as patient in Alzheimer's Disease. *Text* 16/1: 61–90.

Harris, Betty Donley. 1986. I write in order to live. In J. Alexander et al., eds., *Women and Aging*. Corvallis, Oregon: Calyx Books. 82–83.

Hummert, Mary Lee, Wiemann, John M., and Nussbaum, Jon, eds.. 1994. *Interpersonal Communication in Older Adulthood*. Newbury Park, California: Sage.

Labov, William. 1972. Some principles of linguistic methodology. *Language in Society* 1:97–120.

Lubinski, Rosemary. 1981. Language and aging: An environmental approach to intervention. *Topics in Language Disorders* 1: 89–97.

McCloskey, M., and Caramazza, A. 1988. Theory and methodology in cognitive neuropsychology: A response to our critics. *Cognitive Neuropsychology* 5: 583–623.

Moody, H. 1989. Gerontology with a human face. In L.E. Thomas, ed., *Research on Adulthood and Aging*. Albany: SUNY Press. 227–240.

Moerman, Michael. 1996. The field of analyzing foreign language conversations. *Journal of Pragmatics* 26:147–158.

Nelson, E. Anne, and Dannefer, Dale. 1992. Aged heterogeneity: Fact or fiction? *The Gerontologist* 32:17–23.

Nussbaum, Jon F., Thompson, Teresa, and Robinson, James D. 1989. *Communication and Aging*. New York: Harper & Row Publishers.

Obler, Loraine K., and Albert, Martin, eds. 1980. *Language and Communication in the Elderly*. Lexington: Lexington Books.

Randall, Margaret. 1986. From: The Journals. In J. Alexander et al., eds., *Women and Aging*. Corvallis, Oregon: Calyx Books. 127–130.

Tannen, Deborah. 1984. *Conversational Style*. Norwood, New Jersey: Ablex.

Ulatowska, Hanna, Cannito, Michael, Hayashi, Mari, and Fleming, Susan. 1985. Language abilities in the elderly. In H. Ulatowska, ed. *The Aging Brain: Communication in the Elderly.* San Diego, California: College-Hill Press.

Ulatowska, Hanna, ed. 1985. *The Aging Brain: Communication in the Elderly.* San Diego, California: College-Hill Press.

Wiemann, John, Gravell, Rosemary, and Wiemann, Michael. 1990. Communication with the elderly: implications for health care and social support. In H. Giles, N. Coupland, and J. Wiemann, eds., *Communication, Health and the Elderly.* Manchester: Manchester University Press.

Language and Communicative Abilities in Old Age

On the Relationship between Memory and Language in the Dementia Spectrum of Depression, Alzheimer Syndrome, and Normal Aging

V. Olga B. Emery

INTRODUCTION

Depressive dementia is a subclass of the overarching class of pseudodementia, which represents a phenotype approximated by a wide variety of underlying disorders (Emery, 1988, 1992, 1994; Emery and Oxman, 1992, 1994). Some of the disorders which can result in a dementia-like presentation are Ganser syndrome (Arieti and Bemporad, 1974; Sachdev and Kiloh, 1994), mania (Caine, 1981; Casey and Fitzgerald, 1988), schizophrenia (Caine, 1981; Sachdev and Kiloh, 1994), delirium (Kramp and Bolwig, 1980; Sachdev and Kiloh, 1994), dissociative reaction (Sachdev and Kiloh, 1994; Wells, 1979), conversion reaction (Caine, 1981; Wells, 1979), and psychoactive drug reactions (Black and Hughes, 1987), as well as depression (Emery, 1988, 1992, 1994; Emery and Oxman, 1992, 1994; Kral, 1983; Kral and Emery, 1989). Although the prevalence of disorders presenting as pseudodementia remains unclear, what is clear is that depressive dementia, synonomously referred to as major depression with depressive dementia or depressive pseudodementia, is possibly the most prevalent subtype of this broad category (Alexopoulos and Nambudiri, 1994; Emery, 1988; Emery and Oxman, 1992, 1994; Kiloh, 1961). It has long been observed that in the differential diagnosis between dementia and pseudodementia, depressive dementia appears to be the single most difficult disorder to distinguish from the so-called "organic" diagnostic categories, particularly primary degenerative dementia of the Alzheimer type (Jorm, 1995; Jorm et al., 1995; Starkstein et al., 1989).

Historically, dementia has been defined as an acquired, severe, "irreversible" kind of intellectual deterioration secondary to organic brain disease (Bulbena and Berrios, 1986). The attempt to distinguish between "non-reversible" cementing illness and dementia-like presentations that with treatment or passage of time appear to "reverse" dates back to at least the 1800s (Mairet, 1883). The term "vesanic dementia" was used to designate cementing syndromes that appeared "reversible" until it was replaced by Wernicke's term "pseudo-dementia" in the late 1800s (Bulbena and Berrios, 1986; Emery, 1988). The term "vesania" originated from the Latin word "sanus" meaning "sane, sound, healthy." Implied in the conceptualization of both "vesanic dementia" and "pseudodementia" is a non-organic or functional etiology. Then, as now, parameters of irreversiblity-reversibility and structure-function, or put another way, organic versus non-organic, form the core around which the constructs of dementia and pseudodementia are antiposed. Argument has centered around these cross-cutting variables for more than a century without resolution and with pervasive consequences for treatment of the dementia-spectrum disorders. The point of view of this chapter is that a dichotomous approach to cementing and pseudodementing illnesses is not productive and that a continuity framework is more useful for understanding dementia-pseudodementia spectrum disorders. The focus here is on depressive dementia, the reconceptualization of which will challenge the usual dichotomy between pseudodementia as functional-reversible and primary degenerative dementia as organic-irreversible.

To date, the conceptual, empirical, and clinical relationships between depressive dementia and primary degenerative dementia (American Psychiatric Association, 1987, 1994) still are not understood. Both depressive dementia and primary degenerative dementia are age-correlated (Alexopoulos, 1990; Reifler and Sherrill, 1990), and the prevalence rate increases dramatically for persons over eighty years of age (Lobo et al., 1995; Niederehe and Oxman, 1994). For example, prevalence figures for dementia in general indicate that about 8% of persons over the age of sixty-five are demented, with prevalence rates rising to over 22% for persons eighty years of age and older (Kay et al., 1980; McAllister and Powers, 1994; Niederehe and Oxman, 1994). Accordingly, given the increasing numbers and proportions of old people in Western countries (Reeves, 1989; U.S. Department of Health and Human Services, 1984), the understanding of the nature and causes of age-correlated dementing disorders, such as depressive dementia and primary degenerative dementia, ranks high as a research priority.

EMPIRICAL CONTEXT

In the long-term follow-up (4 to 18 years after diagnosis) of 44 elderly patients with depressive dementia (mean age=76.5 years), Kral and Emery (1987, 1989) found 79% of these patients had developed degenerative dementia of the Alzheimer phenotype. The modal pattern of these patients was as follows: (1) several episodes of major depression/unipolar without significant cognitive impairment; (2) one or more episodes of major depression/unipolar during which cognitive functioning was extremely adversely affected with subsequent return to "normal"; (3) an episode of apparent depression during which the patient presented an Alzheimer-type profile, with cognitive symptoms subsequently appearing to "reverse," i.e., depressive dementia. During this phase, before cognitive symptoms "reversed," the depressive dementia patients were disoriented and unable to state correctly where they were or what day, month, or year it was. The cognitive impairments of depressive dementia will be described in greater detail as part of the study reported in this chapter. Then, (4) a presentation with an Alzheimer-like syndrome without remission of cognitive symptoms, and with subsequent progressive deterioration consistent with primary degenerative dementia of the Alzheimer phenotype (Emery, 1988). Where postmortems were permitted (9 patients), neuropathological examination of these nine patients revealed the typical markers of Alzheimer syndrome: neuronal loss, neurofibrillary tangles, and neuritic plaques (Kral and Emery, 1987, 1989). Thus, it would appear that a subset of persons with major depression/unipolar are at risk for depressive dementia, and in turn, the majority of persons with depressive dementia are at risk for progressive degenerative dementia of the Alzheimer phenotype.

The association between depressive dementia and subsequent progressive degenerative dementia has been documented in other longitudinal studies (Alexopoulos and Nambudiri, 1994). Frequency of documented progression of depressive dementia into primary degenerative dementia appears to be related to length of follow-up (Emery and Oxman, 1992, 1994). For example, at one-year follow-up, Murphy (1983) reported 3% of 124 elderly depressives were demented. Rabins and colleagues (1984) reported that 12% of older depressed patients were demented at two-year follow-up. Increasing to a three-year follow-up, Reding and associates (1985) reported that more than 50% of elderly patients diagnosed with depressive pseudodementia demonstrated primary degenerative dementia. And, as discussed above, Kral and Emery (1989) found 79% of cases of depressive dementia devolved into primary degenerative dementia after 4 to 18 years (average 8 years); variability in final follow-up reflects in part how long a patient lived after diagnosis of depressive dementia.

The meaning of these data is a core issue of this chapter. Although there has been clinical interest in the differential diagnosis between depressive dementia and the "organic" dementias for many years (e.g., Kiloh, 1961; Roth, 1986; Wells, 1982), the idea that there might exist some fundamental relation between these nosologically distinct categories is relatively new (Alexopoulos and Nambudiri, 1994; Emery, 1988, 1994; Emery and Oxman, 1992; Kral, 1983; Kral and Emery, 1987, 1989). Historically, the affective disorders have not been conceptualized as having connection with "organic" brain syndromes. The association between major depression without dementia, depressive dementia, and primary degenerative dementia represents a new research focus. In order to begin to know why major depression sometimes progresses to depressive dementia and why, in turn, a substantial proportion of cases of depressive dementia seem to devolve into degenerative dementia, multidimensional studies will be required.

Empirical data focused on the relationship between depressive dementia and Alzheimer syndrome are scarce. Systematic studies comparing cognitive function in these two populations are almost nonexistent (Alexopoulos and Nambudiri, 1994; Emery, 1988, 1994; Emery and Oxman, 1992, 1994). Also, with few exceptions (Cassens et al., 1990; Emery, 1988, 1992; Emery and Breslau, 1989; Hart et al., 1987; Massman et al., 1994; Speedie et al., 1990), investigations addressing similarities and differences in cognitive processing between major depression without dementia and Alzheimer syndrome are rare. And further, there appear to be no reported studies of the interactions of differing cognitive functions in these patient populations; for exception, see Emery (1992) on the relation between memory and language in major depression without dementia. And yet the recent longitudinal findings suggesting depressive dementia might be a "transitional state" (Emery, 1988; Emery and Oxman 1994) between major depression without dementia and an Alzheimer-like syndrome, underscore the importance of systematic comparison of these three points of the depression-dementia spectrum.

Cognitive deficits are at the core of the definition of primary degenerative dementia of the Alzheimer type (American Psychiatric Association, 1987, 1994). Accordingly, investigations of cognitive processing in this population as well as in any populations constituting transitional states in its progression are critical for understanding the process of degenerative cementing. The study to be described in this chapter involves comparisons of language and memory in elderly populations of depressive dementia, major depression/unipolar without dementia, and senile dementia Alzheimer's type (SDAT). Normal elderly constitute a normative baseline. Further, the interaction of language and memory in these populations will be examined. As best we can determine, this is the first study of the interaction of language and memory in depressive dementia.

METHOD

Participants

The study involves a total of 72 participants: 12 elderly with depressive dementia (3 men and 9 women); 20 elderly with major depression/ unipolar (6 men and 14 women); 20 elderly with SDAT (8 men and 12 women); and 20 normal elderly (6 men and 14 women). Demographic variables of age, education, race, occupation, native birth, and native language were statistically equivalent across samples. Mean ages of the depressive dementia, major depressive/unipolar, SDAT, and normal elderly samples were 77.2, 74.9, 76.8, and 78.2, respectively. Median ages for these groups in turn were 78.5, 75.5, 78, and 75. Mean years of education were 10.2 years, 11.6 years, 11.4 years, and 12.3 years for depressive dementia, major depression/unipolar, SDAT, and normal elderly samples, respectively. Median years of education for these samples, in turn, were 11 years, 12 years, 12 years, and 12 years.

Major depression/unipolar was diagnosed on the basis of criteria from the 6 Diagnostic and Statistical Manual of Mental Disorders, Third Edition, Revised (DSM-III-R) (American Psychiatric Association, 1987) and Research Diagnostic Criteria, with the Schedule for Affective Disorders and Schizophrenia (Endicott & Spitzer, 1978) used to obtain information needed for diagnosis. The Hamilton Depression Scale (Hamilton, 1967) was used to determine severity of depression, and the Geriatric Depression Scale (Brink et al., 1982), a self-report measure, was used as a reliability check on the observer rating. Only patients scoring in the depressed range of both these instruments were included in the major depression/unipolar sample. The cut-point between normalcy and depression on the Hamilton Depression Scale is a score of 18, and the cut-point on the Geriatric Depression Scale is 10; on both instruments, the higher the score, the more severe the depression. The mean Hamilton Depression score for the major depression/unipolar sample was 31.3, while the mean Geriatric Depression Scale score was 16.9. The Interview for Psychosis (Kahn et al., 1978) was administered to ascertain presence or absence of psychosis. No depressed person was psychotic at time of interview. Mental status was assessed by the Kahn-Goldfarb Mental Status Questionnaire (MSQ) (Kahn et al., 1960; Kahn and Miller, 1978) and by the Bender Face-Hand Test (FHT) (Bender, 1952; Kahn et al., 1960; Kahn and Miller, 1978). The mean score for elderly with major depression/unipolar on the Mental Status Questionnaire was 11 correct responses or, put another way, a mean error of 2. The mean score of this study's depressed sample on the Face-Hand Test was 15.4 correct responses or .6 mean errors. The MSQ has a 13 point total, with 0–2 errors indicating no or mild brain dysfunction, 3–8 errors indicating moderate dysfunction, and 9 or 10 errors indicating severe dysfunction. The FHT consists of 16 trials (8 with eyes closed; 8 with eyes open) of simultaneous double stimulation to contralateral parts of the body, i.e., face and hands. Although normal persons may make errors on the first few trials, persistent errors appear to indicate organic brain dysfunction. Of a maximal possible score of 16, the mild FHT category of severity is indicated by 3–7 errors, the moderate category of severity involves 8–12 errors, and the severe FHT category is indicated by 13–16 errors (Kahn et al., 1960; Kahn and Miller, 1978).

The depressive dementia sample consisted of persons referred to a medical school-hospital medical center with the presumptive diagnosis of dementia. The patients received a thorough medical workup, including tests of vital signs, complete blood count with tests for venereal diseases, B–12 folic acid, diabetes, thyroid abnormalities. Other procedures included urinalysis, electrocardiogram, chest X-ray, and CT scan. All patients underwent psychiatric, neurological, and internal medicine assessments. Depressive dementia was diagnosed on the basis of medical workup, medical/psychiatric history, onset pattern, as well as by scores on the Schedule for Affective Disorders and Schizophrenia, Hamilton Depression Scale, Geriatric Depression Scale, Interview for Psychosis, Mental Status Questionnaire, and Face-Hand Test. The depressive dementia sample was comprised of patients with an Alzheimer-like presentation who also had a long-standing history of major depression/unipolar. Every subject in the depressive dementia sample had at some previous time in life presented with a dementia profile but had subsequently "recovered." The mean Hamilton Depression Scale score of the depressive dementia sample was 25.2, and the mean Geriatric Depression Scale score was 19.2. On the Mental Status Questionnaire, the elderly with depressive dementia had a mean error score of 6.6 errors, which locates the sample in the moderate cognitive impairment severity category of the MSQ. The major depression sample's mean error score on the FHT was 3.7 errors, locating the group in the mild organic impairment category.

Subjects with SDAT underwent the same screening procedures, assessments, and medical workup as did the other two patient samples. Excluded from the SDAT sample were persons with cardiovascular disease, stroke, tumors, endocrine or metabolic disease, substance abuse, or neurological signs not part of Alzheimer symptomatology. SDAT subjects were required to have an ischemia score of less than 4 to make sure there was no vascular confound (Rosen et al., 1980). Ischemia scales assess variables of cerebrovascular illness; recent research has shown that patients with a broader spectrum of vascular disorders become demented than had hitherto been realized (Emery et al., 1994, 1995, 1996), and that many Alzheimer research samples have a serious vascular confound. First diagnosis was at age sixty-five or later. Age sixty-five establishes the boundary between Alzheimer syndrome early onset and senile dementia Alzheimer type (SDAT) (American Psychiatric Association, 1980, 1987, 1994); the latter constitutes the Alzheimer population of this study. The SDAT sample met the criteria of DSM-III-R (American Psychiatric Association, 1987) for primary degenerative dementia of the Alzheimer type: (1) demonstrable evidence of impairment in short-term and long-term memory, (2) impairment in at least one other category of cognitive function to include abstract thinking, language, judgement, apraxia, agnosia, construction, and/or personality change, (3) significant interference with work or usual social activities and relations, (4) insidious onset with a generally progressive deteriorating course, and (5) exclusion of all other specific causes of dementia by history, physical examination, and laboratory tests. Further, individuals with primary psychiatric disorders other than primary degenerative dementia Alzheimer type (e.g., major depression/unipolar, mania, schizophrenia) were excluded from the Alzheimer sample of our study. SDAT subjects were required to show evidence of cognitive impairment on the Mental Status Questionnaire, Face-Hand Test, and Global Deterioration Scale (Reisberg et al., 1982). In other words, to be included in the SDAT sample, a patient could not score in the normal range of any of these measures. The SDAT sample had 7.5 mean errors on the MSQ and a mean error score of 9.5 on the FHT. The combined assessments of the Mental Status Questionnaire, Face-Hand Test, and Global Deterioration Scale served to locate eight SDAT patients in the mild severity category, nine were in the moderate category, and three patients met criteria for a designation of severe organic brain dysfunction. In contrast, the study required that SDAT patients score in the normal range of the Hamilton Depression Scale and Geriatric Depression Scale in order to prevent a depression confound in our comparisons between depressive dementia and SDAT. Mean Hamilton Depression Scale score for the SDAT sample was 12.4, and mean score on the Geriatric Depression Scale was 7.5. As stated, cut-points between normalcy and depression on these instruments are 18 and 10, respectively.

Normal elderly persons were recruited from the community at large. Participants needed to have non-compromised major organ systems, vital signs within normal range, no chronic illness, and self-sufficiency in everyday living. Measures described above were administered to all participants. Accordingly, elderly scoring outside the range of normalcy on any of the assessments were by operational definition "not normal," and were not included in the normal elderly sample of this study. Mean Hamilton Depression Scale score for the normal elderly was 9.8, and mean Geriatric Depression Scale score was 2.9. The mean error on the Mental Status Questionnaire was .6, and the mean error on the Face-Hand Test was .2 for the normal elderly.

All participants gave informed consent. For SDAT and depressive dementia patients, consent was secured from legal guardians or family members also.

Memory Measures

Eight measures of memory were administered to the 72 subjects: Information, Orientation, Mental Control, Digit Span Forward, Digit Span Backward, Verbal Paired Associates, Story Recall, and Katzman Test for Delayed Recall. The first seven of these measures are from the Wechsler Memory Scale (WMS) (Wechsler, 1973). The test of Information consists of six items of personal and current information, e.g., "How old are you," and "Who is President of the United States." Orientation involves five items of time and place, e.g., "What month is this," and "What is the name of the place you are in." For the measure of Mental Control, the participant is asked to count backward from twenty to one, say the alphabet, and count by three's to the number forty. Digit Span Forward requires the participant to repeat a span of digits after hearing them and goes up to a span of eight digits. Digit Span Backward goes to a span of seven digits and requires that upon hearing the digit span, the numbers be repeated in reverse order. Verbal Paired Associates consists of ten pairs of words to be associated across three trials: six pairs involve commonplace associations, such as "baby-cries," "North-South," "fruit-apple," but four pairs of words consist of non-common associations, such as "cabbage-pen," "crush-dark," "obey-inch." The measure of Story Recall (Logical Memory) consists of a 67-word paragraph, broken up into 24 scoring units, telling the story of a scrubwoman who was robbed and her subsequent plight. The Katzman Test for Delayed Recall (Katzman, 1983), consists of a single sentence ("John Brown lives at 42 Market Street in Chicago, Illinois") and was used to assess recall one hour after administration.

Language Measures

Language processing was assessed by use of the Western Aphasia Battery (WAB) (Kertesz, 1982) and Test for Syntactic Complexity (Emery, 1982, 1985, 1986). The structural language variables assessed were repetition, naming, auditory verbal comprehension, grammatical-syntactic processing, and reading.

Of ten Western Aphasia Battery language subtests administered, eight were oral language subtests and two were reading subtests. The eight WAB oral language assessments to be described tap three formal/structural variables of language: repetition, naming, and auditory verbal comprehension. The WAB Repetition Test requires the repetition of 14 items (e.g., "nose," "banana," "the telephone is ringing," "no ifs, ands, or buts") for a total of 100 points. Points are subtracted for phonemic errors or errors in word sequence.

The four WAB measures for naming dysfunction are Object Naming, Sentence Completion, Responsive Speech, and Word Fluency. The Object Naming Test involves the confrontation naming of twenty objects, such as comb, knife, spoon, elastic, and has a 60 point maximum. Sentence Completion comprises five familiar sentences to complete, e.g., "roses are red, violets are _____." The Responsive Speech Test consists of five simple questions such as, "Where do nurses work?" Both these tests have ten point totals. The Word Fluency Test requires the individual to name as many animals as he or she can; one point per animal named.

The WAB auditory verbal comprehension assessment consists of three tests: Yes/No Questions, Auditory Word Recognition, and Sequential Commands. The Yes/No Questions task has 20 questions ("Is the door closed?") for a 20 point total. Eleven items constitute the Sequential Commands Test ("With the book, point to the comb") for a total of 80 points. And real objects, drawn objects, forms, letters, numbers, colors, body parts, and left-right items require recognition in the Auditory Word Recognition Test (60 point total).

The WAB Reading Commands Test consists of six commands presented on a card which the participant must read, e.g., "Wave goodbye" (20 point total). The WAB Reading Comprehension of Sentences Test has eight items to be answered: the correct answer depends on sentence comprehension, for example, "Shovels and saws are common tools; they have parts made of (farmer, forest, metal, cutting)." The test has a 40 point total.

The Test for Syntactic Complexity (TSC) (Emery, 1982, 1985, 1986) is a 36-item instrument designed to assess processing of various complex syntactic relations which are late to develop in the sequence of language learning (Chomsky, 1979; Dale, 1976). The TSC was devised in such a way that correct linguistic processing, i.e., the correct analysis of meaning, depends directly on correct processing of syntactic complexities. In spontaneous speech and other unstructured linguistic exchange, meaning is often apprehended or communicated through the use of contextual cues or redundancy (Emery, 1985, 1992). The TSC was designed to eliminate any cues external to syntactic structure. The TSC assesses the processing of the following syntactic forms: (1) prepositions of time sequence ("Do you put on your stockings after your shoes?"); (2) passive subject-object discrimination ("The boy is called by the girl; who is called and who did the calling?"); (3) possessive relations of a reversible construction ("What is the relationship of your brother's father to you?")' and (4) communication of narrative action events which are concrete ("John and Mary run to the hospital really fast") versus the communication of abstract and/or logical relations of the same number of words ("John runs faster than George but slower than Humphrey").

Non-Verbal Measures

Two non-verbal measures were also administered. The WAB Apraxia Test consists of twenty commands evenly distributed across apraxia categories of upper limb ("scratch your head"), facial ("put out your tongue"), instrumental ("use a spoon to eat"), and complex ("pretend to drive a car") (60-point total). WAB Calculation has 12 problems of addition, subtraction, multiplication, and division (24 points).

Statistical Measures

Three statistical approaches were used. First, to determine significance of difference in means, a one-way Analysis-of-Variance (ANOVA) was used to compare the four samples. The ANOVA was followed by Scheffe's test. Further, *t*-tests were used to obtain exact *t*-values and alpha levels. Two-tailed tests were used to interpret significance. Second, the Omega Squared statistic was calculated from obtained differences between means using the method described by Hays (1981), and was utilized to determine effect size of tests for purposes of discriminant function and predictive power. Third, Pearson correlations were calculated between all measures of language and memory in order to begin to determine extent and nature of correlatedness and interaction between these two cognitive functions.

RESULTS OF STUDY

The results of the study are organized and presented along the three lines corresponding to statistical approaches outlined above.

Difference of Means

Results from the ANOVA indicate that on all measures, there are significant differences between the four populations at the .0001 level, excepting Digits Forward (.0002), Auditory Word Recognition (.0002),

Apraxia (.0002), and Yes/No Questions (.001). All means for participants with depressive dementia, major depression/unipolar, SDAT, as well as normal elderly on eight measures of memory, nine measures of oral language, two measures of reading, and two non-verbal measures, can be inspected in Tables 1, 2, and 3.

The data suggest a general pattern of results in which the normal elderly have the highest means, with major depression/unipolar with comparable or lower. Elderly with depressive dementia consistently rank third, and the SDAT elderly have the lowest means. Scheffe's tests indicate that all comparisons between normal elderly and elderly with Alzheimer's syndrome are statistically significant. Also, comparisons between patients with major depression/unipolar and SDAT are clear cut; all comparisons are statistically significant. Further, Scheffe's tests show that all comparisons between elderly with depressive dementia and normal elderly are significant.

In contrast, comparisons between patients with depressive dementia and major depression/unipolar are sometimes, but not always, significant. And comparisons between depressive dementia and SDAT are most often not significant. For the remainder of this results section, the focus will be on the variability of depressive dementia in relation to depression and especially in relation to SDAT. This variability lies at the core of the diagnostic issues which are the focus of this chaper. A more detailed analysis of results follows.

Means/Memory:

Looking first at the Information column, one sees that the F-value resulting from the ANOVA is 62.87 (p = .0001); see Table 1 for sample means and standard errors of the means. An analysis of Scheffe's tests involving the t-distribution shows that the t-value resulting from the difference of means between depressive dementia and major depression is 4.02 ($df = 30$, $p = .001$) (Table 4). The difference of means between SDAT and depressive dementia results in a t-value of 1.97 ($df = 30$, $p = .07$) (Table 5).

For Orientation, ($F = 40.50$, $p = .0001$), the follow-up test between depressive dementia and depression yields a t-value of 4.80 ($df = 30$, $p = .0001$); see Table 4. The alpha resulting from the comparison between SDAT and depressive dementia is not significant ($t = 1.30$); see Table 5.

Table 1. Comparison of Means by Sample on Measures of Memory

Measure (maximal score)	Normal Elderly (n = 20)	Major Depression/ Unipolar (n = 20)	Depressive Dementia (n = 12)	SDAT (n = 20)	F
Information (6)	5.65 ± .15	4.85 ± .23	2.33 ± .58	1.10 ± .23	62.87****
Orientation (5)	5.00 ± .00	4.45 ± .25	2.25 ± .43	1.55 ± .33	40.50****
Story Recall (24)	10.90 ± .84	7.00 ± .91	2.73 ± .70	1.15 ± .42	35.35****
Verbal Paired Associates (30)	23.60 ± .89	13.42 ± 2.06	7.36 ± 2.36	4.55 ± 1.38	28.73****
Katzman Delayed (30)	23.00 ± 2.07	14.00 ± 2.82	2.08 ± 2.08	.50 ± .50	26.49****
Mental Control (9)	8.98 ± .03	6.63 ± .45	5.29 ± .79	3.53 ± .74	19.43****
Digits Backward (7)	4.40 ± .28	3.00 ± .39	2.00 ± .48	1.37 ± .43	12.15*****
Digits Forward (8)	7.15 ± .26	5.70 ± .31	4.58 ± .74	4.58 ± .53	7.73 ***

Note: Values reported are the mean plus or minus the standard error of the mean.

**** p is equal to/less than .0001

*** p is equal to/less than .0002

Table 2. Comparison of Means by Sample on Measures of Oral Language

Measure (maximal score)	Normal Elderly ($n = 20$)	Major Depression/ Unipolar ($n = 20$)	Depressive Dementia ($n = 12$)	SDAT ($n = 20$)	F
Test for Syntactic Complexity (36)	29.95 ± 1.16	24.90 ± 1.91	14.09 ± 2.99	8.75 ± 2.03	$27.10{****}$
Word Fluency (20)	$16.40 \pm .89$	11.26 ± 1.66	6.40 ± 1.17	$3.32 \pm .68$	$25.58{****}$
Sequential Commands (80)	$78.00 \pm .66$	72.40 ± 3.41	48.67 ± 9.71	38.40 ± 7.07	$13.20{****}$
Sentence Completion (10)	$10.00 \pm .00$	$10.00 \pm .00$	$9.09 \pm .56$	$6.21 \pm .92$	$12.70{****}$
Responsive Speech (10)	$10.00 \pm .00$	$9.95 \pm .05$	$9.64 \pm .24$	$6.57 \pm .95$	$12.03{****}$
Repetition (100)	95.00 ± 1.82	84.20 ± 2.82	76.36 ± 6.82	59.00 ± 7.12	$11.11{****}$
Confronting Naming (60)	$60.00 \pm .00$	$59.85 \pm .15$	50.67 ± 5.08	44.90 ± 4.14	$9.13{***}$
Auditory Word Recognition (60)	$59.95 \pm .05$	$58.95 \pm .41$	51.18 ± 4.31	47.60 ± 3.21	$7.63{***}$
Yes/No Questions (60)	$60.00 \pm .00$	$59.60 \pm .22$	50.75 ± 4.55	51.60 ± 2.46	$5.83{***}$

Note: Values reported are the mean plus or minus the standard error of the mean.

**** p is equal to/less than .0001

*** p is equal to/less than .001

Table 3. Comparison of Means by Sample on Reading Measures and Non-Verbal Measures

Measure (maximal score)	Normal Elderly (n = 20)	Major Depression/ Unipolar (n = 20)	Depressive Dementia (n = 12)	SDAT (n = 20)	F
Reading					
Reading Comprehension of Sentences (40)	35.20 ± 1.74	37.47 ± 1.07	24.00 ± 4.26	14.56 ± 2.54	26.16****
Reading Commands (20)	20.00 ± .00	20.00 ± .00	16.33 ± 2.06	13.33 ± 1.72	9.90****
Non-Verbal					
Calculation (24)	23.10 ± .34	21.58 ± .89	14.91 ± 2.56	11.06 ± 2.25	14.65****
Apraxia (60)	59.50 ± .19	57.70 ± .64	52.82 ± 3.65	39.65 ± 5.72	7.66***

Note: Values reported are the mean plus or minus the standard error of the mean.
**** p is equal to/less than .0001
*** p is equal to/less than .001

Table 4. Estimates of Effect Size for Depressive Dementia and Major Depression/Unipolar

Measure	t-value	df	p	Omega Squared
Memory				
Information	4.02	30	.001	.32
Orientation	4.80	30	.0001	.41
Story Recall	3.25	28	.003	.26
Katzman Delayed	3.40	30	.003	.25
Mental Control	—	—	NS	—
Verbal Paired Associates	1.86	28	.08	.08
Digits Forward	—	—	NS	—
Digits Backward	—	—	NS	—
Oral Language				
Test for Syntactic Complexity	3.19	29	.003	.23
Word Fluency	2.40	27	.03	.14
Sequential Commands	2.31	30	.04	.12
Confrontation Naming	—	—	NS	—
Sentence Completion	—	—	NS	—
Responsive Speech	—	—	NS	—
Auditory Word Recognition	—	—	NS	—
Yes/No Questions	—	—	NS	—
Repetition	—	—	NS	—
Reading				
Reading Comprehension	3.07	27	.02	.22
Reading Commands	—	—	NS	—
Non-Verbal				
Calculation	2.46	28	.03	.14
Apraxia	—	—	NS	—

Table 5. Estimates of Effect Size for Depressive Dementia and SDAT

Measure	t-value	df	p	Omega Squared
Memory				
Information	1.97	30	.07	.08
Orientation	—	—	NS	—
Story Recall	2.06	29	.05	.10
Katzman Delayed	—	—	NS	—
Mental Control	—	—	NS	—
Verbal Paired Associates	—	—	NS	—
Digits Forward	—	—	NS	—
Digits Backward	—	—	NS	—
Oral Language				
Test for Syntactic Complexity	—	—	NS	—
Word Fluency	2.45	28	.02	.15
Sequential Commands	—	—	NS	—
Confrontation Naming	—	—	NS	—
Sentence Completion	2.68	30	.01	.16
Responsive Speech	3.32	30	.003	.24
Auditory Word Recognition	—	—	NS	—
Yes/No Questions	—	—	NS	—
Repetition	—	—	NS	—
Reading				
Reading Comprehension	2.02	27	.05	.10
Reading Commands	—	—	NS	—
Non-Verbal				
Calculation	—	—	NS	—
Apraxia	1.94	30	.06	.08

The ANOVA for Story Recall results in a F-value of 35.35 (p = .0001). In following up with the Scheffe procedure, the t-test between depressive dementia and major depression/unipolar results in an alpha of .003 (t = 3.25), while the comparison between SDAT and depressive dementia results in an alpha of .05 (t = 2.06).

Results for Verbal Paired Associates (F = 28.73, p = .0001) and Katzman Delayed (F = 26.49, p = .0001), indicate that the difference of means between depressive dementia and major depression on Verbal Paired Associates is not significant (t = 1.86), whereas the difference of means for the Katzman Delayed is significant (t = 3.40, p = .002) (Table 4). The comparison of SDAT with depressive dementia shows neither alpha is significant (Table 5).

On the variable of Mental Control (F = 19.43, p = .0001), there is no significant difference between depressive dementia and major depression/unipolar nor between depressive dementia and SDAT.

Finally, results for Digits Backward (F = 12.15, p = .0001) and Digits Forward (F = 7.73, p = .0002) indicate that neither comparison between depressive dementia and major depression/unipolar is significant (Table 4). Comparisons between depressive dementia and SDAT also are not significant.

Means/Oral Language and Reading:

The ANOVA results for the Test for Syntactic Complexity yield an F-value of 27.10 (p = .0001); see Table 2 for means and standard errors of the means for all oral language tests. The difference of means between depressive dementia and major depression/unipolar results in a t-value of 3.19 (p = .003) (Table 4). The difference of means between depressive dementia and SDAT on the TSC is not significant (Table 5).

On Word Fluency (F = 25.58, p = .0001), the t-test between depressive dementia and depression results in an alpha of .03 (t = 2.40), whereas the t-test between pseudodementia and SDAT results in an alpha of .02 (t = 2.45). Although the focus of this chapter is on depressive dementia and how this disorder compares with the other populations of interest in this investigation, it is interesting to note that the t-test between normal elderly and major depression/unipolar is significant also (t = 2.77, df = 37, p = .01). Other comparisons of normal controls with major depression/unipolar on measures of language that are significant are: Test for Syntactic Complexity (t = 2.26, df = 38, p = .03); Story Recall (t = 3.15, df = 37, p = .005);

Repetition ($t = 3.45$, $df = 38$, $p = .001$); and Sequential Commands ($t = 2.44$, $df = 38$, $p = .02$). For a detailed analysis of differences in language processing between normal elderly and patients with major depression/unipolar which uses different samples than in the present study, see Emery and Breslau (1989).

Looking at Sequential Commands ($F = 13.20$, $p = .0001$), the difference of means between depressive dementia and major depression/unipolar yields a t-value of 2.31 ($p = .04$). The difference of means between SDAT and depressive dementia is not significant (Table 5).

Comparisons between depressive dementia and major depression/unipolar are not significant in either Sentence Completion or Responsive Speech. However, both comparisons between SDAT and depressive dementia are statistically significant, with a t-value of 2.68 ($p = .01$) for Sentence Completion, and a t-value of 3.32 ($p = .003$) for Responsive Speech (Table 5).

The Repetition Test ($F = 11.11$, $p = .0001$) shows there is no significant difference between depressive dementia and major depression/unipolar; nor is the comparison-between SDAT and depressive dementia significant. Similarly, on Confrontation Naming, the comparisons between depressive dementia and major depression/unipolar, as well as comparisons between depressive dementia and SDAT, are not statistically significant.

Finally, for Auditory Word Recognition ($F = 7.63$, p = .0002) and Yes/No Questions ($F = 5.83$, $p = .001$), there is no significant difference between depressive dementia and major depression/unipolar, nor is there a significant difference between SDAT and depressive dementia (Table 5).

For the reading assessments shown in Table 3, on Reading Comprehension of Sentences ($F = 26.16$, $p = .0001$), the difference of means between depressive dementia and major depression/unipolar is significant ($t = 3.07$, $p = .02$), as is the difference between SDAT and depressive dementia ($t = 2.02$, $p = .05$). For Reading Commands ($F = 9.90$, $p = .0001$), neither of the comparisons are significant (Tables 4 and 5).

Means/Non-Verbal:

The assessment for Calculation yielded an F-value of 14.65 across the four groups (Table 3). The comparison between depressive dementia and major depression/unipolar ($t = 2.46$, $p = .03$) is significant, whereas the comparison between SDAT and depressive dementia is not. For Apraxia ($F = 7.66$, $p = .0002$), neither the difference between depressive dementia and major depression nor the difference between SDAT and depressive dementia are significant.

Estimates of Effect Size/Omega Squared Statistic

In this section, the focus is on effect size. The Omega Squared statistic was calculated from obtained differences between means utilizing the method described by Hays (1981), and was used to estimate effect size of tests with the aim of discriminant function and prediction. In other words, which tests discriminate best between the research populations on the cognitive assessments given? On which measures is there the biggest discriminant value? Which measures have the greatest power to differentiate between the patient populations discussed in this chapter?

It can be seen in Table 6, that in the category of memory tests, strength of statistical association decreases in the following order for depressive dementia when distinguished from major depression/unipolar: Orientation (.41), Information (.32), Story Recall (.26), Katzman Delayed (.25), and Verbal Paired Associates (.08); the remaining measures of memory had no discriminant power at all. In the category of oral language, discriminant function between depressive dementia and major depression/unipolar is best accomplished by Test for Syntactic Complexity (.23), Word Fluency (.14), and Sequential Commands (.12). Reading Comprehension (.22) distinguishes between depressive dementia and major depression/unipolar almost as well as the TSC.

In addressing the key question of which measures best differentiate between SDAT and depressive dementia, one finds that of all measures of memory, oral language, reading, and non-verbal, only seven measures appear to distinguish between these two populations at all. Among measures of memory, one finds the modest Omega Squared values of .10 (Story Recall) and .08 (Information). The strongest power of discrimination occurs with Responsive Speech (.24). Sentence Completion and Word Fluency show effect sizes of .16 and .15. Finally, Reading Comprehension yields an Omega Squared value of .10 and Apraxia results in an Omega Squared value of .08.

Table 6. Comparison of Omega Squared Patterns

Measure	SDAT and Major Depression/ Unipolar	Depressive Dementia and Major Depression/ Unipolar	Depressive Dementia and SDAT
Oral Language			
Test for Syntactic Complexity	.45	.23	—
Word Fluency	.33	.14	.15
Sequential Commands	.31	.12	—
Confrontation Naming	.30	—	—
Sentence Completion	.29	—	.16
Responsive Speech	.25	—	.24
Auditory Word Recognition	.24	—	—
Repetition	.20	—	—
Yes/No Questions	.19	—	—
Reading			
Reading Comprehension of Sentences	.65	.22	.10
Reading Commanands	.27	—	—
Non-Verbal			
Calculation	.33	.14	—
Apraxia	.18	—	.08
Memory			
Information	.77	.32	.08
Orientation	.55	.41	—
Story Recall	.46	.26	.10
Katzman Delayed	.35	.25	—
Mental Control	.23	—	—
Verbal Paired Associates	.18	.08	—
Digits Backward	.17	—	—
Digits Forward	—	—	—

In comparing patterns of effect size in the research populations, it is of interest to see that even though the magnitudes of the Omega Squared values differ substantially, the pattern of discriminability between depressive dementia and major depression/unipolar follows the pattern of discriminability between SDAT and major depression/ unipolar. In contrast, the pattern of discriminability between depressive dementia and SDAT appears to reverse the rank ordering of discriminant power between SDAT and major depression/unipolar as well as that of depressive dementia and major depression/unipolar (Table 6). Thus, it would appear that depressive dementia and SDAT share a commonality related to cognitive processing vis-à-vis major depression/unipolar. In terms of patterning of effect size, the data point to some fundamental resemblance between depressive dementia and SDAT, based on a common relation to major depression/unipolar. Put another way, when A is to C, as B is to C, then some similarity obtains between A and B. This similarity is at the crux of the questions explored in this chapter, i.e., What is the fundamental nature of depressive dementia? Is the similarity between SDAT and depressive dementia, in essence, "pseudo," or does there exist some basic commonality between the two populations that approaches identity? It appears that the common factor of dementia between depressive dementia and SDAT has more explanatory power than does the common factor of depression between depressive dementia and major depression/unipolar.

Correlations Between Memory and Language

The significant Pearson correlation coefficients between memory and language for the four samples can be inspected in Table 7. For the normal elderly, the statistical relation between memory and language is generally not significant. There are only 6 significant correlations out of a possible 88 coefficients between memory and language.

Turning to the data for the elderly with major depression/unipolar, one finds 20 significant correlations beeween memory and language. Looking next at the number of significant correlations between the two cognitive functions for the patient group with depressive dementia, one sees that the number increases again, and that there are 25 significant correlations out of the possible 88. Further, not only does the number of significant correlations increase, but the degree of relatedness also reliably increases. Ninety-two percent of the significant correlations in the depressive dementia group show strength of correlatedness greater than .60 in contrast to the 5% for patients with major depression/unipolar. And the percentage of correlatedness at the .01 significance level or less is greater in depressive dementia (44%) than in major depression/unipolar (15%) (Table 7). A further distinction found in the two groups is that of the 20 significant correlations in major depression/unipolar, only half are shared with the depressive dementia patients. Put another way, of significant correlations in the depressive dementia sample, only 50% of the major depression/unipolar group's significant correlations are also part of the depressive dementia sample's significant correlations. Thus, the two groups have quite a different pattern profile in terms of which memory and language tests are significantly correlated for each sample (Table 7).

Finally, looking at the Pearson correlations between memory and language in the SDAT sample, data show 59 significant correlations out of the possible 88. Thus, again, with increased sample organicity, there is an increase in number of significant correlation coefficients between memory and language.

To summarize, for normal elderly, major depressed/unipolar, depressive dementia, and SDAT patients, results show the percentages of significant correlations between memory and language are 7%, 23%, 28%, and 67%, in turn. Further, the data suggest that as number of significant correlations between memory and language increase with sample organicity, there is also an increase in strength of correlatedness.

DISCUSSION

We have seen there are notable differences between the four samples on all measures of memory and language. All comparisons between normal elderly and depressive dementia patients are significant as are all comparisons between normal elderly and SDAT patients. Also, all comparisons between elderly persons with major depression/unipolar and SDAT are significant. However, significance varies when depressive dementia is compared to major depression/unipolar or to SDAT.

Memory Processing

The greatest discriminant function between depressive dementia and major depression/unipolar occurs with Orientation. The test that

Table 7. Significant Pearson Correlation Coefficients Between Language and Memory for Each Sample

	Info	Orient	MentalC	DigitsF	DigitsB	StoryR	PairedA	KatzmanD
Normal Elderly								
ReadingComp	—	—	—	—	—	—	—	—
ReadingComm	—	—	—	—	—	—	—	—
TSC	—	—	—	—	.47*	.52*	—	—
SeqCommands	—	—	.55*	.78***	—	—	—	—
WordFluenc/Un	—	—	—	—	.46*	—	—	.48*
RespSpeech	—	—	—	—	—	—	—	—
SentCompletion	—	—	—	—	—	—	—	—
ConObNaming	—	—	—	—	—	—	—	—
Yes/NoQuest	—	—	—	—	—	—	—	—
AudWordRec	—	—	—	—	—	—	—	—
Repetition	—	—	—	—	—	—	—	—

Note: * p equal/less than .05 ** p equal/less than .01 *** p equal/less than .001

Table 7 (*continued*)

	Info	Orient	MentalC	DigitsF	DigitsB	StoryR	PairedA	KatzmanD
Major Depression								
Unipolar								
ReadingComp	.52*	—	—	—	—	—	—	—
ReadingComm	—	—	—	—	—	—	—	—
TSC	.47*	—	.57*	—	.46*	.56*	.49*	—
SeqCommands	—	—	.51*	—	—	—	.53*	.54*
WordFluenc/Un	.48*	—	.54*	—	.46*	—	—	.52*
RespSpeech	—	.52*	—	—	—	—	—	—
SentCompletion	—	—	—	—	—	—	—	—
ConObNaming	—	.52*	—	—	—	—	—	—
Yes/NoQuest	.65*	—	—	—	—	—	—	—
AudWordRec	.47*	—	.49*	—	.45*	—	—	—
Repetition	—	—	.59***	—	—	—	.53*	—

Note: * *p* equal/less than .05   ** *p* equal/less than .01   *** *p* equal/less than .001

Table 7 (*continued*)

	Info	Orient	MentalC	DigitsF	DigitsB	StoryR	PairedA	KatzmanD
Depressive Dementia								
ReadingComp	—	—	—	—	—	.73**	—	—
ReadingComm	.63*	—	—	.71**	—	—	.62*	—
TSC	—	—	—	.58*	.80**	—	.79**	—
SeqCommands	.65*	—	—	.69*	.75**	.75**	.72**	—
WordFluenc/Un	.72**	.64*	—	—	.72**	.73**	—	—
RespSpeech	—	—	—	—	—	—	—	—
SentCompletion	—	—	—	—	—	—	—	—
ConObNaming	—	—	—	—	—	—	—	—
Yes/NoQuest	.60*	—	—	—	—	—	—	.68*
AudWordRec	.61*	—	.63*	.76**	.61*	.58*	—	—
Repetition	—	—	.62*	—	.66*	—	—	—

Note: * *p* equal/less than .05   ** *p* equal/less than .01   *** *p* equal/less than .001

Table 7 (*continued*)

	Info	Orient	MentalC	DigitsF	DigitsB	StoryR	PairedA	KatzmanD
SDAT								
ReadingComp	.77***	.61**	.80***	.68***	.78***	.55*	—	—
ReadingComm	.86***	.71***	.62**	.61**	.61**	—	—	—
TSC	.61**	.56*	.76***	.60**	.54*	.51*	.68***	—
SeqCommands	.78***	.64**	.80***	.58**	.63***	—	.49*	—
WordFluenc/Un	.85***	.72***	.80***	.68***	.73***	.52*	.59**	—
RespSpeech	.76***	.56*	.65**	—	.52*	.46*	.51*	—
SentCompletion	.70***	.55*	.65**	—	.59**	—	.47*	—
ConObNaming	.67**	.63**	.69***	.74***	.51*	—	—	—
Yes/NoQuest	.59**	.48*	.61**	—	.49*	—	—	—
AudWordRec	.51*	.54*	.51*	.53*	—	—	—	—
Repetition	.60**	.52*	.53*	—	—	—	.65**	—

Note: * p equal/less than .05   ** p equal/less than .01   *** p equal/less than .001

differentiates the two populations second best is Information. This same effect size pattern is seen for the discrimination of SDAT from major depression/unipolar; Orientation and Information have the greatest power to distinguish between these two groups. Measures of Orientation, Information, and Mental Control are characterized by combinative information processing requirements, predominantly those of tertiary memory which refers to well-known, overlearned material of both a personal nature (e.g., name, date of birth) and of a general nature (e.g., alphabet, President of country). Depressive dementia and SDAT are distinguished by the relative failure of these patients to process simple, well-known overlearned material as compared to patients with major depression/unipolar.

But what measures distinguished depressive dementia and SDAT? Greatest discrimination between these two populations on memory measures is with Story Recall. Story Recall is a measure of secondary memory (Poon, 1985), which requires new learning. Thus, this particular finding as well as the overall data from this investigation point to the idea that although depressive dementia and SDAT share similar effect patterns based on their common factor of dementia, patients with depressive dementia are somewhat less cognitively deteriorated than are SDAT patients and thus can still learn somewhat better.

These findings do not map neatly onto any of the existing conceptual frameworks for memory. Nevertheless, three theoretical systems are sufficiently relevant to mention.

First, our findings may be interpreted through information processing theory (Kaszniak, Poon, and Reige, 1986; Poon, 1985) with the following trends identified: (1) all study populations have greatest difficulty with measures of secondary memory, that is, with the acquisition and/or retrieval of new information, i.e., Story Recall and Katzman Delayed; (2) in SDAT, primary memory (limited capacity memory store that precedes entry into secondary memory) is best preserved, i.e., repetition (Digits Forward); (3) in major depression/unipolar and normal aging tertiary memory (overlearned material, personal material, cliches, stereotypes) is best preserved, i.e., Orientation, Information, Mental Control; and (4) depressive dementia falls between SDAT on the one hand and major depression/unipolar and normal aging on the other, with greatest and almost equal preservation of primary memory (repetition/Digits Forward) and tertiary memory (alphabet/Mental Control). However, overall the deficit in memory for depressive dementia is closest to SDAT.

Second, the distinction between memory processing of old information and new information (Light and Burke, 1993) suggests a parallel of information processing theory. The greatest qualitative and quantitative difference in memory between SDAT and major depression/unipolar or normal aging revolves around the SDAT decrement in tertiary memory (Orientation, Information, Mental Control). Unlike the normal aged or patients with major depression/unipolar, SDAT patients had difficulty remembering old information, especially items of personal history and/or non-personal, overlearned, heavily enculturated material from the remote past, i.e., tertiary memory. It appears that the disease process of degenerative dementia progressively destroys a person's information base of old, overlearned material, even when that material is personal. Although tertiary memory is significantly worse in depressive dementia than in major depression/unipolar, it is significantly better than in SDAT. Thus the measure of Information, which tests mainly old information, is useful for distinguishing depressive dementia in its intermediate position between major depression/unipolar and SDAT.

The third memory framework that provides a context for study findings revolves around the distinction between explicit and implicit processing (Light and Burke, 1993; Moscovitch, 1982), and although the paradigm was developed for memory research, it is relevant also for the understanding of language processing (Emery, 1982, 1985, 1992, 1993, 1996) and will be discussed in the section that follows.

Language Processing

We can look now at the domain of oral language. For all study samples, the greatest decrement by far occurs with the two most complex oral language measures, the Test for Syntactic Complexity and Word Fluency. The TSC (see pages 34–35 and Emery, 1982, 1985, 1986, 1993) requires explicit interpretation of complex syntactic structures, and Word Fluency (see page 34 and Emery, 1996; Emery and Breslau, 1988, 1989) represents what we have termed a meta-naming or meta-morphological task that is far more complex than naming tasks per se (see page 34). While within-sample findings indicate that each group has most difficulty with these two complex measures, the performance level for each sample was different enough from each of the other samples to result in statistical significance between all groups, except between depressive dementia and SDAT. This fact is reflected in effect size patterns which indicate that depressive dementia is best discriminated from major depression/unipolar, as is SDAT, by these two most complex measures. Conversely, depressive dementia is best distinguished from SDAT by two of the three least complex oral language tests, Responsive Speech and Sentence Completion; both of these tests are comprised of simple naming questions, e.g., "Where do nurses work," "Roses are red, violets are what?"

In previous research I found that performance decrement in SDAT is positively correlated with complexity and that the explicit processing requirement increases complexity (Emery, 1982, 1985, 1988, 1993, 1996; Emery and Breslau, 1989). Data from the present study suggest a corollary. Although complex tasks are first and most severely affected in SDAT, the degenerative process of the disease disproportionately impacts also on tasks of lesser complexity that require only implicit processing when compared to depressive dementia. In other words, the organic degeneration of SDAT impacts even the simplest of language tasks; these simplest language tasks are better preserved in depressive dementia. If we want to cast a broader net, the data indicate that depressive dementia is best distinguished from SDAT with a combination of naming tasks and meta-naming tasks (see Table 6 and Emery, 1988).

The Relation Between Memory and Language

The positive relation between memory and language increases with an increase in sample organicity. In other words, the less severe the organic decrement of the sample, the fewer the positive correlations between memory and language. Thus, it would appear that severity of organic decrement is an intervening variable in the positive relation between language and memory.

In theoretical terms, how can one begin to conceptualize the relation between language and memory? To begin to understand the correlation matrix from the present study, one must ferret out the theoretical connection between "semantic memory" and the "semantic" rank of the semiotic hierarchy. This connection does not appear to have been addressed previously.

We can start by looking at the linguistic properties of "semantics." The semiotic system is hierarchical, going from simple to more complex units of language, with categorical ranks of phonology, morphology, syntax, and semantics (Chomsky, 1979; DeSaussure, 1966; Huck and Ojeda, 1987; Yngve, 1986). Phonology refers to sound without reference to meaning, whereas morphology involves the smallest units of meaningful signalling (parts of words and words). Syntax refers to the structure of phrases and sentences. Semantics refers to the analysis, organization, and interpretation of meaning. But, whereas phonology, morphology, and syntax form a true hierarchy, semantics cross-cuts both morphology and syntax (Emery, 1982, 1985, 1988). Semantics requires one to render meaningful a string of parts of words/words, phrases, sentences, paragraphs, including the concepts inherent in these linguistic units, through processes of comprehension, analysis, organization, and interpretation. Semantic processing at the level of the part of word/word is less complex than at the level of larger aggregates of words (Emery, 1982, 1985, 1986).

Semantics as a dimension of language presupposes normative memorial function and once normative language skills have been attained, developmental linguistic processing assumes that the linguistic forms being processed will first of all be "remembered." A person cannot render meaningful parts of words/words if the normative denotation and connotation of these basic units are not "remembered" or otherwise accessed. Similarly, semantic processing cannot take place for aggregates of words if rules of normative phrases and sentence structure are not "remembered."

Looking at it another way, one can ask if memory depends on normative linguistic processing. There do appear to be forms of memory that are not linguistically based (e.g., in animals). Also, the pre-verbal infant has sensory memory function (e.g., visual, auditory, olfactory) that is not linguistic in nature. However, categories of memory that are essentially defined or characterized as based on words, ideas, concepts are, by definition, linguistically based and depend on semantic processing. Therefore, I would propose that "semantic memory" and linguistic processing at the "semantic" level are "systemically interconnected." The systemic interconnection of these cognitive activities only becomes apparent in the context of pathology. As long as normative levels of processing exist for both these higher cortical activities, each activity represents what appears to be an independent and specialized function. A prototype might be found in the more tangible body organs, e.g., heart, lungs. So long as these organs function within a normative range, each organ has its specialized activities. However, severe dysfunction of any one organ impacts on the function of others. Thus, semantic memory might presuppose normative semantic-linguistic processing and semantic-linguistic processing might presuppose normative semantic memory.

Thus it follows that the Pearson correlations between language and memory were negligible for the normal elderly of this study. A normal adult, by definition, has both normative language and memory processing, thus fulfilling the underlying requirement for both these higher cortical activities. In contrast, organic deterioration of either of these cognitive activities impacts on the synergistic, codependent function. Thus, the correlation matrix of the present study reflects this interaction with the increasing number of positive correlations between language and memory as severity of sample organicity increases.

CONCLUSION

This chapter has focused on the degree and kind of deficits in memory and language in populations of major depression without dementia, depressive dementia, SDAT, and normal aging. In comparisons between normal elderly and the patient populations, the normal elderly scored consistently and significantly better, and the impact of the disease process of SDAT was significantly greater than that of major depression/unipolar. In contrast, comparisons between depressive dementia and SDAT reach significance on only a few measures. Overall, the pattern of deficits in language and memory for depressive dementia patients is closer to SDAT than it is to major depression/unipolar. Discriminant function analyses have been carried out and results have been presented in this chapter indicating which combination of measures best discriminate depressive dementia from the other populations.

The positive relationship between memory and language appears to increase with the increase in severity of population organicity. This chapter has proposed that "semantic memory" and "semantic linguistic processing" are "systemically interconnected" and that this interconnection only becomes apparent in the context of pathology.

The data suggest that organic deterioration is best viewed as continuous. The dichotomous approach to organic deterioration is less productive for understanding the research results. A spectrum approach to major depression/unipolar, depressive dementia, and primary degenerative dementia is proposed. The utility of such a spectrum approach is underscored by recent findings from structural neuroimaging studies and neurochemical studies (Alexopoulos and Nambudiri, 1994; Arora et al., 1991; Dobie and Raskind, 1990; Emery and Oxman, 1992, 1994), indicating, for example, that there exists a dementia spectrum of depression.

Whereas the cognitive findings of the study are consistent with the interpretation that depressive dementia is a transitional state in a long-term degenerative cementing process, a full understanding of the spectrum of depression-dementia can only be acquired by repeated assessments on the same individuals over time. Future research must include the systematic longitudinal study of the depression-dementia spectrum. A long-term approach is necessary in order to answer basic questions that the present investigation has brought into focus.

REFERENCES

Alexopoulos, G. 1990. Clinical and biological findings in late-onset depression. In *Review of Psychiatry,* Volume 9, edited by A. Tasman, S.M. Goldfinger, and C.A. Kaufman. Pp. 249–262. Washington, D.C.: American Psychiatric Press.

Alexopoulos, G., and Nambudiri, D.E. 1994. Depressive dementia: Cognitive and biologic correlates and the course of illness. In *Dementia: Presentations, Differential Diagnosis, and Nosology,* edited by V.O.B. Emery and T.E. Oxman. Pp. 321–336. Baltimore: Johns Hopkins University Press.

American Psychiatric Association. 1980. *Diagnostic and Statistical Manual of Mental Disorders,* third edition. Washington, D.C.: Author.

American Psychiatric Association. 1987. *Diagnostic and Statistical Manual of Mental Disorders,* third edition revised. Washington, D.C.: Author.

American Psychiatric Association. 1994. *Diagnostic and Statistical Manual of Mental Disorders,* fourth edition. Washington, D.C.: Author.

Arieti, S., and Bemporad, J. 1974. Rare, unclassifiable, and collective psychiatric syndromes. In *American Handbook of Psychiatry,* edited by S. Arieti and E. Brody. Pp. 710–722. New York: Basic Books.

Arora, R., Emery, V.O.B., and Meltzer, H.Y. 1991. Serotonin uptake in the blood platelets of Alzheimer's disease patients. *Neurology 41,* 1307–1309.

Bender, M. 1952. *Disorders in Perception.* Springfield, Illinois: Charles C. Thomas.

Black, K., and Hughes, P. 1987. Alzheimer's disease: Making the diagnosis. *American Family Physician 36,* 196–202.

Brink, T., Yesavage, J., Lum, O., Heersma, P., Aday, V., and Rose, T. 1982. Screening tests for geriatric depression. *Clinical Gerontologist 1*, 37–44.

Bulbena, A., and Berrios, G. 1986. Pseudodementia: Facts and figures. *British Journal of Psychiatry 148*, 87–94.

Caine, E. 1981. Pseudodementia. *Archives of General Psychiatry 38*, 1359–1364.

Casey, D., and Fitzgerald, B. 1988. Mania and pseudodementia. *Journal of Clinical Psychiatry 49*, 74–84.

Cassens, G., Wolfe, L., and Zola, M. 1990. The neuropsychology of depressions. *Journal of Neuropsychiatry 2*, 203–213.

Chomsky, C. 1979. The *Acquisition of Syntax in Children from 5 to 10*. Cambridge, Massachusetts: M.I.T. Press.

Dale, P. 1976. *Language Development: Structure and Function.* New York: Holt, Rinehart, and Winston.

DeSaussure, F. 1966. *Course in General Linguistics.* New York: McGraw-Hill.

Dobie, D., and Raskind, M. 1990. Biology in geriatric psychiatry: Diagnostic implications. In *Review of Psychiatry,* Volume 9, edited by A. Tasman, S.M. Goldfinger, and C.A. Kaufman. Pp. 232–249. Washington, D.C.: American Psychiatric Press.

Emery, V.O.B. 1982. *Linguistic Patterning in the Second Half of the Life Cycle.* Doctoral Dissertation. The University of Chicago, Department of Behavioral Sciences, Committee on Human Development, Chicago, Illinois.

Emery, V.O.B. 1985. Language and aging. *Experimental Aging Research Monograph Series 11* (1).

Emery, V.O.B. 1986. Linguistic decrement in normal aging. *Language Communication 6*, 47–62.

Emery, V.O.B. 1988. *Pseudodementia: A Theoretical and Empirical Discussion.* Western Reserve Geriatric Education Center Interdisciplinary Monograph Series, edited by R. Hubbard and J. Kowal. Cleveland: Case Western Reserve University School of Medicine.

Emery, V.O.B. 1992. Interaction of language and memory in major depression and senile dementia Alzheimer's type. In *Memory Functioning in Dementia,* edited by L. Backman. Pp. 175–204. Advances in Psychology Series. Amsterdam: Elsevier Science Publishers.

Emery, V.O.B. 1993. Language and memory processing in senile dementia Alzheimer's type. In *Language, Memory, and Aging,* edited by L. Light and D. Burke. Pp. 221–243. New York: Cambridge University Press.

Emery, V.O.B. 1994. The interaction of memory and language in depressive dementia. In *Dementia: Presentations, Differential Diagnosis, and*

Nosology, edited by V.O.B. Emery and T.E. Oxman. Pp. 298–321. Baltimore: Johns Hopkins University Press.

Emery, V.O.B. 1996. Language functioning. In *Cognitive Neuropsychology of Alzheimer-Type Dementia,* edited by R.G. Morris. Pp. 166–192. Oxford: Oxford University Press.

Emery, V.O.B., and Breslau, L.D. 1988. The problem of naming in SDAT: A relative deficit. *Experimental Aging Research 14,* 181–193.

Emery, V.O.B., and Breslau, L.D. 1989. Language deficits in depression: Comparisons with SDAT and normal aging. *Journal of Gerontology 44* 85–92. -

Emery, V.O.B., Gillie, E.X., and Randev, P.T. 1994. Vascular dementia redefined. In *Dementia: Presentations, Differential Diagnosis, and Nosology,* edited by V.O.B. Emery and T.E. Oxman. Pp. 162–195. Baltimore: Johns Hopkins University Press.

Emery, V.O.B., Gillie, E.X., and Ramdev, P.T. 1995. Noninfarct vascular dementia. In *Treating Alzheimer's and Other Dementias,* edited by M. Bergener and S. Finkel. Pp. 184–204. New York: Springer Publishing Company.

Emery, V.O.B., Gillie, E.X., and Smith, J.A. 1996. Reclassification of the vascular dementias: Comparisons of infarct and noninfarct vascular dementias. *International Psychogeriatrics 8,* 33–66.

Emery, V.O.B., and Oxman, T.E. 1992. Update on the dementia spectrum of depression. *American Journal of Psychiatry 149,* 305–317.

Emery, V.O.B., and Oxman, T.E. 1994. The spectrum of depressive dementia. In *Dementia: Presentations, Differential Diagnosis, and Nosology,* edited by V.O.B. Emery and T.E. Oxman. Pp. 251- 277. Baltimore: Johns Hopkins University Press.

Endicott, J., and Spitzer, R. 1978. A diagnostic interview: The schedule for affective disorders and schizophrenia. *Archives of General Psychiatry 35,* 837–844.

Hamilton, M. 1967. Development of a rating scale for primary depressive illness. *British Journal of Social and Clinical Psychology 6,* 278–296.

Hart, R.P., Kwentus, J.A., Hamer, R., and Taylor, J.R. 1987. Selective reminding procedure in depression and dementia. *Psychology and Aging,* *2,* 111–115.

Hays, W. 1981. *Statistics.* New York: Holt, Rinehart, and Winston.

Huck, G., and Ojeda, A. 1987. *Syntax and Semantics.* New York: Academic Press.

Jorm, A.F. 1995. The epidemiology of depressive states in the elderly: Implications for recognition, intervention, and prevention. *Social Psychiatry and Psychiatric Epidemiology 30,* 53–59.

Jorm, A.F., MacKinnon, A.J., Henderson, A.S., Scott, R., Christensen, H., Korten, A.E., Cullen, J.S., and Mulligan, R. 1995. The Psychogeriatric Assessment Scales: A multi-dimensional alternative to categorical diagnoses of dementia and depression in the elderly. *Psychological Medicine 25,* 447–460.

Kahn, R., Goldfarb, A., Pollack, M., and Peck, A. 1960. Brief objective measures for determination of mental status in the aged. *American Journal of Psychiatry 117,* 326–328.

Kahn, R., Kodish, A., and Emery,V.O.B. 1978. *Interview for Psychosis.* Chicago: The University of Chicago School of Medicine.

Kahn, R., and Miller, N. 1978. Assessment of altered brain function in the aged. In *Clinical Psychology in Gerontology,* edited by M. Storandt, I. Siegler, and M. Elias. New York: Plenum Press.

Kaszniak, A.W., Poon, L., and Reige, W. 1986. Assessing memory deficits: An information processing approach. In *Handbook for Clinical Memory Assessment of Older Adults,* edited by L. Poon. Pp. 168–189. Washington, D.C.: American Psychological Association.

Katzman, R. 1983. *Biological Aspects of Alzheimer's Disease.* Cold Spring Harbor, New York: Cold Spring Harbor Laboratory.

Kay, D., and Bergmann, K. 1980. Epidemiology of mental disorders among the aged in the community. In *Handbook of Mental Health and Aging,* edited by J. Birren and B. Sloane. Pp. 34–56. Englewood Cliffs, New Jersey: Prentice-Hall.

Kertesz, A. 1982. *Western Aphasia Battery.* New York: Grune and Stratton.

Kiloh, L. 1961. Pseudodementia. *Acta Psychiatrica Scandinavica 37,* 336- 351.

Kral, V. 1983. The relationship between senile dementia (Alzheimer type) and depression. *Canadian Journal of Psychiatry 28,* 304- 306.

Kral, V., and Emery, V.O.B. 1987, August. Depressive Pseudodementia in the Aged. Paper presented at the Third Congress of the International Psychogeriatric Association, Chicago, Illinois.

Kral, V., and Emery, V.O.B. 1989. Long-term follow-up of depressive pseudodementia. *Canadian Journal of Psychiatry 35,* 445–447.

Kramp, P., and Bolwig, T. 1980. Electroconvulsive therapy in acute delirious states. *Comprehensive Psychiatry 22,* 368–371.

Light, L., and Burke, D. 1993. Patterns of language and memory in old age. In *Language, Memory, and Aging,* edited by L. Light and D. Burke. Pp. 244–273. New York: Cambridge University Press.

Lobo, A., Saz, P., Marcos, G., Dia, J.L., and DeLaCamara, C. 1995. The prevalence of dementia and depression in the elderly community of a southern European population. *Archives of General Psychiatry 52,* 497–506.

Mairet, A. 1883. *De la demence melancholique.* Paris: G. Masson.

Massman, P., Butters, N., and Delis, D. 1994. Some comparisons of verbal learning deficits in Alzheimer dementia, Huntington disease, and depression. In *Dementia: Presentations, Differential Diagnosis, and Nosology,* edited by V.O.B. Emery and T.E. Oxman. Pp. 232–249. Baltimore: Johns Hopkins University Press.

McAllister, T.W., and Powers, R. 1994. Approaches to the Treatment of Dementing Illness. In *Dementia: Presentations, Differential Diagnosis, and Nosology,* edited by V.O.B. Emery and T.E. Oxman. Pp. 355–384. Baltimore: Johns Hopkins University Press.

Moscovitch, M. 1982. A neuropsychological approach to perception and memory in normal and pathological aging. In *Aging and Cognitive Processes,* edited by F.I.M. Craik and S.Trehub. Pp. 55–78. New York: Plenum Press.

Murphy, E. 1983. The prognosis of depression in old age. *British Journal of Psychiatry 142,* 111–119.

Niederehe, G.T., and Oxman, T.E. 1994. The dementias: Construct and nosologic validity. In *Dementia: Presentations, Differential Diagnosis, and Nosology,* edited by V.O.B. Emery and T.E. Oxman. Pp. 19–46. Baltimore: Johns Hopkins University Press.

Poon, L.W. 1985. Differences in human memory with aging: Nature, causes, and clinical implications. In *Handbook of the Psychology of Aging,* edited by J. Birren and R.W. Schaie. Pp. 427–462. New York: Van Nostrand Reinhold.

Rabins, P., Merchant, A., and Neseadt, G. 1984. Criteria for diagnosing reversible dementia cuased by depression: Validation by 2-year follow-up. *British Journal of Psychiatry 144,* 488–492.

Reding, M., Haycox, J., and Blass, J. 1985. Depression in patients referred to a dementia clinic. *Archives of Neurology 42,* 894-896.

Reeves, A.G. 1989. Aging brains: Some observations. *Seminars in Neurology 9,* 1–4.

Reifler, B., and Sherrill, K. 1990. Dementias: Reversible and irreversible. In *Review of Psychiatry,* Volume 9, edited by A. Tasman, S.M. Goldfinger, and C.A. Raufman. Pp. 220–231. Washington, D.C.: American Psychiatric Press.

Reisberg, B., Ferris, S.H., DeLeon, H., and Crook, T. 1982. The Global Deterioration Scale (GDS): An instrument for assessment of primary degenerative dementia. *American Journal of Psychiatry 139,* 1136–1139.

Rosen, W., Terry, R., Fuld, P, Katzman, R., and Peck, A. 1980. Pathological verification of ischemic score in differentiation of dementias. *Annals of Neurology 7,* 486–488.

Roth, M. 1986. Differential diagnosis of psychiatric disorders in old age. *Hospital Practice 67,* 111–125.

Sachdev, P., and Kiloh, L.G. 1994. The nondepressive pseudodementias. In *Dementia: Presentations, Differential Diagnosis, and Nosology,* edited by V.O.B. Emery and T.E. Oxman. Pp. 277–298. Baltimore: Johns Hopkins University Press.

Speedie, L., Rabins, P., Pearlson, G., and Moberg, P. 1990. Confrontation naming deficit in dementia of depression. *Journal of Neuropsychiatry 2,* 59–63.

Starkstein, S., Rabins, P., Berthier, M., Cohen, B., Folstein, M.F., and Robinson, R. 1989. Dementia of depression among patients with neurological disorders and functional depression. *Journal of Neuropsychiatry 1,* 59–63.

United States Department of Health and Human Services. 1984. *Report of the Secretary's Task Force on Alzheimer's Disease.* Washington, D.C.: U.S. Government Printing Office.

Wechsler, D. 1973. *Wechsler Memory Scale: A Standardized Memory Scale for Clinical Use.* New York: The Journal Press.

Wells, C. 1982. Refinements in the diagnosis of dementia. *American Journal of Psychiatry 139,* 621–622.

Yngve, V. 1986. *Linguistics as a Science.* Bloomington, Indiana: Indiana University Press.

CHAPTER 3

Written Input to Enhance Comprehension in Dementia of the Alzheimer's Type

Loraine K. Obler
Lorraine Obermann
Ina Samuels
Martin L. Albert

INTRODUCTION

At times Alzheimer's disease would seem to be more difficult for the family members and caretakers than for the individuals who have it; patients with Alzheimer's disease may appear oblivious to the disease, but the people who care for them see the "shell" of their loved-ones remain while their "inner person" seems to be slipping away. One characteristic feature of language dissolution in Dementia of the Alzheimer's Type (DAT) is progressive loss of comprehension abilities. For the caretaker, the question becomes "How can I 'make' this person understand?"

In this study, we asked how one can enable patients with Alzheimer's disease to understand better. Our method was one employed by speech-language pathologists; first we used our clinical observations that sometimes putting questions in written form helped our patients. Then we set out to test this observation. We gave patients comprehension materials from a standardized test for language breakdown in adults—the Boston Diagnostic Aphasia Examination (Goodglass and Kaplan, 1972)—in different modalities (written only, oral only, and both together). We calculated the number of items the patients got right under each condition and whether these were significantly different. Before discussing our results, however, let us look at what was known about comprehension in patients with Alzheimer's disease before we undertook our study.

In the earliest stages of DAT, problems with oral comprehension are not as prominent as problems of remembering and saying the names of things. However, in later stages impairments of oral comprehension become more obvious, even to the casual observer. Indeed patients with DAT come to eventually resemble patients with Wernicke's aphasia-that form of language disturbance resulting from brain-damage (e.g., from a stroke) in which patients' speech sounds normal from a distance but is quite devoid of content, and comprehension of spoken and written language is quite poor. In the end stages of DAT, *oral comprehension* is restricted to occasional words and phrases (Obler and Albert, 1984) with no or virtually no observable comprehension.

We refer here to the natural history of *oral* comprehension in DAT because so little work has been done on *written* language comprehension in dementia. Rather, in what few studies there have been, the focus has been on how patients with DAT are able to read aloud relatively well. Schwartz et al. (1980) have reported the case of WHLP, who was able to read aloud but with no apparent comprehension. Sevush (1984) described the retained ability to read aloud in the face of poor reading comprehension in their demented patients. Patterson et al. (1994) have demonstrated that reading aloud is relatively but not completely spared in DAT, in that reading of irregularly spelled words in English (e.g., *yacht*) does start to decline in the middle stages of the disease.

In our clinical practice, however, we have observed that families and caretakers of demented patients rarely spontaneously use writing to explicitly enhance comprehension. One family does use a very large calendar, and when speaking with the patient by phone, they tell her to write the material onto the calendar so she can recall it later, but this is more of a memory aid. In a hospital one of us has worked in, health-care workers will put up signs for demented patients indicating the way to their bed, but these serve more as a guide to spatial location. These cues, we note, take advantage of a potential for spared written language abilities in DAT patients. Moreover, it is standard practice with patients with Wernicke's aphasia (whom, as mentioned above, DAT patients strongly resemble in the mid-late stage; see Obler and Albert, 1984) to write out information in order to enhance their comprehension (Kennedy, 1983).

While the language behavior of patients in certain middle stages of Alzheimer's dementia may resemble that of Wernicke's aphasics, the therapeutic approaches might conceivably differ given the different underlying etiologies and concomitant deficits. After all, the patients with DAT have cellular changes throughout their brains and have cognitive problems (with memory, problem solving, etc.) in addition to the language problems, while the patients with Wernicke's aphasia have brain-damage restricted to a more limited area, and their problems are primarily language related.

In the light of our observations of successful use of written cues with DAT patients, we hypothesized that written input would enhance language comprehension for those patients, at least for certain forms of stimulus material, because written material may compensate for the attentional deficits of DAT in ways in which auditory input cannot. To address this question of immediate therapeutic interest we presented materials to our patients in three ways: written only, auditory only, and combined written plus auditory.

METHODOLOGY

Subjects

Nine subjects with probable DAT were evaluated in this clinical pilot study. Diagnoses in each case conformed to the research diagnostic criteria established by the NIH-ADRDA working group (McKhann et al., 1984). All subjects were in the early-middle to middle stages of the syndrome according to our linguistic criteria (Obler and Albert, 1984). That is, remembering the names of things was no longer the predominant problem. In addition to these "name" problems, the patients now had marked problems comprehending what people said to them, and when they spoke their speech contained some meaningless words and many empty words and phrases (e.g. "things," "they," "those ones"). Our subjects first presented symptoms within the prior five years, with a mean of 2.5 years since reported onset. Ages ranged from fifty-eight to eighty-six years with a mean of sixty-three years. Mean level of education was 13 years with a range from 9 to 17 years. Five of the subjects were female and four were male. Hearing and vision were normal or were adjusted to normal by means of a hearing aid and/or prescription eyeglasses. All subjects were native speakers of English with no bilingual history, and all but one were right handed.

Procedure

The *materials* we used were the 13 comprehension subtests of the Boston Diagnostic Aphasia Exam (Goodglass and Kaplan, 1972) presented with examples in Table 1. These tests include a variety of comprehension questions and require a variety of responses. In some the patient must point to the picture that a spoken or written word refers to; in others the patients must listen to (or read) a sentence or paragraph, and answer "yes" or "no" to questions about it (e.g. "Is a hammer good for cutting wood?").

All materials were presented three times to each of our nine subjects, once each in the written only, auditory only, and written plus auditory conditions. Order of conditions was random, with at least two days intervening between testings. Thus we overrode the possibility that it could have made a difference which condition came first, and we precluded the possibility that subjects might remember an item from one condition and thus do better on subsequent ones as they might conceivably have done had we given all three conditions on the same day.

All stimuli in the written and combined conditions were presented on laminated 4" x 6" index cards with enlarged type. The majority of the subtests required a simple yes/no response or a gesture, as in Commands and Body-Part Identification. In order to respond to stimuli with multiple-choice answer sets, subjects either stated their response or selected it from a set of choices on an answer card. In instances where written multiple choice answers were required for our testing but not available as part of the original Boston Diagnostic Aphasia Examination, sets of choices were created. For example, "The lion was killed by the tiger" is followed by the question "Who's dead?" when presented in the auditory modality in the Boston Diagnostic Aphasia Examination. For presentation in both written modalities in the current experiment, a response card was constructed offering the choice, "Lion-Tiger" and the subject was instructed to either respond verbally or point to the correct answer.

When subjects did not respond within ten seconds, they were prompted with "Tell me which answer you think is best." If subjects appeared to have difficulty comprehending the nature of the task but attempted to respond, they were cued as in the following examples: "Answer yes or no," "Please move the penny," and, "Please point with

Table 1. Boston Diagnostic Aphasia Exam Subtests

Prepositions of Location-e.g., "Put the penny under the cup."

Before-After-e.g., "Is noon time *before* evening?"

With-To Pointing-e.g., "Point to the fork, then to the pen; now please pick up the pen. Now, point to the pen with the fork."

Passive Subject-Object Discrimination-e.g., "If I tell you 'the lion was killed by the tiger,' which animal is dead?"

Comprehension of Possession-e.g., "Suppose I point to someone across the street and say 'that person is my wife's brother.' Am I looking at a man or a woman?"

Subject of Verb Complement-e.g., "John asked his father to mail the letter and he did. Who mailed the letter?"

Word Discrimination-e.g., The patient sees a choice of 5 items and must show the examiner the object, letter, form, action, color, or number mentioned.

Body-Part Identification-e.g., The patient must point to each of 18 items, from ear to index finger.

Right-Left Discrimination-e.g., The patient is asked to point to 8 items, right ear to left cheek.

Commands-e.g., 1. "Make a fist," 5. "Tap each shoulder twice with 2 fingers keeping your eyes shut."

Complex Ideational Material I-e.g., "Will a cork sink in water?"

Complex Ideational Material II-e.g., The patient is read a brief story and asked for questions about it. The questions are paired, albeit not consecutively, to offer mutually exclusive choices: "Was the clerk suspicious of this guest? Did the clerk trust this guest?"

Comprehension of Sentences and Paragraphs-The patient hears or reads an item and has multiple choice response, e.g., a dog can talk, bark, sing, cat. The tenth item is a three-sentence paragraph with phrase length choices.

your finger." Subjects who responded correctly after one cue were given credit for a correct answer, but count was made of the number of cues required for each subject for each subtest in each condition. At no time was the stimulus material repeated auditorily; in the written conditions, however, the patients had the material in front of them for as long as they needed it.

Scoring

Each correct response was given one point, with a total of 111 possible correct responses for all 13 subtests combined. The number of correct responses for each subject on each subtest under each of the three conditions was calculated and then converted to percentage correct. The percentages correct for each subject across all 13 subtests in each condition were summed and averaged; these scores were subjected to a two-way subject-x-condition ANOVA to determine significant differences among the three conditions for the nine subjects. Percentages correct for each subtest across the nine subjects in each condition were also summed and averaged. These scores were then subjected to a two-way subject-x-condition ANOVA to determine significant differences among the three conditions of presentation for each of the 13 subtests. Further analyses were conducted by paired *t*-tests for significant main effects as is standardly done to see exactly where significance lies once an ANOVA has documented it.

Results

Pertinent results are summarized in Table 2. There were no significant subject effects, which is to say, the pattern of behavior across all subjects was what was of interest.

Results for the 13 subtests across all subjects under the three conditions of presentation are presented in Table 3. The following subtests were the ones with significant main effects for condition, that is, where subjects as a group performed significantly better in one condition than the others: *With-To Pointing, Passive Subject/Object Discrimination, Body-Part Identification, Commands, Complex Ideational Material II,* and *Comprehension of Sentences and Paragraphs.* On two additional subtests significance was approached ($p < .10$): *Comprehension of Possession,* and *Complex Ideational Materials I.*

Table 2. Percentage Correct Across All Subtests for Each Subject Under Each Condition

Subject	Auditory	Written	Combined
1	74.7	89.2	76.5
2	78.4	74.8	80.2
3	75.6	76.5	74.7
4	73.9	82.9	82.9
5	80.2	87.4	93.7
6	72.1	75.6	81.1
7	87.4	90.0	90.0
8	90.0	84.7	86.5
9	63.1	68.5	75.6
Mean	77.37	81.1	82.6

Table 3. Mean Percentage Correct Across Subjects on All Subtests for the Three Conditions of Presentation

	Auditory	Written	Combined	
Prepositions of Location	85.2	85.4	85.2	$F = .02$, n.s.
Before-After	55.5	59.2	55.5	$F = .4$, n.s.
With-To Pointing	77.8	69.1	78.5	$F = 4.25, p < .05*$
Subject/Object Discrimination	55.5	63.0	74.0	$F = 5.11, p < .05*$
Comprehension of Possession	62.2	55.5	66.7	$F = 1.48$, n.s.
Word Discrimination	96.3	97.6	97.2	$F = 1.64$, n.s.
Body-Part Identification	79.6	90.7	85.1	$F = 25.32, p < .001*$
Right-Left Discrimination	87.2	88.9	83.3	$F = 2.76$, n.s.
Commands	68.9	66.7	57.8	$F = 6.46, p < .01*$
Complex Ideational Material I	75.0	63.9	69.4	$F = 3.31, p < .10$
Complex Ideational Material II	68.5	75.0	77.8	$F = 4.83, p < .05*$
Comprehension of Sentences and Paragraphs	53.3	68.9	71.9	$F = 15.75, p < .001*$

* See Table 4 for *t*-tests and significance

Table 4. T-tests on Subtests with Significant Conditional Effects

Subtest	T-test by conditions		
With-To Pointing	A/C $t = .36$, n.s.	A/W $t = 4.14, p < .005$	C/W $t = 4.47, p < .005$
Subj/Obj Discrim.	W/A $t = 2.65, p < .01$	C/W $t = 3.59, p < .005$	C/A $t = 5.96, p < .005$
Body Part I.D.	C/A $t = 2.91, p < .01$	W/C $t = 4.14, p <. 005$	W/A $t = 6.49, p < .005$
Commands	A/W $t = .56$, n.s.	W/C $t = 2.4, p < .02$	A/C $t = 3.0, p < .005$
Compl. Ideat. II	W/C $t = 1.0$, n.s.	W/A $t = 3.89, p < .005$	C/A $t = 5.16, p < .005$
Sent. and Paragraphs	W/C $t = 1.03$, n.s.	W/A $t = 7.8, p < .005$	C/A $t = 8.35, p < .005$

A=Auditory   W=Written   C=Combined

As Table 4 indicates, in five of the six tests for which significant condition differences were found, the combined presentation—both hearing and reading together—was superior to at least one of the single conditions. (Only for commands was it the worst mode of presentation.) In three of those tests the combined condition was significantly better than the written only condition; in four it was significantly better than auditory only condition.[1]

As to the two subtests that approached significance, the combined presentation was best for Comprehension of Possession, and written only was worst, whereas for Complex Ideational Material I the auditory only condition resulted in the best performance, and the combined written resulted in the worst.

Further inspection of the individual data in Table 2 compared the individuals' ranked performance under the three conditions. For six subjects the auditory only condition was worst; for one subject it was best. For eight subjects, then, either the written or the combined condition was best; for two subjects they were virtually equal; for two the written only was best, and for four the combined was best.

Discussion

Although conducted with a small number of subjects, this study supports the clinical impression that written input, either alone or in combination with auditory input, can be helpful in aiding comprehension for early-mid to mid-stage patients with dementia of the Alzheimer's type. Eight of our nine subjects benefitted overall in the BDAE Comprehension Subtests either by the addition of written materials to auditory input or in the written only condition. Of the six tasks that showed significant main effects for condition, in five either the written or the combined conditions elicited the best performances for our group of subjects.

For what specific comprehension activities is written input most or least likely to benefit? Most striking is the difference between the commands and with-to pointing, on the one hand, for which auditory only is the best modality, and the four tests for which combined or written are more helpful. With-to pointing in fact involves command structure (e.g. "Point to the . . . "), and it is rare that we are asked to respond to commands in writing. In addition to Complex Ideational Materials I, discussed below, the other task on which auditory input was actually easiest, and significantly so, was the command subtest. On screening tests of aphasia, written commands are given to the subjects, who are often unable to respond. Thus it appears not particularly helpful to use writing to convey commands to DAT patients. Rather, when we are telling the patient to do something, this should be done orally as is so common in daily life. When we want to get information in and ask the patient a question about it, however, written material appears more helpful.

Consider also the comparison between Complex Ideational Materials I and Complex Ideational Materials II. For Complex Ideational Materials I, with single sentences requiring simply a "yes" or "no" response (such as "Will a good pair of rubber boots keep water out?"), performance in the auditory only condition was significantly better than performance in either the written or the combined conditions. Performance in the combined condition was significantly better than performance on the written only condition. By contrast, on Complex Ideational Materials II, where questions were asked regarding complete paragraphs that the patients had heard, performance in the auditory only condition is significantly worse than performance in either written or combined conditions, which did not differ significantly from each other.

Comparison between these two tests strongly suggests that it is for longer messages that DAT patients benefit most with written materials. We suspect that underlying attentional and memory deficits (e.g., Chertkow and Bub, 1990) account for the enhancement of DAT patients' comprehension abilities via written materials. In the written format, the subjects have the material continually in front of them, whereas in the auditory condition, stimulus materials stream by.

In the literature on comprehension in Wernicke's aphasics, whom, as we have said, DAT patients resemble in the mid-to-late (4th) stage (Obler and Albert, 1984), one finds patients for whom written comprehension is better than auditory comprehension and other patients for whom the converse is true (e.g., Hecaen and Albert, 1978; and Sevush et al., 1983). Indeed, we may infer that these two sorts of Wernicke's aphasics occur in relatively equal numbers, because Hartje and Poeck (1978) reported no significant differences for their Wernicke's aphasics (or indeed any other aphasic group) between oral and written presentation of the Token Test, a test developed by two aphasiologists to provide a scaler measure of comprehension abilities (De Renzi and Vignolo, 1962). That is to say, one could argue that the effects of their patients' performing better on one or the other task were washed out by simply averaging across the group. For the demented patients in our sample, by contrast, the substantially larger group is that for whom written input enhanced comprehension. No doubt the differences in the underlying etiology of what otherwise appears to be very similar symptomatology account for the different distribution. That is, in the Wernicke's aphasics the comprehension deficits are due more strictly to disturbances of language resulting from damage to auditory processing areas of the brain, whereas for the DAT patients, we speculate, the underlying attentional and memory problems cause functional deficits that mimic these language disturbances.

Our finding that written input is useful for eight out of nine subjects with DAT does not contradict the findings of Schwartz et al. (1980) and of Sevush (1984). Both studies reported their DAT patients were substantially and more able to read aloud than to read for comprehension. Yet in neither study were auditory comprehension scores compared to written comprehension scores. Thus it is conceivable that their patients' auditory comprehension for similar materials would have been even poorer than was their written comprehension. Alternatively, it is possible that their patients were more advanced in the progression of demented language dissolution, and that indeed our patients may reach a stage at which written comprehension will no longer be beneficial. For patients in the early to mid-stages of the disease, however, we would recommend substantial experimentation with written input in order to enhance comprehension.

Any time it is necessary to give information to the patient, that material could be written out in short sentences, preferably typed on a word processor (unless perhaps the patient was used to reading an individual's handwriting before the onset of the Alzheimer's Dementia). The family member, clinician, or home-care worker could then point to the materials, read them along with the patient, perhaps pointing to each word as it is read, and then ask the patient questions about the material, perhaps asking the same question in several different ways to assure that the answer is consistent.

NOTE

1. Consistent with these indications of the inadequacy of the auditory only condition was the mean number of cues required in each condition. The mean was 9 for the auditory only condition which was non-significantly greater than either the written (at 5.8) or combined (at 6.3) conditions.

REFERENCES

Chertkow, H., and Bub, D. 1990. Semantic memory loss in Alzheimer's Type Dementia. In M. Schwartz, ed., *Modular Deficits in Alzheimer Type Dementia*. Cambridge, Mass: MIT Press.

De Renzi, E., and Vignolo, L. 1962. The Token Test: a sensitive test to detect receptive disturbances in aphasics. *Brain*, 85, 655–678.

Goodglass, H., and Kaplan, E. 1972. *Boston Diagnostic Aphasia Exam*. Philadelphia: Lea and Febiger.

Hartje, W., and Poeck, K. 1978. Token-Test-Leistung aphasischer Patienten bei vokaler und visueller Testanweisung, *Nervenarzt*, 49, 654–657.

Hecaen, H., and Albert, M. L. 1978. *Human Neuropsychology*, New York: J. Wiley and Sons.

Kennedy, J. 1983. Treatment of Wernicke's aphasia. In W. Perkins, ed., *Language Handicaps in Adults*, New York: Thieme-Stratton.

McKhann, G., Drachman, D., Folstein, M., Katzman, R., Price, D., Stadlan, E.M. 1984. Clinical diagnosis of Alzheimer's disease: report of the NINCDS-ADRDA Work Group under the auspices of Department of Health and Human Services task force on Alzheimer's disease. *Neurology*, 34, 939–944.

Obler, L., and Albert, M. 1984. Language in Aging. In M.L. Albert, ed., *Clinical Neurology of Aging*, New York: Oxford University Press, 245–253.

Patterson, K., Graham, N., and Hodges, J. 1994. Reading in Dementia of the Alzheimer Type: a preserved ability? *Neuropsychology*, 8, 395–407.

Schwartz, M., Saffran, E., and Marin O. 1980. Fractioning the reading process in dementia: evidence for word specific print-to-sound associations. In M. Coltheart, K. Patterson, and J. Marshall, eds., *Deep Dyslexia*. London: Routledge and Kegan Paul, 259–269.

Sevush, S., Roltgen, D., Campanella, D., Heilman, K. 1983. Preserved oral reading in Wernicke's aphasia. *Neurology*, 33, 916–920.

Sevush, S. 1984. Oral versus semantic reading in Alzheimer's disease, paper presented at American Academy of Neurology, Boston, March.

CHAPTER 4

Language-Related Factors Influencing Naming in Adulthood[1]

Barbara A. Barresi
Loraine K. Obler
Rhoda Au
Martin L. Albert

INTRODUCTION

Research suggests that there is an age-related decline in naming pictures of objects (Borod, Goodglass, and Kaplan, 1980; Nicholas, Obler, Albert, and Goodglass, 1985; Au, Obler, Joung, and Albert, 1990) and actions (Nicholas et al., 1985; Au et al., 1990). Vocabulary definition remains stable with age (Bayles and Kaszniak, 1987), while naming pictured objects decreases from age thirty; most significantly between the ages of seventy and eighty (Nicholas et al., 1985). While there is a sharp decline in the ability to respond on a pictured naming task among seventy-year-olds as a group, some individuals in this age group performed as well as younger adults (Nicholas et al., 1985; Borod et al., 1980). Reasons for this variability are unclear.

One explanation for age-related naming variability is the effect of education. Research evidence demonstrates a relation between education level and ability to perform on the Boston Naming Test (Borod et al., 1980; Bayles and Kaszniak, 1987). The Boston Naming Test is commonly used to assess object naming in normal and language-impaired adults and children. It is composed of 85 (Kaplan, Goodglass, and Weintraub, 1976) or 60 (Kaplan, Goodglass, and Weintraub, 1983) line drawings of objects, very common ones at the beginning of the test (e.g. "bed") and increasingly less common ones as the test progresses (e.g. "abacus"). Farmer (1990), however, reported no significant correlation between education and naming in her study of responses on the 60-item version of the Boston Naming Test (Kaplan et al., 1983) in 125 men aged twenty to sixty-nine years with 8 to 22 years of education.

It is unlikely that educational level alone accounts for all the variability in naming, since many older adults whose naming ability was well preserved did not have the opportunity to further their education for socio-economic reasons. We suspect that other factors, apart from age and education, may exert an influence on naming abilities. Considering that naming is a verbal language task, it is possible that at least some of these factors may be associated with ways in which people use various forms of language in their daily lives.

Aphasic individuals benefit from treatment that enhances their ability to speak and to comprehend (Sparks, Helm, and Albert, 1974; Helm and Barresi, 1980; Helm-Estabrooks, Fitzpatrick, and Barresi, 1981; Helm-Estabrooks, Fitzpatrick, and Barresi, 1982). If stimulation of language can improve language performance in a brain-damaged, aphasic population, one might expect that normal elderly people who have been stimulated by language-related activities in their daily lives might demonstrate better naming performance on formal test measures than those who used language less. Moreover, Obler and Albert (1977) reported that for bilingual or polyglot aphasic patients who evidenced differential impairment in their language abilities (i.e. one language recovered better or sooner than another despite their being equally well known prior to the onset of aphasia), it was the language they had been using at the time of the aphasia-producing event that was most likely to recover best. This observation suggested that language "practice" or language use preserves or primes the system. Conversely, those individuals who are *not* engaged in a variety of language-related activities might be expected to perform worse. To our knowledge, there are no previous studies examining how the ways in which people use language in their daily lives may influence their performance on object-naming tests once their formal education has ended.

We designed a study asking if there are language-related activities associated with object-naming ability across the adult lifespan. In defining "language-related activities," we began with a broad definition to include factors that may be both directly and indirectly related to naming abilities. These included personality characteristics (e.g., sociability, shyness, wittiness, etc.), participation in such language activities as conversing, reading, and writing in native and, where applicable, second languages, and an array of tasks such as listening to the radio, watching television, attending movies, rote memorization (e.g. poems, song lyrics, prayers, etc.), and memory for details.

METHOD

Participants

The participants in this study were selected from a larger pool of adults who are undergoing a variety of cognitive and language tests in an on-going, longitudinal study of Language in the Aging Brain at the Boston Veterans Administration Medical Center. We were able to contact 62 adults who had been taking part in the study for 10 years. Fifty-seven of them completed a questionnaire designed to explore a wide selection of language-related activities. The participants responded to the questionnaire from three to four years after completing the third round of naming testing. Testing individuals for the longitudinal project began in 1978 and was conducted approximately every three years thereafter. For this study, data were analyzed for all 40 of those adults for whom three test scores of the Boston Naming Test (Kaplan, Goodglass, and Weintraub, 1976) were available over the course of the past decade. (For object- and action-naming results on the entire population see Nicholas et al., 1985).

Adults ranged in age from forty to eighty-three years and in education from 7 to 25 years. There were 16 men and 24 women from four age groups: forties, sixties, seventies, and eighties. There were no adults in their fifties who had taken part in three rounds of testing in the longitudinal study. Therefore, this age group was missing from the present study. Eleven adults were in each of the three younger age groups: forties, sixties, and seventies, and seven were in their eighties. In order to reduce variables that might influence language performance and to keep the groups as homogeneous as possible, all participants had been screened to rule out left-handedness, a history of neurological or psychiatric disorder, uncorrected hearing or visual problems, and alcoholism. See Table 1 for demographic data on the entire study population as well as on participants by age group.

Table 1. Mean Ages and Years of Education for All Subjects and for Subjects by Age Group

	Age		Education	
$N = 40$	64.9 (14.7)		13.6 (3.2)	
	Range = 40 to 83 years		Range = 7 to 25 years	
	40s	60s	70s	80s
$N =$	11	11	11	7
Age	44.0 (3.0)	64.2 (3.4)	76.1 (3.5)	81.4 (1.0)
Education	15.8 (1.3)	12.5 (2.5)	12.4 (2.4)	13.7 (5.5)

Questionnaire

A questionnaire was constructed with the assistance of an epidemiologist experienced in the administration of questionnaires and piloted with four elderly volunteers, three women and one man, comparable in age and educational levels to those of the two oldest groups of adults in the Language in the Aging Brain project. The purpose of the pilot study was to ensure that the questions were stated clearly and that older adults could complete the questionnaire without difficulty. Minor revisions in wording were made, and the questionnaire used in the study reported here consisted of 56 questions that explored a wide range of language-related activities to ascertain how adults use language in their daily lives. Many question types had multiple subsets of items such as the questions about reading and television viewing described below.

The questionnaire included a diverse group of question types. Some questions required general estimates (e.g., "On average, how many hours per week do you read now?") and specific answers (e.g., "Including yourself, how many people live in your household presently?"). Other types of questions required a *yes* or *no* response (e.g., "In the past two years have you memorized any of the items listed below?" poems, song lyrics, prayers, etc.). More often, responses on a three-point scale were required (e.g. never, sometimes, or often for "How often do you read the following?" classics, romance, novels, etc. or very good, average, or poor for "How good are you at remembering the following details?" names of actors and actresses, names of acquaintances, telephone numbers, etc.). A question about television viewing ("How often do you watch the following television programs per week?") required responses on a four-point scale (0, 1 to 5, 6 to 10, or more than 10 hours per week of watching interview shows, quiz shows, soap operas, situation comedies, etc.). A five-point response scale (daily, weekly, monthly, yearly, never) was presented for questions regarding the frequency of engaging in various conversations with adults and children, reading for pleasure and business, writing for pleasure and as part of one's work, watching television, listening to the radio, attending movies or the theater, giving lectures, editing text, speaking on the telephone, typing, using a word processor, working on computer programming, singing, and praying.

Procedure

The participants were telephoned to acquaint them with the study and to elicit their cooperation. If they could not be reached by telephone, they were sent a letter describing the study and asking them to return a postcard with their consent. Questionnaires were mailed to those people who agreed to participate, and they were paid when the questionnaires were returned. Participants who omitted questions or who provided ambiguous responses received a follow-up telephone call to complete the information requested.

Analyses

Statistical analyses were performed using the Statistical Package for Social Sciences (SPSS-X). Means and standard deviations were calculated for 123 questionnaire items, and those items with floor or ceiling effects were eliminated from further analysis. Such effects indicated that all, or nearly all, participants responded to some items in the same way, at the bottom or the top of the response scale, revealing no variability for that particular item. Thus, no meaningful comparisons could be made for those items. For questions with multiple items, data were collapsed to yield 18 scales of questions. A statistical test of reliability was computed for each scale to determine the consistency and dependability of the scale to measure equivalent items. Five scales of questions achieved acceptable reliability ratings of .70 or above and were retained for further analyses. These scales were: (1) work-related language use, (2) second language use, (3) television viewing, (4) memory for details, and (5) keyboard activities.

Questions from scales that did not reach a criterion of .70 were considered in a series of factor analyses using varimax rotation. This statistical measure is designed to group a large amount of data that may overlap (common in questionnaire studies) into smaller clusters to make it easier to interpret the findings. These items included personality characteristics, writing diversity, reading (newspapers and other materials), and conversation. The factor analyses revealed one conversation and three reading factors with reliability scores of .70 or greater. The remaining factors with a reliability criterion less than .70 were not considered reliable. See Table 2 for the results of these factor analyses.

Table 2. Results of Factor Analysis: Factors Extracted with Varimax Rotation

Description of Item	Component Loading	M (SD)
Factor 1: Leisure Reading		
Reading recipes	.87	0.92 (.66)
Reading style pages in the newspaper	.76	0.82 (.74)
Reading arts and leisure in the newspaper	.65	1.20 (.66)
Factor 2: Reading News		
Reading national news	.88	1.80 (.46)
Reading international news	.78	1.69 (.52)
Reading news about people	.38	1.72 (.45)
Factor 3: Professional Reading		
Reading texts	.66	0.66 (.58)
Reading technical/business materials	.61	0.80 (.76)
Reading financial news	.60	1.08 (.66)
Reading magazines	.46	1.60 (.54)
Factor 4: Conversations		
Discussions about people	.94	1.50 (.56)
Discussions about politics	.76	1.32 (.47)
Discussions about ideas	.64	1.40 (.54)
Joking	.44	1.45 (.50)

Thus, a total of nine scales had internal consistency, indicating that the questions within those scales were reliable. These scales were: (1) work-related language use (e.g., proofreading, lecturing/teaching, research, writing, reading aloud, acting, singing, filling out forms, mathematical calculation, sales, computer programming, typing, speaking English with foreigners, and translation); (2) second language use (understanding, speaking, reading, and writing); (3) television viewing (e.g., interview shows, quiz shows, situation comedies, news, films/movies, religious programs, educational TV, sports, concerts, and mysteries); (4) memory for details (e.g., names of actors and actresses, names of acquaintances, telephone numbers, facts about friends, sports statistics, the way people look, and details in general); (5) keyboard activities (e.g., typing, using a word processor, and computer programming); (6) conversations (e.g., discussions about politics, discussions about people and activities, discussions about ideas, and joking); (7) professional reading (e.g., textbooks, magazines, technical/business materials, financial news); (8) leisure reading (e.g., recipes, style pages, and arts and leisure); and (9) reading news (e.g., national news, international news, and news about people). Data analysis also included four single questions that were not part of a scale with multiple items such as the average number of hours per week spent reading, the number of people living in the home, the number of adult education courses taken within the past three years, and the frequency of listening to the radio. Refer to Table 3 for means, standard deviations, and ranges of these data.

The experimental version of the Boston Naming Test (Kaplan et al., 1976) had been administered to these participants three times over the course of a decade. This version consists of 85 black-and-white line drawings of objects presented with increasing order of naming difficulty (from *tree* to *trellis*). For this study a mean of the three individual test scores was computed to arrive at a single composite score representing the participants' naming abilities over the decade. To determine the stability of naming over time in our adult population as a group, paired t-tests were computed. Comparisons of BNT scores for all three test sessions revealed no significant differences between the means at any of the three testings, t (39) = .88, p = .38 between Test 1 and Test 2, t (39) = .41, p = .68 between Test 2 and Test 3, and t (39) = 1.27, p = .21 between Test 1 and Test 3. Furthermore, there were strong intercorrelations between each of the three testings, r = .80 between

Table 3. Means, Standard Deviations, Ranges, and Highest Possible Scores for Language-Related Factors

Language-Related Factors	M (SD)	Range	Highest Possible
Work-related language use	9.20 (5.11)	0–22	28
Second language use	1.91 (2.06)	0–7	8
Television viewing	9.40 (3.42)	1–21	30
Memory for details	14.90 (2.73)	11–21	21
Keyboard activities	2.25 (3.20)	0–11	12
Conversations	5.68 (1.60)	3–8	8
Professional reading	4.12 (1.85)	1–8	8
Leisure reading	3.00 (1.72)	0–6	6
Reading news	5.20 (1.15)	1–6	6
Number of reading hours/week	11.82 (6.79)	2–35	open
Number of people in the home	2.38 (1.39)	1–6	open
Number of adult education courses	1.95 (2.18)	0–6	open
Listening to the radio	3.70 (0.76)	0–4	4

Test 1 and Test 2, $r = .76$ between Test 2 and Test 3, and $r = .76$ between Test 1 and Test 3. Thus, over the course of a decade, there was no significant overall variation in confrontation naming, indicating that, as a group, the adults in this study generally had similar results for all three testings.

Correlation analyses initially were performed to examine the relationships between the composite BNT score and questionnaire data. A hierarchical multiple regression analysis then was performed to determine which of the factors that correlated significantly with the composite Boston Naming Test score accounted for a significant proportion of naming while controlling for participants' age and education.

RESULTS

To answer the question of what factors influence naming in adulthood, Pearson Product Moment Correlations were performed, revealing significant negative correlations between the composite BNT score and age, $r = -.42$, and television viewing, $r = -.52$. This suggested that better naming was associated with younger adults and less television viewing. There were significant positive correlations between naming and education, $r = .48$, professional reading, $r = .38$, the number of adult education courses taken, $r = .37$, work-related language use, $r = .34$, keyboard activities, $r = .47$, and the number of people living in the home, $r = .39$. This suggested that better naming was associated with higher levels of education, more professional reading, a greater number of adult education courses taken, more work-related language use, more keyboard activities, and more people living in the home. The remaining factors (second language use, memory for details, conversations, leisure reading, reading news, the average number of hours per week spent reading) did not correlate significantly with naming ability.

We then reviewed correlation analyses to determine the association between age and education and to determine if age and education were possible confounding variables that could account for naming. Significant negative correlations were found between age and education, $r = -.34$, and between age and number of people living in the home, $r = -.38$, conversation, $r = -.40$, and keyboard activities, $r = -.32$. This indicated that older adults had fewer years of education, lived with fewer people at home, had fewer conversations, and engaged in keyboard activities less frequently than younger adults. Significant positive correlations were found between education and number of people living in the home, $r = .31$, work-related language use, $r = .38$, professional reading, $r = .56$, number of adult education courses taken, $r = .32$, and keyboard activities, $r = .34$. This result suggested that adults with more years of education lived with more people at home, used more work-related language, did more professional reading, took more adult education courses, and engaged in keyboard activities more frequently than adults with fewer years of education. A significant negative correlation was found between education and number of reading hours per week, $r = -.32$, indicating that adults with more years of education read fewer hours per week than adults with fewer years of education. Thus, age and education were identified as potential confounding variables.

In order to examine the relationship between naming and those questionnaire variables we predicted would influence naming while controlling for age and education, we performed a hierarchical multiple regression analysis. Age and education were entered into the equation first, followed by television viewing, work-related language use, and professional reading. The regression analysis revealed that age accounted for a significant 17% of the variance in naming, F (1, 38) = 8.00, $p < .01$, $R^2 = .17$; education accounted for an additional 13% of the variance in naming, F (2, 37) = 8.14, $p < .01$, $R^2 = .30$; and television viewing accounted for another 16% of the variance in naming, F (3, 36) = 10.12, $p < .001$, $R^2 = .46$. Work-related language use, F (4, 35) = 8.12, $p < .001$, $R^2 = .48$, and professional reading, F (5, 34) = 6.60, $p < .001$, $R^2 = .49$, added only 2% and 1% respectively to a proportion of the variance in naming. Thus, age, education, television viewing, work-related language use, and professional reading together contributed to 49% of the variance of the BNT scores. Among them, however, only television viewing made a significant, unique contribution to naming beyond age and education. See Table 4.

Table 4 . Results of the Multiple Regression Analysis

	Beta	t	Significance
Age	–0.25	–1.91	.06
Education	0.18	1.16	.25
Television viewing	–0.41	–3.30	.002*
Work-related language use	0.14	1.08	.28
Professional reading	0.12	0.88	.38
F (5, 34) = 6.60; $R^2 = .49$			

Note. *significant

To explain the unique contribution of television viewing to naming, we compared the 13 questionnaire factors and demographic data of 5 participants who watched the least amount of television with 7 participants who watched the most. Those adults who watched the least television had significantly higher BNT scores, t (10) = 3.56, $p < .01$, more years of education, t (10) = 3.63, $p < .01$, greater number of people living in the home, t (10) = 2.35, $p < .05$, and engaged in more keyboard activities, t (10) = 4.58, $p < .001$, than those adults who watched the most television. The seven adults who watched the most television had significantly better memory for details, t (10) = –3.18, p < .01, than the adults who watched the least television. Two of the five adults in the least-television-viewing group were retired, while five of the seven adults in the most-television-viewing group were retired. There were no significant differences between groups for age, work-related language use, professional reading, second language use, conversation, leisure reading, reading news, the number of reading hours per week, the number of adult education courses, public speaking, or radio listening. The age range was virtually the same for both groups (forty-two to eighty-two years in the least-television-viewing group and forty-three to eighty-two years in the most-television-viewing group).

DISCUSSION

In this group of adults we observed an age-related decline in naming ability consistent with previously published analyses of the data set from which these longitudinally tested participants were selected (Nicholas et al., 1985; Au et al., 1990) and with the findings of other studies (Borod et al., 1980; Farmer, 1990). Furthermore, as others have reported (Borod et al., 1980; Bayles and Kaszniak, 1987; but see Farmer, 1990), education correlated with naming ability. However, age and education were not the only factors contributing significantly to naming ability in adulthood. Television viewing, in this study, had a significant negative impact on naming ability.

Higher naming scores were associated with watching less television, work-related language use (e.g., proofreading, lecturing/teaching, filling out forms, etc.), professional reading (e.g., texts, magazines, technical and business material, and financial news), number of adult education courses taken, keyboard activities, and number of people living in the home. However, examination of the results revealed that number of people living in the home and keyboard activities were associated with both age and education as well as with naming. Therefore, we cannot conclude that these factors influence naming independently of age and education. Similarly, adults with more years of education were likely to have more work-related language use, more professional reading, and to have taken a greater number of adult education courses. Moreover, a hierarchical multiple regression analysis revealed that when age, education, television viewing, work-related language use, and professional reading were entered into an equation in that order, only television viewing made a significant independent contribution to naming. Furthermore, these findings suggest that television viewing exerts a strong influence on naming since 16% of the variance in naming scores could be attributed to this factor while controlling for age and education.

We are left, then, with the difficult challenge of having to explain the significant result that increased naming ability is associated with decreased television viewing. One might have thought that age alone could account for this finding; that is, perhaps as people grow older they watch more television. However, age did not approach a significant correlation with television viewing. Alternatively, one might have posited that education alone could account for the observed correlation between naming and television viewing. This, too, is not the case, since there was no significant correlation between education and television viewing. Furthermore, our multivariate regression analysis revealed that age and education were not confounding variables.

Clearly, then, what stands out in this study is that less television viewing is associated with better naming and that neither age nor education can account for the correlation. While causal explanations cannot be made from our analyses, it is, nevertheless, tempting to speculate about reasons for this finding. Information processing theory poses a distinction between passive and active processes with vocabulary definition tasks (that is, the ability to define words) considered "passive" and confrontation naming tasks (that is, the ability to name pictured items) "active" (Salthouse, 1988). We propose that adults who watch more television have more opportunity to practice passive processes and less opportunity to practice active lexical access processes. This speculation is strengthened by the fact (revealed by our analysis of the adults at the extreme tails of the television viewing continuum) that adults who watched the most television were more likely to be retired and to be living alone. We suggest that adults who want to maintain their word-finding abilities throughout their lifespans should be encouraged to engage in more "active" language activities. It is less clear from our study, however, what constitutes these "active" language activities.

NOTE

1. This work was supported by VA Merit Review Grant 001 and by an Emerson College pre-doctoral assistantship awarded to the first author and by an Emerson College Faculty Research Grant awarded to the second author.

The authors would like to thank the following people for their contributions to the design and interpretation of this study. The members of the Language in the Aging Brain lab at the Boston VA Medical Center collected the naming data for our longitudinal study; the Spring 1990 Language in Aging class at the City University of New York collected data for the original pilot study of this project; Debra Savage and Sally Ziegler helped in the construction of the questionnaire; and Kathy Flannery and T. J. Rosen assisted us in the statistical analyses and interpretation of our data. Address correspondence to Barbara A. Barresi, VA Medical Center (12A), Building 9, Room 321, 150 So. Huntington Avenue, Boston, MA 02130.

REFERENCES

Au, R., Obler, L. K., Joung, P. C., and Albert, M. L. 1990. Naming in normal aging: Age-related differences or age-related changes? *Journal of Clinical and Experimental Neuropsychology, 12,* 30.

Bayles, K. A. and Kaszniak, A. W. 1987. *Communication and Cognition in Normal Aging and Dementia.* Boston: Little, Brown.

Borod, J., Goodglass, H., and Kaplan, E. 1980. Normative data on the Boston Diagnostic Aphasia Examination, Parietal Lobe Battery, and Boston Naming Test. *Journal of Clinical Neuropsychology, 2,* 209–215.

Farmer, A. 1990. Performance of normal males on the Boston Naming Test and the Word Test. *Aphasiology, 4,* 293–296.

Helm, N. A. and Barresi, B. 1980. Voluntary control of involuntary utterances: A treatment approach for severe aphasia. *Clinical Aphasiology Conference Proceedings,* Minneapolis: BRK Publishers.

Helm-Estabrooks, N., Fitzpatrick, P. M., and Barresi, B. 1981. Response of an agrammatic patient to a syntax stimulation program for aphasia. *Journal of Speech and Hearing Disorders, 46,* 422–427.

Helm-Estabrooks, N., Fitzpatrick, P. M. and Barresi, B. 1982. Visual action therapy for global aphasia. *Journal of Speech and Hearing Disorders, 47,* 385–389.

Kaplan, E., Goodglass, H., and Weintraub, S. 1976. *The Boston Naming Test,* Experimental Edition.

Kaplan, E., Goodglass, H., and Weintraub, S. 1983. *The Boston Naming Test,* Philadelphia: Lea & Febiger.

Nicholas, M., Obler, L., Albert, M., and Goodglass, H. 1985. Lexical retrieval in healthy aging. *Cortex, 21,* 595–606.

Obler, L.K., and Albert, M. L. 1977. Influence of aging on recovery from aphasia in polyglots. *Brain and Language, 4,* 460–463.

Salthouse, T. A. 1988. Effects of aging on verbal abilities: Examination of the psychometric literature. In L. L. Light and D. M. Burke, eds., *Language, Memory and Aging.* New York: Cambridge University Press.

Sparks, R., Helm, N., and Albert, M. 1974. Aphasia rehabilitation resulting from melodic intonation therapy. *Cortex, 10,* 303–316.

CHAPTER 5

Inferences in Processing of Text in Elderly Populations[1]

Hanna K. Ulatowska
Sandra Bond Chapman
Julene Johnson

INTRODUCTION

There is considerable controversy as to whether or not aging has deleterious effects on language, particularly at a discourse or text level. A number of studies have documented age-related changes in quantity and quality of discourse information retained whereas other studies have found minimal differences across age groups (Craik and Rabinowitz, 1984; Dixon, Hultsch, Simon, and von Eye, 1984; Hartley, 1988; Hultsch and Dixon, 1984).

The disparity among discourse findings may be explained, in part, by sociological and biological factors. Sociological factors such as level of education, recent exposure to learning environments, and verbal ability as measured by vocabulary tests have been shown to account for discourse differences across age groups (Meyer and Rice, 1983; Poon, Krauss, and Bowles, 1984; Taub, 1979). With regard to biological factors, there is growing evidence that a generalized slowing of the neurologic system occurs with aging. It has been suggested that this produces some "slowing" of cognitive processing abilities that may lead to a reduction or inefficiency of information processing (Cohen, 1988; Hartley, 1988; Klatzky, 1988; Salthouse, 1988).

Despite the equivocal findings in the literature on age-related differences in discourse processing, one of the most promising avenues for illuminating age effects on discourse appears to be related to depth of processing. The prediction is that tasks requiring "deeper" levels of information processing should be more sensitive to age effects (Cohen, 1988; Light and Burke, 1988). This viewpoint is motivated by two beliefs related to discourse processing. One is that processing demands are increased on tasks that require "deeper" levels of text processing. The second one is that processing resources are compromised with increased age.

Support for a deficit in depth of processing with increased age comes from findings that implicit textual information is processed more poorly than explicit information (Cohen, 1979, 1981; Light and Capps, 1986; Light, Zelinski, and Moore, 1982). This pattern suggests that processing of explicitly stated textual information may be preserved with age since this requires only superficial processing. In contrast, processing of implicit information may be more vulnerable to age effects. However, these findings must be interpreted cautiously since the differences in implicit versus explicit processing appear to inadequately explain age-related changes. Other studies did not confirm the pattern of greater age differences for implicit information (Belmore, 1981; Till, 1985).

The primary focus of this chapter is to describe one possible method for examining depth of processing in neurolinguistic studies of aging. Whereas depth of processing has been defined in various ways, it is defined in this chapter by the nature of the inference generated in transforming the textual information from a particular stimulus. Inferences have been characterized by researchers in a number of disciplines including linguists, psychologists, and cognitive psychologists. Consequently, the use of inference provides a theoretical framework for investigating depth of processing. In the final section of this chapter, a preliminary study will be briefly summarized to illustrate the utility of the theoretical framework of inference generation in examining discourse change throughout the life span. The method utilizes fables as a particular narrative genre for tapping different levels of processing. As described below, fables provide a rich resource for investigating different levels of inferencing due to the organization and content inherent in most fables.

DEPTH OF PROCESSING

Definition

Originally, the term "depth of processing" was used by cognitive psychologists to refer to processing stages in text comprehension. An increased depth of processing implied a greater number of steps of semantic or cognitive analysis (Craik and Lockhart, 1972). Initially, the levels of processing concept was offered as a framework for predicting what information would be recalled from a particular text. It was postulated that information processed at a deeper level was more likely to be retained than superficially or shallowly processed information. Baddeley (1982) modified the concept of levels of processing by broadening the scope of "levels" to the construct of "domains" of processing. He suggested that information may be processed simultaneously within a number of domains rather than in a linear or hierarchical sequence of processes as implicated by the "level" of processing framework. However, Baddeley himself (1982) remarked that the concept of domains of processing was not testable in any simple way. Cohen (1979, 1988) and Cohen and Faulkner (1981, 1984) defined depth of processing using the contrast between processing surface content and processing information that required the listener to make inferences. Specifically, shallow processing was represented by processing text that required only straightforward reproduction of the surface form of the text. In contrast, deep processing was defined by information processing that required inference construction.

Cohen (1988) defines inferencing as the ability to understand information that is implied but not explicitly stated. In order to construct inferences, information must be integrated with the rest of the textual information as well as related to world knowledge (i.e., previously acquired and stored information) and personal experience. Thus, inference construction requires that the listener build bridges among intact knowledge structures. Cohen and colleagues laid the groundwork for using an inferential framework as a feasible method for testing depth of processing.

Age Effects on Depth of Processing

The empirical evidence suggests that many of the individual knowledge systems underlying discourse processing are minimally affected as a function of age. In particular, the linguistic rules governing well-formed sentences, an important but not essential component for supporting discourse structure, remain relatively impervious to age-related decline (Bayles and Kaszniak, 1987). Additionally, the world knowledge system appears to be well preserved into old age (Baltes, 1993).

Nonetheless, recent investigations show that age-related deficits are prevalent, particularly on complex discourse comprehension tasks. The general assumption is that age effects become more prominent as the task difficulty increases due to an excessive burden placed on inferential processing and working memory (Cohen, 1988; Klatzky, 1988). That is, discourse processing may be intact at shallow levels of processing as manifested by preserved ability to comprehend and remember explicitly stated textual information. One commonly offered explanation for the relative preservation in the processing of explicit information in old age is that explicit information processing minimizes the demands on working memory.

However, deeper levels of processing may be more vulnerable to aging effects because integration and construction of discourse information is necessary for accurate encoding. Cohen (1988) concludes that old people are especially impaired on answering questions or on verifying conclusions that require inferencing, possibly because inferences place high demands on working memory.

Elderly individuals may experience difficulties in constructing a unitary, meaningful representation of a text because they have difficulties integrating information across knowledge systems. Thus their ability to engage in "deeper" levels of processing may be diminished (Burke and Harrold, 1988; Klatzky, 1988). Despite the growing evidence of impaired inferential processing in elderly populations, there is some concern over methodological factors that may produce results that do not generalize to processing in real-life discourse tasks. Some of the concerns are discussed below.

Limitations of Previous Studies

On-line Versus Off-line. Researchers have utilized various methods for testing depth of processing, some using on-line and others using off-line procedures. On-line inferential processes are measured during the processing of a text, while off-line inferences are generated after listening to or reading the text (Magliano and Graesser, 1991). Whereas some inferences are activated by specific or local elements in the text, other inferences are more global in nature and occur at the end of a passage. These latter inferences can only be made using off-line procedures. Examples of global type inferences include making judgments or interpretations regarding the theme, the lesson, or the author's intent.

To date, the majority of studies have used on-line measures to tap depth of processing; however, there is growing support for off-line measures. Magliano and Graesser (1991) offer a number of arguments against on-line procedures. One argument suggests that on-line designs may encourage superficial processing of text. For example, a commonly used on-line procedure is a lexical decision task. In the lexical decision task, an individual is presented a text one sentence at a time. After each sentence a letter string (e.g., either *jump* or *pujm*) is presented and the individual is to decide whether or not the letter string is a word. Since individuals tend to comprehend a passage only as deeply as the task requirements necessitate, a lexical decision task may encourage processing texts at a surface level rather than at a deeper, semantic level. Another shortcoming of on-line measures is that they are often disruptive to normal processing, since many on-line tasks interrupt the flow of information processing and require interpreters to process the information one word or one sentence at a time.

Artificiality of Experimental Texts. Magliano and Graesser (1991) address a number of shortcomings related to experimental texts commonly adopted to examine inferential processing. For one, they suggest that it is virtually impossible to generate two versions of a text (a control version and an experimental version) and maintain the same meanings across the texts. For example, a control text typically contains explicitly stated information, whereas the experimental text is designed in an attempt to convey the same information in an implicit form requiring the reader to make inferences. Any differences between populations may be explained by the awkwardness of the control version, since the manipulation of the textual content often results in a pointless, incoherent text with unintended changes in meaning.

A second shortcoming arises from the use of artificial, experimenter-generated texts instead of naturalistic ones. While experimenter-created texts provide a means of examining a specific type of inference, these artificial texts seldom contain the dimensions and components found in naturalistic texts that contribute significantly to processing. For example, narratives have a well-defined information structure with content directed at conveying some message, point, or moral. Without this underlying structure, individuals may react to the uninteresting nature of the content.

Finally, experimental texts are often very short, comprised of only one or two sentences. Magliano and Graesser (1991) contend that short passages are basically content-deprived in that they do not provide sufficient context to allow normal inferential processing. In the next section, fables are offered as a text genre that is useful in examining depth of processing as well as able to overcome some of the shortcomings of artificial texts. Specifically, the narrative genre of fables provides a rich, naturalistic text that can be utilized as an off-line measure for inferential processing.

FABLES: A NATURALISTIC GENRE

Characterization of Fables

Fables are a particular narrative genre with a cognitive-linguistic representation of complex situations and actions encountered in everyday life. The function or intent of fables is to convey a lesson or a moral based on conventionalized, cultural truths (Abramowska, 1991). Therefore, the content of a fable is typically built around characters, actions, and goals that result in some lesson being conveyed. The lesson not only applies to the fable characters but also generalizes to people in everyday situations. As a result of these two levels of application for the lesson, fables can be interpreted at a surface level (i.e., a lesson for the specific fable characters) and at a deep level (i.e., a generalized lesson that applies to people in real-life situations). For full interpretation of a fable to be achieved, the generalized lesson (deep level) of the fable must be encoded. Thus, a fable represents a verbal puzzle or verbal problem-solving task that requires grasping the generalized moral or lesson as the solution (Ulatowska, Sadowska, Kordys, and Kadzielawa, 1993).

Metis in Fables

The lesson of a particular fable is typically conveyed to the listener by manipulating different types of "metis." Metis involves the practical application of intelligence by the main character to achieve his desired goal. The main character of a fable typically carries out an unconventional scheme to obtain his end using deceit or trickery. The scheme may succeed or fail. For example, the Fox and Raven fable (see Appendix) illustrates successful metis in that the fox achieves his goal of getting food by using flattery to trick the raven. An example of failed metis is apparent in the Raven and Pigeons fable where the raven pretends to be something he is not, losing chances to get food both from others and from his own kind. Metis may unfold through the actions of the fable's characters as in the Fox and Raven fable or through the use of language as in the Woman and Doctor fable.

Role of Animal and Human Characters

Structurally, fables have a paradigmatic set of characters that are clearly identifiable and possess the power to perform certain actions. While some fables have human actors, the majority of fables contain animal characters. There are two reasons why fables with animal characters are prevalent: (1) lessons can be transmitted to a culture/group without indicting "guilty" parties; (2) many animals have generalized characteristics that are well-known to most cultures, making animals uniquely suited for expressing certain lessons (e.g., sly as a fox, quick as a fox, dumb as a donkey, stubborn as a mule, gullible as a goat, cocky as a rabbit). Thus, the animals in a particular fable are carefully selected so that their stereotypic, yet culturally dependent, characteristics match their role in the story, increasing the predictability and plausibility of the situation. A sample fable with animal characters (i.e., Fox and Raven) is presented in the Appendix. In certain fables, the human actors are depicted in social roles common to certain scripts based on real life situations as exhibited by the Woman and Doctor or Farmer and Sons fables (see Appendix), while other human characters perform actions common to mankind in general. Scripts are knowledge structures consisting of stereotyped action sequences of actions that define a well-known situation, e.g., patient and doctor script (Schank and Abelson, 1977). The selection of fables with human characters may enhance comprehension if the characters' actions are consistent with script knowledge. On the other hand, impaired comprehension may result if the actions are inconsistent with script knowledge.

Fables provide a relatively short, naturalistic text with simple language and a clearly delineated story structure. Consequently, fables may be utilized with a wide variety of geriatric populations with linguistic and/or cognitive deficits because of the inherent semantic and structural features.

Processing of Fables

As stated above, fables provide appropriate texts for studying depth of processing since they convey a message at a surface level and at a deep level. As with most texts, a "deep" understanding of fables involves inference generation. The processing of fables entails different types of inference construction.

Types of inferences. In this section, inferences necessary for interpreting the deep meaning of fables are outlined. As will be discussed, inference construction provides a theoretical framework for exploring whether or not a given individual grasps the central meaning of a fable. One possible approach for determining the necessary inferences will be discussed with exemplification using two groups of normal elderly and one group of aphasic individuals. The underlying assumption is that the success of an individual's performance can be evaluated by tapping which inferences are produced and by examining the specificity of the response. Earlier studies on inferential processing in adult populations focused on comprehension requiring minimal responses to probe questions, for example, yes-no questions or requests for specific factual information. The present framework examines comprehension through production by soliciting responses that require interpretation and manipulation of the whole text content, such as manifested in producing summaries or giving morals.

Table 1 outlines the categories of inference-type relevant to the present study with example inferences. These categories were adopted from the work of Magliano and Graesser (1991). The inference types are classified along two dimensions, *intratextual* and *extratextual.* Intratextual inference constructions are those that isolate and integrate certain textual information with other textual information. Extratextual inference constructions are those reflected in responses that integrate textual information with more generalized world knowledge and personal experiences. Extratextual inference strategies reflect deeper levels of integration and generalization.

Discourse comprehension is achieved through a wide range of processing strategies involving inference construction. The primary issue in this chapter concerns how processing strategies invoke different types of inferences as various comprehension tasks are performed. While a variety of tasks can be used to investigate inference construction, the ones utilized in this research were selected to take advantage of the semantic and structural components of fables. The specific tasks used to evaluate depth of processing and inference construction in processing fables include: (1) retelling the fable, (2) summarizing the fable, (3) identifying the perceived main character with justification, (4) giving the main idea or gist, and (5) deriving the moral from the fable.

Table 1. Examples of Inference Types According to Intratextual and Extratextual Responses Reflective of Depth of Processing for the *Fox and Raven Fable*

Type of inference	Examples of Inference	
	Intratextual	Extratextual
State Trait	Fox is hungry.	People can be deceptive.
	Fox is sly/smart.	People can be gullible.
	Raven is not smart.	
Superordinate goal	The Fox wanted to get the Raven's cheese.	People may take advantage of others to get something from them.
Instrument	The Fox used flattery to get the Raven's cheese.	People may use flattery to manipulate you.
Causal consequence	The Raven lost his cheese because he opened his beak to "show off his voice."	You will lose in the end if you believe everything you hear.
Theme	The Raven was tricked.	The use of flattery to achieve one's own end.
Author's intent/deep meaning	If you're a raven, don't listen to the words of a fox.	Don't be deceived by flattery.

Categories from Magliano and Graesser, 1991.

The various types of inferences that may contribute to formulating a response to each particular task are described below. However, the main focus of this chapter is on response strategies for the "gist" and "moral" tasks since these two tasks appear to be the most revealing in examining depth of processing.

Definition of Task and Potential Inferences Generated

Retelling a fable. Retelling involves reproducing or transforming a text after a complete model (written or verbal) has been provided. Since fables are relatively short and expressed in language that is simple both lexically and syntactically, they can be retold with minimal transformations of information. Retelling can be accomplished primarily through simple deletion and paraphrasing of the original story content. Typically, minimal inferencing is required for retelling short fables, particularly if memory is preserved. Of all the tasks outlined above, retelling is cognitively the simplest.

Summarizing a fable. Summarizing a fable involves selectively reducing the content of the fable while preserving the most important information. The actual production of a summary can reflect various levels of inference generation. In a very simple process, a summary can be produced by simple deletion of information. Deletion of information is one of three macrorules of text transformation defined by van Dijk (1980). In order to produce a summary by simply deleting information, a listener/reader must generate inferences that allow him/her to comprehend the "trick" and the cause or reason for the trick's success or failure. Inference construction related to comprehending the "trick" allows the listener to interpret a character's plan of action or motivation behind an action, which in the case of fables is a trick. Causal inferences relate to comprehending the explicit actions of the characters, allowing listeners to make predictions about future events. Both "trick" inferences and causal inferences can be made by integrating particular textual information with other textual information which represents an intratextual strategy.

In a more complex process of inference generation, a summary can be produced by application of the macrorules of construction and generalization (van Dijk, 1980). Construction is the replacement of specific information with a more global concept. Generalization occurs when specific information is replaced with more generalized information. Summaries produced by the strategies of construction and generalization require making inferences and integrating textual knowledge and real world knowledge. This type of response represents an extratextual strategy. The listener must infer the superordinate goals of the characters. Additionally, world knowledge permits the listener to infer the author's message or intent in writing the fable.

Identification and justification of the main character. In order to identify the main character and justify the choice, the listener may make minimal inferences that involve primarily intratextual inference construction. For example, the main character may be identified on the basis of sheer frequency of mention. Alternatively, the listener may select the main character based only on his own personal evaluation of the character independent of the character's role in the story. This latter type would be exemplified in a choice of a "dog" over a "fox" with the justification that "I like dogs" or "Dogs are nice." In this personalized type of response, the responder gives only his personal evaluation and fails to build inferences between textual and personal life experiences. The personal evaluation is inappropriate to the inferential demands of the main character justification task.

Reflecting a deeper level of processing, the main character may be selected on the basis of the character's role in teaching or learning a lesson. Thus, the main character can be either a winner who "teaches" the other a lesson or a loser who "learns" a lesson. The identification and justification of a particular choice of main character according to one who teaches or learns a lesson involves a number of inference constructions, including causal, trait, instrumental, and superordinate goal inferences (see Table 1). For example, a correct identification and appropriate justification of the fable's main character requires proper inference construction as to which character is the instigator of the event sequence planned to achieve a goal (superordinate goal inference) as well as the character who is responsible for the outcome (i.e., causal inference). For example, in the Fox and Raven fable, the fox devises and carries out a scheme that allows him to trick the raven out of his cheese. Additionally, inferences related to understanding the means by which a character achieves his goal (i.e., instrumental inference) are important to appropriate selection of the main character (e.g., the use of flattery by the fox to get the cheese from the raven). Comprehenders also use trait inferences to determine who is the main character or hero in the story by inferring characteristics based on an actor's actions (e.g., the sly fox because he devised a scheme to trick the raven or the gullible raven because he fell for flattery).

In summary, identification of the main character may reflect only shallow level processing as suggested by decisions based on sheer frequency or personal evaluations. Nonetheless, the appropriate response for justification for one's choices of main characters typically involves integrating textual with extratextual knowledge. Bridging inferences between the fable's content and knowledge about the real world reflects deeper levels of processing due to the inference constructions required across knowledge systems.

Gist and moral. Grasping the gist and the moral of the fable appears to be the most revealing of the tasks described herein. This task reveals whether or not individuals can make inferences from the fable content to real world knowledge systems. The ability to tie textual information to real world knowledge is a strategy referred to as extratextual and reflects deeper levels of processing. The gist and the moral of fables can be expressed at different levels of generalization.

However, both of these tasks are more likely to elicit an extratextual response by normal individuals as compared to the other tasks of retelling, summarizing, or identifying and rationalizing the main character.

At the most concrete or shallow level, the gist may be expressed as a shorter version of the summary achieved through simple deletion of information and produced using only the explicit fable content (intratextual response). This level of gist interpretation results from the comprehender making inferences so that he or she realizes the "trick" or metis expressed in the fable. Thus, the trick is appreciated through making inferences across the superordinate goal (e.g., the fox's scheme to get the cheese), the instrument to achieve the goal (e.g., flattery), and the outcome of the goal (e.g., the fox gets the cheese by flattering the raven and causing him to open his beak and drop the cheese).

At a deeper level or more abstract level, the gist can be expressed in the form of a moral. When a moral-type response is produced for the gist, it suggests that the comprehender not only made the inferences mentioned above (the superordinate goal, the instrument and the causal consequence) but also made inferences regarding the theme and underlying intent of the story. Thematic and underlying intent inferences are derived from the characters' goals and plans, representing the foundation of the didactic component of fables. For example, the theme for the Fox and Raven fable is the diversion of the raven's attention from his cheese by the fox's flattery. The underlying intent in fables is to convey a lesson that applies to real world situations. In the Fox and Raven fable the lesson could be expressed as: "Don't lose sight of your goals by falling prey to flattery."

Similar to gist responses, morals may also be expressed at various levels of generalization. Certain moral responses reflect that the inferences made are restricted primarily to the textual content. For this type of moral response, the moral would pertain specifically to the characters in the fable (e.g., the raven should not have listened to the flattery of the fox and opened his beak to sing in the Fox and Raven fable). Inference construction necessary for producing this intratextual moral would include superordinate goal, instrument, and causal consequence inferences. More appropriately, however, the expression of the moral reflects an integration of the important intratextual inferences (i.e., superordinate goal, instrument, and causal consequence or outcome inferences) with extratextual information, (e.g., thematic and author intent inferences). As a result, a lesson is derived that has a broader level of application to life in general (extratextual inference construction).

Differences occur in the probability of eliciting extratextual type inferences for the gist and moral tasks across populations. For healthy adults, the range of responses is greater for gist responses than for moral responses. This occurs because the moral task is more likely to result in an extratextual type lesson. Indeed, the nature of the moral task has an inherent requirement of a generalized, extratextual response. In contrast, the gist task does not have the same restrictions as the moral task since an intratextual or extratextual response is equally acceptable.

A PRELIMINARY STUDY USING FABLES

The final part of this chapter summarizes an exploratory study of inferential processing as manifested in gist and moral responses for fables in three adult populations. The three groups of 15 subjects each included two healthy groups differing in age, an older middle-age group (fifty to seventy years) and an old elderly group (>eighty years), and a neurologically-impaired group with a single, left cerebral vascular accident resulting in aphasia (forty-six to seventy-five years). Aphasic patients with single strokes were selected to preclude a more progressive disease process. Each subject received a battery of standardized cognitive and linguistic measures. The battery was designed to evaluate relevant behaviors necessary to performing the experimental battery. Since the fables were presented simultaneously in verbal and written form, language tests were administered to assess auditory comprehension and reading comprehension. The cognitive measures included selected subtests from the Wechsler Adult Intelligence Scale-Revised (Wechsler, 1981), i.e., picture arrangement, block design, and similarities. These tests were given to assess logical sequencing of information, problem solving, and abstracting semantic information, all of which are prerequisite abilities to transforming information from fables in the form of retelling, summarizing, and producing gists and morals.

This study illustrates the importance of using contrastive groups to illuminate differences and similarities in discourse processing between normal aging adults and aging adults with various neurologic deficits. We were interested in whether inferencing differences would be demonstrated across various tasks according to (a) age effects and/or (b) linguistic problems associated with aphasia. By utilizing naturalistic tasks that allow individuals to freely exhibit their inferential processing tendencies, an examination can be made of how linguistic or cognitive deficits are manifested in various groups processing of texts at a deeper or more abstract level.

Rationale for Contrastive Groups

Contrasts between different aging populations are essential for understanding changes in language as a function of age since characteristic features of a particular population become more apparent when compared against performances of other normal or pathological populations (Ulatowska and Chapman, 1991). In the present preliminary study, two healthy adult groups were investigated to examine whether or not differences exist in depth of processing for fables as a function of age. Based on the empirical evidence suggesting that depth of processing is altered in aging, the hypothesis was that the old-elderly group would have difficulty making inferences that required the mixing or integration of textual knowledge with real world knowledge. Mild to moderately-impaired aphasic patients were evaluated on the same measures to determine how linguistic disturbances would affect inferential ability as reflected in gist and moral responses. The prediction was that aphasic patients would also have difficulties making inferences across textual and extratextual knowledge systems. This study sought to characterize what type of strategies the two groups would adopt when faced with difficult inferential processing tasks.

Tasks and Procedures

Tasks. A theoretical framework utilizing the intratextual and extratextual inferences described above was adapted to examine differences across groups in depth of processing. The tasks in the present experiment tap different degrees of inference construction in that some tasks require minimal inferencing and others require making inferences across textual content and integrating this information with world knowledge. The stimuli used to assess depth of processing consisted of six Aesop's fables. The fables were presented in written form to each subject and were read aloud by the examiner while the subject followed along. (Sample fables are presented in the Appendix.) Following the presentation of each story, the subjects were asked to generate texts/responses to the following tasks: (1) retell the story, (2) summarize the story, (3) specify a hero and provide a justification, (4) give the main idea or gist of the story, (5) formulate a moral or a lesson, and (6) provide a title.

Analyses. The analyses for the gist and moral tasks involved matching the information contained in the responses against the information contained in the stimulus text. The analyses yielded a dichotomy of responses into intratextual and extratextual categories according to different degrees of adherence to the stimulus text. Intratextual responses were derived primarily from making inferences using the information contained in the fable, whereas extratextual responses involved bridging inference construction using a mixture of the stimulus text information and information based on world knowledge.

Results and Discussion

Performance patterns for older middle-age, old-elderly and aphasic groups on the tasks of gist and moral are shown in Figure 1. The bar graphs show the percentage of extratextual responses for the three groups. For the gist task, the older middle-age and old-elderly subjects produced a majority of extratextual responses (57% and 64%, respectively) for fables. The tendency toward extratextual responses on the gist task provides evidence that the ability to bridge inferences is well preserved into old age. The support for this argument is provided by the fact that the old-elderly subjects tended to produce an extratextual response on the gist task, a task which does not require this bridging of inferences. As stated previously, an intratextual or extratextual response for the gist task is equally acceptable. In contrast, the aphasic patients gave only 30% extratextual responses for the gist tasks indicating a strong tendency toward intratextual responses.

The bias toward extratextual responses on the moral task was even greater than on the gist task for both the older middle-age and the old-elderly groups (96%). It is interesting to note that both older middle-age and old-elderly groups occasionally produced multiple morals for one fable. Similar to the response pattern on the gist task, aphasic patients persisted in their tendency to give intratextual responses even for the moral task (Figure 1). The tendency toward intratextual responses by aphasic patients is more aberrant for the moral task than for the gist task. This is so because the nature of providing a moral requires a

Figure 1. Mean Percentage of Extratextual Responses on Gist and Moral Tasks Across Six Fables in Three Populations

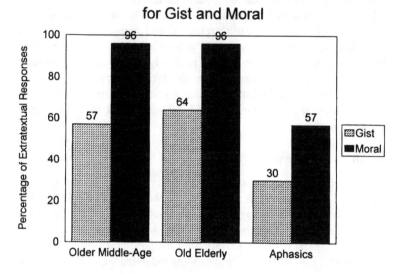

generalized response involving inference construction based on the textual content and an extratextual, real world application. It is important to note the increase in percentage of extratextual responses on the moral task (57%) by aphasic patients as compared to the percentage of extratextual responses for gist (30%), suggesting an awareness of the differences in task requirements. Their performance, nonetheless, was markedly impaired on the moral task.

Counter to expectations, the results did not support our original prediction that the old-elderly group would show more difficulties than the older middle-age group on tasks requiring greater depth of processing. Indeed, the old-elderly group performed at a similar level (96%) as the middle-age group on producing appropriate, generalized morals. Based on the success of the old-elderly group in producing extratextual morals, it appears that they were able to build inferences across the textual and real world knowledge systems.

The relative preservation of inferential processing in this population of octogenarians may be explained, in part, by their high level of linguistic and communicative ability. Evidence for preserved linguistic ability is apparent in their use of metaphoric and proverbial language as well as their facility with complex syntactic structures. Examples of metaphorical and proverbial responses include the following responses from old-elderly individuals: (For the Raven and Pigeons fable)—"To be true blue, don't change your colors"; "He cut off the limb he was sitting on"; "Birds of a feather flock together"; (For the Woman and Doctor fable)—"Don't steal people blind"; (For the Fox and Goat fable)—"Watch out for the fox, the fox will outfox you" and "Look before you leap." An example of complex syntax is evident in the following response: "Don't even think for one little minute that you've reached the top on account that there's somebody there that's just a little bigger than you" (for Two Roosters Fable).

Evidence for preserved communicative ability is provided by the numerous instances of abstract and succinctly-stated responses of old-elderly. Producing abstract responses in a succinct form suggests that old-elderly are able to optimally select language in order to convey a message. When the communicative situation demanded a succinct response, old-elderly individuals in the study were able to produce an appropriate, concise response.

Although the old-elderly subjects in the present study did not differ from the middle-age group on the selected measures, it is important to note that some problems in inferencing were exhibited by both old-elderly and middle-age individuals. The problems became evident on the more complex stories, such as the Woman and Doctor fable. This story is more complex because it has two parallel plot lines, one according to the doctor's plan and the other based on the woman's actions. Additional complexity arises from the fact that the trick involves metaphoric use of language. In this particular story, some subjects seemed to base their interpretations more on script knowledge than on the specific textual information, indicating incomplete inference construction. Some examples of responses from old-elderly individuals include: "When you go to the doctor, make sure his treatment is helping you"; "Don't pay the doctor until you are through with the treatment"; and "Be sure you have a contract with your doctor as to what he's going to do before you have it done." Since the Woman and Doctor fable was more difficult for some individuals, this story provided a means of illuminating what processing strategies individuals might adopt when incomplete inferencing occurred. One reason this particular story elicited responses based more on script than on textual knowledge is likely due to the salience of a patient and doctor scenario for older adults.

As predicted, the aphasic individuals did indeed exhibit difficulty making the appropriate inference construction for textual and extratextual knowledge systems. Nonetheless, it is important to note that many aphasic patients did produce extratextual responses, particularly for the moral task. While the finding of intratextual response tendency in aphasic patients is not surprising, the underlying mechanism for the difficulties in aphasic patients is not necessarily straightforward. It is tempting to attribute the problems in inference construction in aphasic patients to language impairment. However, the tendency toward intratextual responses cannot be completely accounted for by the patients' linguistic deficits. Some aphasic patients produced syntactically complex responses but nonetheless produced responses that appeared to be text-bound in that most inferences were restricted to textual information (e.g., "If you're a raven, don't open your mouth if you have cheese"). Moreover, these same patients scored relatively high on the language measures (80th percentile or better). In contrast, other patients with impaired language were able to produce extratextual responses, suggesting inference construction across textual and extratextual knowledge systems. The point is that aphasic patients' ability to produce responses indicative of inference construction across knowledge systems does not correspond directly to linguistic abilities. Additionally, the correlations between performances on the cognitive measures and ability to produce generalized moral responses were unimpressive.

Some aphasic patients exhibited problems in the level of specificity of their responses, some being too specific and some being nonspecific. The specific responses were exemplified by intratextual responses with interpretation tied directly to the specific situation. Many of the responses for the gist and moral tasks contained primarily explicitly stated information from the original story, suggesting lack of inferential processing. The aphasic response, "The fox ran away with cheese" on the gist task for the Fox and Raven fable simply restates the outcome of the story. This is not to say that aphasic patients failed to engage in inferential processing. Some responses did indicate inference construction as seen in responses signaling the lesson from the character's viewpoint. An example of this latter response is "If you're a raven, don't open your mouth."

On the other hand, some aphasics showed the opposite pattern from overspecificity, in that they tended to produce overgeneralized or nonspecific responses that applied to numerous fables. Examples of overgeneralized morals include: "Don't be greedy" given for the Raven and Pigeons fable and the Farmer and Sons, or "Be aware" for the Fox and Raven and Fox and Goat fables.

CONCLUSION

Based on this exploratory study, it appears that aphasic patients, the two healthy groups of old-elderly and middle-age adults form a continuum in their response patterns. All three populations produced intra- and extratextual responses indicating different types of inference construction. The three groups did, however, show quantitative differences with the aphasic group producing more intratextual responses even on a task (i.e., moral task) for which extratextual responses were required. Despite the continuum of responses, it appears that the ends of the continuum tend to differentiate the populations. At one end, metaphorical or proverbial morals and even multiple morals were produced by the old-elderly and middle-age adults but rarely by aphasic patients. At the other end of the continuum, responses consisting of explicitly stated information with minimal rephrasing were produced by aphasic patients.

With the present study, there are some issues pertaining to inferential processing that need additional consideration. It is not possible to specify which inferences are made since the responses may result from a number of inferences. While it is our belief that off-line tasks requiring different levels of processing are necessary for tapping levels of inference construction, perhaps additional information could be probed to determine which inferences are and are not successfully made. There appears to be a hierarchy of abstractness for responses related to different types of inferences. However, the precise hierarchy remains to be established. The use of more complex fables may reveal different patterns from the optimistic one of this present study. It is possible that these results do not generalize to the old-elderly population as a whole. Rather, the findings may be related to the specific characteristics of the group studied, i.e., a group of well-educated and active individuals.

We believe, however, that a more in-depth profile of insight into inferential processing abilities and disabilities for various elderly populations can be obtained using different tasks, such as the ones described in the present chapter. In particular, we recommend using tasks that require an individual to process the central meaning at various levels of generalization placing different demands on inferential processing. For normal aging populations, texts containing more information than the short fables described herein may place greater demands on the inferential system. Moreover, some tasks will be more informative than others in allowing for clear interpretation of intactness in deep levels of inferential processing. For the present study, the tasks of producing gists and morals were the most revealing. The task of identification of the main character with justification provided supportive information to verify the focus on the central meaning. The task of retelling was used to determine whether individuals were capable of holding the information in short-term memory long enough to retell the information. Clearly, if individuals are unable to hold the story content in working memory, they will be at a great disadvantage in transforming the central information in the form of either a gist or a moral.

The significance of the present approach in understanding linguistic ability in elderly populations is that the framework explores linguistic ability within the broader context of cognitive function as reflected in inferential processing. In contrast, studies that examine language in the old-elderly from a narrow context related to lexical or syntactic abilities may lead to false assumptions regarding their facility in manipulating larger chunks of information. Thus, we propose that an approach that examines inferential processing will allow us to come closer to characterizing the important aspects of linguistic and cognitive function relevant to communicative competence in the elderly.

NOTE

1. This work is supported by a grant from the Texas Higher Education Coordinating Board, Division of Research, Planning, and Finance—009741–013; and by grant AG09486 from the National Institute on Aging. The authors also acknowledge the contribution of Research Assistant, Carmen Branch, in data analysis and manuscript preparation.

REFERENCES

Abramowska, J. 1991. *Polska bajka ezopowa*. [Polish Aesop's fable]. Poznan: Wydawnictwo Naukowe Uniwersytetu im. Adama Mickiewicza.

Baddeley, A. D. 1982. Domains of recollection. *Psychological Review, 89*(6), 708–729.

Baltes, P. B. 1993. The aging mind: Potential and limits. *Gerontologist, 33*(5), 580–596.

Bayles, V. A., & Kaszniak, A. W. 1987. *Communication and Cognition in Normal Aging and Dementia.* London: Taylor and Francis.

Belmore, S. M. 1981. Age-related changes in processing explicit and implicit language. *Journal of Gerontology, 36,* 316–322.

Burke, D. M., & Harrold, R. M. 1988. Automatic and effortful semantic processes in old age: Experimental and naturalistic approaches. In L. L. Light & D. M. Burke, eds., *Language, Memory, and Aging.* New York: Cambridge University Press. 100–116.

Cohen, G. 1979. Language comprehension in old age. *Cognitive Psychology, 11,* 412–429.

Cohen, G. 1981. Inferential reasoning in old age. *Cognition, 9,* 59–72.

Cohen, G. 1988. Age differences in memory for texts: Production deficiency or processing limitations? In L. L. Light & D. M. Burke, eds., *Language, Memory, and Aging.* New York: Cambridge University Press. 171–190.

Cohen, G., and Faulkner, D. 1981. Memory for discourse in old age. *Discourse Processes, 4,* 253–265.

Cohen, G., and Faulkner D. 1984. Memory for text: Some age differences in the nature of the information that is retained after listening to texts. In H. Bouma and D. Bouwhuis, eds., *Attention and Performance: X. Control of Language Processes.* Hillsdale, New Jersey: Lawrence Erlbaum. 501–513.

Craik, F. I. M., and Lockhart, R. S. 1972. Levels of processing: A framework for memory research. *Journal of Verbal Learning and Verbal Behavior, 11,* 671–684.

Craik, F. I. M., and Rabinowitz, J. C. 1984. Age differences in the acquisition and use of verbal information. In H. Bouma & D. Bouwhuis, eds., *Attention and Performance: X. Control of Language Processes.* Hillsdale, New Jersey: Lawrence Erlbaum. 471–499.

Dixon, R. A., Hultsch, D. F., Simon, E. W., and von Eye, A. 1984. Verbal ability and text structure effects on adult age differences in text recall. *Journal of Verbal Learning and Verbal Behavior, 23,* 569–578.

Hartley, J. T. 1988. Aging and individual differences in memory for written discourse. In L. L. Light and D. M. Burke, eds., *Language, Memory, and Aging.* New York: Cambridge University Press. 36–57.

Hultsch, D. F., and Dixon, R. A. 1984. Memory for test materials in adulthood. In P. B. Baltes and O. G. Brim, eds., *Life-span Development and Behavior: 6.* Orlando, Florida: Academic Press. 77–108.

Klatzky, R. L. 1988. Theories of information processing and theories of aging. In L. L. Light and D. M. Burke, eds., *Language, Memory, and Aging.* New York: Cambridge University Press. 1–16.

Light, L. L., and Burke, D. M. 1988. Patterns of language and memory in old age. In L. L. Light and D. M. Burke, eds., *Language, Memory, and Aging.* New York: Cambridge University Press. 244–271.

Light, L. L., and Capps, J. L. 1986. Comprehension of pronouns in young and older adults. *Developmental Psychology, 22,* 580–585.

Light, L. L., Zelinski, E. M., and Moore, M. 1982. Adult age differences in reasoning from new information. *Journal of Experimental Psychology: Learning, Memory, and Cognition, 8,* 435–447.

Magliano, J. P. and Graesser, A. C. 1991. A three-pronged method for studying inference generation in literary text. *Poetics, 20,* 193–232.

Meyer, B. J. F., and Rice, G. E. 1983. Learning and memory from text across the adult life span. In J. Fine and R. O. Freedle, eds., *Developmental Studies in Discourse.* Norwood, New Jersey: Ablex. 291–306.

Poon, L. W., Krauss, I. K., and Bowles, N. L. 1984. On subject selection in cognitive aging research. *Experimental Aging Research, 10,* 43–49.

Salthouse, T. A. 1988. Effects of aging on verbal abilities: Examination of the psychometric literature. In L. L. Light & D. M. Burke, eds., *Language, Memory, and Aging.* New York: Cambridge University Press. 17–35.

Schank, R. C., and Abelson, R. 1977. *Scripts, Plans, Goals and Understanding: An Inquiry into Human Knowledge Structures.* Hillsdale, New Jersey: Lawrence Erlbaum.

Taub, H. A. 1979. Comprehension and memory of prose materials by young and old adults. *Experimental Aging Research, 5,* 3–13.

Till, R. E. 1985. Verbatim and inferential memory in young and elderly adults. *Journal of Gerontology, 40,* 316–332.

Ulatowska, H. K., and Chapman, S. B. 1991. Neurolinguistics and aging. In D. Ripich, ed., *Handbook of Geriatric Communication Disorders.* San Diego, CA: College-Hill Press. 21–37.

Ulatowska, H. K., Sadowska, M., Kordys, J. and Kadzielawa. 1993. Selected aspects of narratives in Polish speaking aphasics as illustrated by Aesop's Fables. In H. Brownell and Y. Joanette, eds., *Narrative Discourse in Normal Aging and Neurologically Impaired Adults.* San Diego, California: Singular.

van Dijk, T. A. 1980. *Macrostructures: An Interdisciplinary Study of Global Structures in Discourse, Interaction, and Cognition.* Hillsdale, New Jersey: Lawrence Erlbaum.

Wechsler, D. 1981. *Wechsler Adult Intelligence Scale-Revised.* New York: Psychological Corporation.

APPENDIX: AESOP'S FABLES

Farmer and Sons

A farmer worked in a vineyard and became rich. He wanted his sons to be just like him. On his deathbed the farmer told his sons that there was a great treasure buried in the vineyard. After the farmer died, the sons went to the vineyard and dug up the soil. They could not find a buried treasure. At harvest time, the vineyard produced the best grapes ever. Now the sons understood the meaning of the treasure.

Fox and Goat

Once upon a time a fox was chasing a rooster. He did not notice a well in the ground, and so he fell into it. The well was very deep, and the fox could not get out. He looked up and noticed a goat standing at the edge of the well. The fox then lowered his head and pretended that he was drinking water. He began saying how good the water tasted, making the goat want some of it. The goat jumped in the well and began drinking. This is what the fox was waiting for. The fox climbed on the goat's back, jumped out and ran away. Later that night the goat was rescued by the farmer.

Fox and Raven

A raven was sitting on a tree holding a piece of cheese in his beak. A fox saw him and decided he wanted the cheese. He stood under the tree and began to praise the raven. He told the raven that he was a very beautiful bird and that he should become a king. The fox said that he would like to hear the raven's voice to be sure that the raven could give orders. Then the raven decided to show off his voice. He opened his beak and the cheese fell out onto the ground. The fox grabbed the cheese and ran away.

Raven and Pigeons

A hungry raven saw that pigeons in the pigeon coop had a lot of food. He painted his feathers white to look like them. But when he started to crow, they realized that he was a raven and chased him away. So he returned to his own kind. But the other ravens did not recognize him because he had his feathers painted white, so they also chased him away.

Two Roosters

Two roosters were fighting over the chicken yard. The one who was defeated hid in the corner. The other rooster flew to the top of the roost and began crowing and flapping his wings to boast of his victory. Suddenly an eagle swooped down, grabbed the rooster and carried him away. This was good luck for the defeated rooster. Now he could rule over the roost and have all the hens that he desired.

Woman and Doctor

A certain old woman suffered from a disease of the eyes. She called a doctor. The doctor came every day and rubbed some ointment on her eyes. When the old woman had her eyes closed, the doctor secretly carried her belongings out of her house. When he finished his treatment, he demanded a payment. The old woman refused. The doctor took her to court. In court, the old woman said that her vision was worse because before the treatment she saw all of her belongings, but after the treatment she could not see any of them. This is why she refused to pay.

CHAPTER 6

Facilitating Conversation with an Alzheimer's Disease Sufferer Through the Use of Indirect Repair

Steven R. Sabat

INTRODUCTION

Among the many problems that result from Alzheimer's disease (A.D.) is that as a result of insults to areas of the brain which involve the ability to recall, pronounce, and organize words, the speech of the sufferer is compromised (Irigaray, 1973; Bayles, 1979; Obler, 1981; Appell et al., 1982; Kempler, 1984; Shuttleworth and Huber, 1988). As a result, the sufferer can often be looked upon as being confused, be seen as not having coherent thoughts, and not be taken seriously by others. In such situations, the sufferer and caregivers experience great frustration, anger, and depression. The focus of the present chapter will be on the development of a strategy that may aid caregivers and sufferers in the communicative process. Specifically I will attempt to show how caregivers can aid themselves and the sufferer so as to make clearer the latter's meanings and intentions. The specific strategy which will be explored has been shown to be effective in enhancing communication with people who have suffered from a type of language disorder other than that caused by Alzheimer's disease, non-fluent aphasia.

Researchers have shed light upon a strategy to facilitate communication between aphasics and caregivers. The study (de Bleser and Weisman, 1986) involved an examination of the impact of the behavior of non-aphasics on conversational ability under conditions of pre-arranged model dialogues of non-fluent aphasics. The authors discovered that (1) non-aphasics used more dialogue remediation strategies when conversing with aphasics than when conversing with non-aphasics; (2) such strategies included the use of indirect forms of repair. Examples of indirect repair are questioning the intention of the aphasic in his or her speech and the use of questions that are marked by their intonation patterns rather than by interrogatives. In addition, the listener can restate his or her understanding of the afflicted person's speech in such a way as to allow the latter to confirm the correctness of the listener's understanding—i.e., one can say, "So you're saying that . . ." or "Let me see if I understand what you mean . . . " followed by the listener's understanding of what the afflicted speaker has said. Indirect repair was seen as a means whereby the non-aphasic partner could check as to whether or not he or she understood the other's point correctly. A third finding was that there was no evidence that non-aphasic partners used more direct repair mechanisms with aphasics than with non-aphasics, direct repair being overt corrections of pronunciation or of the words chosen, i.e., "red" as opposed to "green" in describing an object's color.

The authors found no evidence to support the idea that the aphasic person had lost the ability to engage in dialogue despite the fact that under experimental conditions in which standardized tests were used, the aphasics showed marked deficiencies in all linguistic components such as syntax, semantics, and phonology in all modalities (reading, writing, aural comprehension, and spoken production). The authors attributed the lack of disturbance in dialogue to (1) the cooperative attitude of the non-aphasic partner, and (2) the idea that aphasia involves a disturbance in the basic instrumentalities, or elements, of language as they are measured in standard tests rather than in the condition of its use in natural conversation.

Indirect repair is but one means whereby the non-afflicted partner can exhibit a cooperative attitude in a conversation. The authors also refer to the fact that non-aphasic partners did not monopolize the conversation through the use of their superior linguistic ability but did show evidence of accommodation. "A finer linguistic analysis would additionally reveal that the unimpaired partner also adjusts non-intrusively by using shorter and simplified sentence structures, which are easy for the aphasic to understand and use as a model for his production" (p. 284). Even though the aphasic person was clearly impaired in linguistic expression, he or she was still able to make valuable contributions to conversations if the non-aphasic partner used such forms of cooperation.

Another study (Sabat, 1991) involved the adaptation of de Bleser and Weisman's approach to an A.D. sufferer and showed that indirect repair was an extremely useful means of facilitating natural, spontaneous conversation. To wit, by checking my understanding of the afflicted person's utterance, I provided her with the opportunity to confirm my understanding and/or elaborate upon that understanding. The former allowed the conversation to continue smoothly, whereas her elaboration allowed me to understand further what she was trying to say. Specifically, the use of indirect repair allowed for an exchange of information that led to her describing her frustration in dealing with new people in unfamiliar places, along with the difficulty she experienced in holding on to her thoughts. In addition, she was able to communicate the reasons for her dissatisfaction with her support group, her desire not to undergo further standardized testing ("I know what's wrong with me"), and her desire to have reciprocal social relationships. Without my cooperation, which involved the use of indirect repair and which stemmed from my wish to understand her views, the afflicted person's speech could easily have been seen as disjointed, rambling, stilted, and confused and the same adjectives could easily have been used to describe her thoughts themselves. Thus, incorrect inferences could easily have been made about her and about the effects of A.D. on language.

A number of authors have supported the use of cooperative strategies in facilitating conversation. Rommetveit (1974) saw social dynamics such as the identities of the interlocutors, the time available to converse, and the purpose of the conversation as determining factors in the nature of conversation. In addition, Goodwin and Heritage (1990) proposed that particular attributes of the speaker, such as body movement and how events and objects are made the focus of joint attention, can have a great impact upon the conversation's form, and Goodwin (1980) indicated that a variety of behaviors on the part of the listener, such as participation displays, can affect the behavior of the speaker.

Gumperz and Tannen (1979) also proposed that the characteristics of the participants in conversation can have an effect upon the discourse. For instance, if the interlocutors do not share characteristics such as, for example, age, gender, location (nursing home vs. independent living), to name a few, it is possible that the listener can make incorrect inferences about the speaker which lead either to the development or confirmation of incorrect stereotypes. In the present case of a linguistic impairment, it would be incorrect to infer that the A.D. sufferer cannot think coherently or engage in meaningful conversation. Such an inference would be especially likely to occur if the listener did not consider his or her own behavior as having an effect upon that of the A.D. sufferer (Hamilton, 1994; Sabat, 1994).

Because the Sabat study involved only one afflicted person, it would be difficult to generalize from the findings. The case study method is an example of "intensive design" (Sabat and Harre, 1994) in which a phenomenon is exemplified in detail without trying to support a generalization. Individual cases might be representative of many, but further empirical research is required to establish how far what is demonstrated in the individual case can be generalized. Thus, the present study was undertaken to establish whether or not the above findings could be extended to yet another A.D. sufferer.

In the present study, the views of the above authors and the use of indirect repair were brought to bear in order to explore their effects upon natural, spontaneous conversation with an A.D. sufferer.

SUBJECT

The subject was a male A.D. sufferer (Dr. B.), age sixty-eight, who had suffered from A.D. for four years. According to standardized tests, he was considered moderately (Stage 4, Global Deterioration Scale, Reisberg et al., 1982) to severely (score of 5, Mini-Mental State Test, Folstein et al., 1975) afflicted, and he satisfied NINCDS-ADRDA criteria (a set of criteria established by the National Institute of Nervous and Communicative Diseases and Stroke along with the Alzheimer's Disease and Related Disorders Association by McKhann et al., 1984) for probable A.D. He was unable to dress himself, had moderate to severe word-finding problems, could not orient himself in time, had difficulty in naming objects and with recall. His signature showed great variability in form from week to week, and he had tremendous difficulty with writing in general. He was a scientist who held a Ph.D. degree and he referred to our work together as "The Project."

PROCEDURE

I met with Dr. B. approximately twice a week, for two hours at a time, for approximately ten months at an adult daycare center which he attended two to three times a week. Our association began with me explaining that I wanted to understand A.D. from the point of view of the sufferer and that I needed his help in that effort. Each conversation proceeded naturally (there were no pre-arranged dialogues) according to the wishes and consent of the interlocutors and was tape recorded. I have selected portions of those conversations from among the many which are relevant to the use of indirect repair mechanisms and the theoretical positions outlined earlier. In the transcripts that follow, indirect repairs are in italics and followed by a number in parentheses to facilitate subsequent references.

I have chosen to present extended transcripts so that readers can have an idea of the nature of the conversations themselves, including the points of view, concerns, emotions, and thoughts of the afflicted person. In this way, the A.D. sufferer might come alive, as it were, and not be represented solely by a set of impersonal data.

CONVERSATIONAL TRANSCRIPTS

Conversation 1

This was part of the second conversation I had with Dr. B. In addition to discussing relevant family background material, Dr. B. was explaining some of the situations that he encountered at the daycare center, and then I began to discuss with him the views of some researchers concerning the A.D. sufferer as a way to explain to him what I was interested in studying.

Dr. B.:   Sometimes I have to tow, kowtow to people outside, um, that I feel I'm, you know, more superior.

S.R.S.:   That must be very frustrating.

Dr. B.:   Well it must be for you too. Um, anyway, (director's name) and his wife are very, very wonderful. Um, and I don't know how much more. There are things that trigger more information.

S.R.S.:   Do you remember how old you were when you met your wife?

Dr. B.:   We, both of us were about the same age.

S.R.S.:   Were you in your twenties?

Dr. B.:   Yeah.

S.R.S.:   What did you admire most about her?

Dr. B.:   Um, she has a very tight meaner of picking up, I think, information to sort of pull it pack and forth.

S.R.S.:   *So you could discuss intellectual things with her very easily.* (1)

Dr. B.:   Oh yeah.

S.R.S.:   *Seems that you have a great deal of respect for her mind.* (2)

Dr. B.:   Of course I should. I think we're just about equals and . . .
          right now somebody's coming at the door.

(A staff member enters to invite Dr. B. to play a game with the group,
which he politely declines.)

S.R.S.:   It was interesting for me last week when I asked you about
          what you thought—they were playing some games in the next
          room and I asked you what you thought of that, and you said,
          "it's filler."

Dr. B.:   Uh, okay, oh yeah, that was information. It's, it is filler, okay.

S.R.S.:   *Do you mean it's nonsense and doesn't amount to much and
          just passes the time?* (3)

Dr. B.:   Yeah, but certainly don't want this to embarrass because if it
          gets out. Sometimes, um, I will be picking up information and
          uh, never know whether it's gonna come or not. I'd like to
          keep talking, but, uh, is mine important enough at this stage or
          something? I think you're bored.

S.R.S.:   I'm not bored for a microsecond. You're important.

Dr. B.:   Why?

S.R.S.:   There are people who do research who talk about A.D.
          sufferers as people who have lost themselves—the loss of the
          self, and I don't believe that.

Dr. B.:   Well I agree—I gree that uh even if I find, uh, if I'm a
          problem or something or has even if I go up before my wife
          first, she does that everyday, doing that, but I, it comes in and
          do it easily.

S.R.S.:   You don't think that you've lost your sense of self now do
          you?

Dr. B.:   In what respect?

S.R.S.:   You know who you are.

Dr. B.:   Yeah, definitely. I know who I am. And sometimes I have to
          fake, um, as to people that I deal with back and forth.

S.R.S.:   What do you have to fake?

Dr. B.:   Uh, I uh fake for uh, uh, course I feel I could, could have done
          more. Um, can I do better now? I don't know.

S.R.S.:   I don't know either.

Dr. B.:   I don't know either.

S.R.S.: *But when you say you have to fake, are you saying that —is that part of kowtowing to people?* (4)

Dr. B.: Oh, yeah. And uh, it's a slick game.

S.R.S.: *Slick game?* (5)

Dr. B.: That's the only way I think, sometimes, uh, that I find, yeah, I find slick games.

S.R.S.: *When you say that you fake things does that mean that you have thoughts about what's going on and you don't say anything or try to appear to be different than you are?* (6)

Dr. B.: Ya, or being different. The staff, I love them very dear, very very much. Uh, I don't necessarily need what's, what's, what's in the room.

Conversation 2

Conversation 2 is part of the ninth conversation I had with Dr. B. The subject had to do with his experience of learning new things and being unable to recall that information soon after but being able to retrieve it at a later time.

S.R.S.: Some people think that A.D. sufferers can't learn new things.

Dr. B.: Oh that's not so. I have pieces, portions of, that I grab as I work and that's it.

S.R.S.: That's important because many family members of A.D. sufferers think that the person with the disease can't learn anything new.

Dr. B.: No. That's a no-no. I, I know either whether I anticipate it, something, um, or not, or um, I can anticipate it again, you know, think very hard. Alzheimer's . . . far as I'm concerned, Alzheimer's is, is, are pieces. I'm learning pieces. Does that mean anything?

S.R.S.: Yes it does. You see, you're able to learn and retain

Dr. B.: That I can do.

S.R.S.: different parts of things.

Dr. B.: Different parts of things.

S.R.S.: If I thought that you could learn nothing new, I wouldn't try to teach you anything new, right?

Dr. B.: Ya.

S.R.S.: Not only would I not try to teach you, but I might not engage you in a way that I would engage a person in conversation if I thought that the person would remember what I said.

Dr. B.: But I pick up. No, better still, um, I pick pieces of information and I can't try *or* and then another two weeks ago of going back, I can pick up the whole thing again. Does this help you?

S.R.S.: *Yes, yes. Let me see if I understand correctly. You can pick up pieces of information and you know you have that information, but then it gets mixed up. But some time later it can come back. (7)*

Dr. B.: Oh ya. That's a pattern. Does it help?

S.R.S.: *Yes, because there may be times when you try like crazy to remember something and you can't. But then some time later, out of nowhere, the information comes back to you. (8)*

Dr. B.: Oh I get a lot of things like that.

S.R.S.: I thought so, but I didn't know for certain.

Dr. B.: I had started taking notes. Now here's all notes with X's which means these are—I had a sensitive area and I couldn't do it. Here is something that is a sort of a problem. I take project material and it sort of gets out of my head as it is very fast, uh, like my wife will want to go someplace or something like that so it was too difficult. I had started this before we actually started talking. Um, I found that I was, uh, doing um, I was, I was, I would make a very important information to me and I kept losing this information. As a matter of fact, (he reads) "lost of information while working." I'm losing things fast, however. When I started over with this thing (keeping notes) I could retrieve, I can retrieve information and it's three X's are strong—I can maintain the material. I can get information and hold it for some time in the evening. What happens if things erode? I didn't want, but I just, I go through a piece of material, a newspaper, uh, anything else, and I can keep it up, I keep it up, and then about five minutes, ten minutes, that information, that material that I talk to you that I had, gets away from me. *But* then I was talking at home and um, I was able to retrieve some things. So I get quantity. Is this very important? I didn't even look for names, but I lost something. That is, I, I was talking to myself, or thinking about it, and, and, it, it, uh, failed. I just came down lost.

S.R.S.   *So there was something that you were thinking about, and suddenly you felt like you lost track of what it was?* (9)

Dr. B.:   Yeah, in a way. Then every so often with all the papers, and I forgive you, forgive me for all the things that were here because I'm trying to do—this is information, this is lost, um but I don't know what is the quantity or the quality that we're forgetting. I, uh, I, it popped into my head in the morning, in early morning. You know this was what I was doing.

S.R.S.   *When you say it popped into your head, you mean that something that you had thought you had lost popped into your head?* (10)

Dr. B.:   Ya, I slaw, I lost something and retrieved most of it, most of it.

Conversation 3

Conversation three is part of the tenth conversation I had with Dr. B. Here he is speaking about his experience of the daycare center, its plethora of activities, and how the pace of activities interferes with his ability to have prolonged conversations with the program director.

S.R.S.:   The other day you mentioned that you had some problem with (name of program director). Does that strike any familiar notes?

Dr. B.:   Every so often I, I get uh, frustrated with him.

S.R.S.:   This is (name)—with the mustache?

Dr. B.:   Yeah, yeah. I like him very much. I like him very, very much. Um, he, he goes to a, let's see how could I do it? I'm certy not nasty with him at all whatsoever and but uh, every so often, uh, uh, the uh, Barnum and Bailey—it's the Barnum and Bailey that I don't like.

S.R.S.:   *You mean it's like a circus around here?* (11)

Dr. B.:   Oh yeah. It's a big, tremendously big circus. Um, I have uh, even during the dinner this evening and uh, it gets uh, sorta screwed up.

S.R.S.   *All of the chaos becomes very difficult for you to deal with?* (12)

Dr. B.:   Yeah. I, uh, and I uh, would not necessarily lie and it, it sort of a nuisance for somebody like you is, um, trying to get you some good material back and forth, and uh, the, it turns out sometimes to a mickey mouse system.

S.R.S.: *You mean in here.* (13)
Dr. B.: In here and (name of director).
S.R.S.: *So some of the things that happen here are pedestrian for you.*
         (14)
Dr. B.: No, the well, what I, what I want to uh, grab, it's counterv, uh,
         worth, it uh, counterworth material in the sense uh, that it
         should not be being.
S.R.S.: *So there are things at the center that are counterproductive.*
         (15)
Dr. B.: Right. That's what I come in once in a while. Nothing of big,
         big deal.

RESULTS

Table 1 presents summary data for relevant aspects of all three
conversations. Total time of talk was measured by subtracting the
pauses in each turn in which they occurred, thus referring to the time
during which the interlocutors were actually speaking. Pauses and time
spent talking were measured with a stopwatch.

Table 1. A Summary of the Data for the Three Conversations

| | Conversations | | | | | |
| | 1 | | 2 | | 3 | |
	Dr. B.	S.R.S.	Dr. B.	S.R.S.	Dr. B.	S.R.S.
time at talk (seconds)	256.9	85.1	611.8	98.3	149.9	34.7
number of utterances	315	223	501	223	186	70
number of turns	18	17	11	11	7	7
median time at talk/ turn (secs.)	15.3	3.5	12.5	8.2	17.9	2.3
number of turns with indirect repairs		6		4		5
percent of turns with indirect repairs		35.3		36.4		71.4

In conversation 1, Dr. B. spoke for 256.9 seconds, whereas I spoke
for 85.1 seconds. Dr. B. produced 315 utterances in 18 turns, whereas I
produced 223 in 17 turns. The median time of a turn was 15.3 seconds
for Dr. B. and 3.5 seconds for me. Of the 17 turns belonging to me, 6
(35.3%) involved the use of indirect repairs. Indirect repairs 1 and 2

could be characterized as further probes, in which I provided some specific elaboration on what he said, whereas in the cases of 3, 4, 5, and 6, I was drawing connections between a number of his previous statements and probing to see whether or not I understood what he was trying to communicate. That I was somewhat successful in these attempts can be seen in that indirect repair 1 was followed by his saying, "Oh yeah"; 2 was followed by his saying, "Of course"; 3 was followed by his saying, "Yeah" and elaborating; 4 by his saying, "Oh yeah"; 5 by his confirming my statement, "That's the only way I think sometimes . . ."; and 6 by his saying "Ya."

In conversation 2, Dr. B.'s total time at talk was 611.8 seconds, whereas I spoke for 98.3 seconds. Dr. B. produced 501 utterances in 11 turns, whereas I produced 223 in 11 turns. The median time per turn was 12.5 seconds for Dr. B. and 8.2 seconds for me. The number of turns in which I made indirect repairs was 4, or 36.4% of my turns. Each direct repair was followed immediately by confirmation: 7 by "Oh ya"; 8 by "Oh I get a lot of things like that"; 9 by "Yeah, in a way"; and 10 by "Ya.." followed by his restating his point positively.

In conversation 3, the total time at talk was 149.9 seconds for Dr. B. and 34.7 seconds for me. Dr. B. produced 186 utterances in 7 turns and I produced 70 in 7 turns. The median time per turn was 17.9 seconds for Dr. B. and 2.3 seconds for me. The number of turns in which indirect repairs were made was 5 (71.4% of my turns). In the instances of indirect repairs, 11 was followed by his saying, "Oh yeah," and then elaborating on what I had said; 12 was followed by his saying "Yeah" and adding another thought; 13 was followed by his repeating my comment and adding to it; 14 was followed by his disconfirming my interpretation of what he had said ("No") followed by further elaboration; and 15 was followed by his confirming my comment by saying, "Right" along with some further comment.

In all three conversations, 15 indirect repairs were followed (1) by agreement or confirmation by Dr. B., (2) by further elaboration, or (3) in one case, by disagreement with what I had said followed by a statement which helped to clarify the issue.

DISCUSSION

The results of the present study confirm in a number of ways, for an A.D. sufferer engaging in spontaneous conversation, the previous findings of de Bleser and Weisman with non-fluent aphasics under conditions of pre-arranged model dialogues that indirect repair can be used to enhance communication between healthy individuals and those who have suffered disturbances in language function. The present results also support previous findings obtained with another A.D. sufferer engaging in spontaneous conversation (Sabat, 1991), indicating that the use of indirect repair may be a promising method by which to gain a deeper understanding of the thoughts of A.D. sufferers and showing that such a method can, indeed, enhance conversation and communication between A.D. sufferers and healthy interlocutors.

For example, I was able to check my understanding of the A.D. sufferer's comments and provide him with a chance to confirm my understanding as correct or to let me know that I did not understand his point and then attempt again to make his point. His confirmation of my understanding allowed the conversation to continue smoothly, and his elaborations allowed for an enhanced understanding on my part. As a result, Dr. B. was able to feel confident that he was being understood. At times, I checked my understanding of his comments by announcing my intent clearly through the use of utterances such as "Let me see if I understand correctly," whereas on other occasions, I simply made a statement which seemed to me to be a restatement of what he had said. In the latter case, he then had the opportunity to respond by confirming my understanding or disconfirming by saying either "yes" or "no." This allowed him to comment without having to make lengthy statements which, for him, were very effortful. For example, in the first conversation (repeated from above), he was describing his wife:

Dr. B.:   Um, she has a very tight meaner of picking up, I think, information to sort of pull in back and forth.
S.R.S.:   So you could discuss intellectual things with her very easily.
Dr. B.:   Oh, yeah.
S.R.S.:   Seems that you have a great deal of respect for her mind.
Dr. B.:   Of course, I should. I think we're about equals.

Also in the first conversation, the use of indirect repairs allowed Dr. B. to communicate how he feels about the program of activities at the daycare center and how he keeps himself at a distance from them:

S.R.S.:   But when you say you have to fake, are you saying that, is that part of kowtowing to people?
Dr. B.:   Oh yeah. And uh, it's a slick game.

S.R.S.: Slick game?

Dr. B.: That's the only way I think sometimes, uh, that I find, yeah, I find slick games.

S.R.S.: When you say fake things, does that mean you have thoughts about what's going on and you don't say anything or try to be different?

Dr. B.: Ya, or being different. The staff, I love them, very dear, very, very much. Uh, I don't necessarily need what's, what's what's in the room.

In the second conversation, the use of indirect repairs allowed me to understand Dr. B.'s experience of being unable to retrieve information soon after having had an experience but being able to do so at some later time:

Dr. B.: But I pick up, no, better still, um, I pick up pieces of information and I can't try or and then another two weeks ago of going back, I can pick up the whole thing again. Does this help you?

S.R.S.: Yes, yes. Let me see if I understand correctly. You can pick up pieces of information and you know you have that information, but then it gets mixed up, but two weeks later it can come back.

Dr. B.: Oh ya, that's a pattern.

In this conversation, Dr. B. was able to communicate some aspects of his experience as an A.D. sufferer. The above dialogue occurred during a conversation which began with his describing A.D. as follows: "Alzheimer's..far as I'm concerned, Alzheimer's is, is, are pieces. I'm learning pieces. Does that mean anything?" Frequently, Dr. B. would ask such a question, or ask whether what he just said is of help to me. He wanted, given his career as a scientist, to provide useful information, and our conversations were far more meaningful to him than were the ongoing activities.

In the third conversation, the use of indirect repairs led to an understanding of Dr. B.'s view of how the activities stood in relation to what he felt was more important (work on "The Project," discussions with the program director), to his frustration concerning the "buzzing, blooming confusion" (to borrow from William James) of the daycare activities.

In these three conversations, the use of indirect repairs led to my enhanced understanding of Dr. B.'s thoughts and feelings and to his satisfaction at being understood. Even though my linguistic abilities were not compromised, I did not dominate the conversations, for Dr. B. in each case had far more total time-at-talk (1,018.6 seconds vs. 218.1 seconds) and produced far more utterances (1002 vs. 516). My turns were not replete with direct repairs. In each conversation, my median time-at-talk per turn was less than that of Dr. B. My comments were shorter in duration and were made for the purpose of understanding more clearly what Dr. B. was saying and to help him understand that I was interested in what he had to say. Dr. B. was thus able to make substantive contributions to the conversations. These results mirror the findings of de Bleser and Weisman with aphasics as well as extend those from earlier work with another A.D. sufferer (Sabat, 1991).

Also in agreement with these authors, it seemed that even though Dr. B. had experienced severe linguistic problems as described by the results of standard neuropsychological tests, such problems were far more related to the instrumentalities of speech than to the condition of its use. Dr. B. was able to engage in spontaneous conversations, to communicate ideas that related to emotional and intellectual aspects of life. He was able to understand my comments, elaborate upon some of them, and correct me where I was mistaken in my understanding of his points. Again, there seems to be a yawning gap between this A.D. sufferer's use of language on test items and his use of language for the purpose of communicating in a meaningful exchange of ideas (see also Hamilton, 1994; Sabat, 1994).

The present results also lend support to Rommetveit's (1974) idea of social dynamics as the determing factors which govern conversational events. Rommetveit referred to certain implicit "contractual aspects" which characterize every conversation and which are governed by factors such as who the interlocutors happen to be, the purpose of the conversation, the time available, and the location of the conversation. My contributions to the conversations reported herein were the result of (1) my desire to understand clearly what Dr. B. was saying, and (2) my awareness of his difficulty in using the mechanics of linguistic production. Such social dynamics include the particular attributes of the speakers (Goodwin and Heritage, 1990). Such attributes, then, can have great bearing upon the form of conversations. In the absence of my cooperation and the use of indirect repairs, Dr. B.'s speech easily could have been viewed as rambling, disjointed, and confused, and these adjectives could then have been applied to his thoughts as well. If such inferences had been made, they would have been patently false. Such faulty inferences can easily lead to further uncooperative behavior on the part of the non-afflicted partner in conversation, to further validation of the initial faulty inference, and to the generation of an incorrect stereotype of the A.D. sufferer. The stereotype itself would then provide the foundation for future uncooperative behavior in conversation as has been explored by Sabat and Harre (1992).

Finally, because Dr. B. had thoughts and feelings to share about a number of issues (as evidenced in the transcripts), it would seem important that the non-afflicted person heed Gumperz and Tannen (1979) and keep the characteristics of the other person in mind. Specifically, the authors found that misunderstandings can occur between members of different ethnic groups and that such misunderstandings can involve innocent inferences made by the listener based on the latter's cultural background. One can perhaps extend such an analysis to members of different groups based on health, such that there are "patients" and "normals" and the latter can be making innocent inferences about the former. Such behavior on the part of the non-afflicted person can position the afflicted person (Sabat and Harre, 1992) as someone with whom it is (or is not) possible to exchange ideas, who has (or hasn't) something to say, and who can (or cannot), indeed, communicate in meaningful ways. In other words, the assumptions that we make about a person affect the way we view and treat the person—we can position the person as incompetent and treat the person accordingly, or we can assume a degree of understanding and act accordingly. One such assumption is that the afflicted person does indeed have something to say and on that assumption, the non-afflicted interlocutor seeks to clarify what is not immediately clear to him or her. One effective way to achieve clarification is with indirect repair. Note that in the conversations reported herein, a large proportion—35.3%, 36.5%, and 71.4%—of my turns involved attempts to clarify for myself what Dr. B. was saying, and such attempts allowed for the mutual exchange of ideas despite Dr. B.'s linguistic problems. The present study indicates that the A.D. sufferer can communicate far more effectively than would be assumed solely on the basis of standardized tests of language and cognition and that the cooperation of the non-afflicted interlocutor, via use of indirect repairs, can facilitate that communicative ability.

REFERENCES

Appell, J., Kertesz, A., and Fisman, M. 1982. A study of language functioning in Alzheimer patients. *Brain and Language*, 17, 73–91.

Bayles, K.A. 1979. Communication profiles in a geriatric population. Unpublished Ph.D. dissertation.

de Bleser, R., and Weisman, H. 1986. The communicative impact of non-fluent aphasia on the dialogue behavior of linguistically impaired partners. In F. Lowenthal and F. Vandamme, eds., *Pragmatics and Education*. New York: Plenum Press.

Folstein, M.F., Folstein, S.E., and McHugh, P.R. 1975. Mini-mental state. *Journal of Psychiatric Research*, 12, 189–198.

Goodwin, C. 1980. Processes of mutual monitoring implicated in the production of descriptive sequences. *Sociological Inquiry* 50, 303–317.

Goodwin, C., and Heritage, J. 1990. Conversation analysis. *Annual Review of Anthropology*, 19, 283–307.

Gumperz, J., and Tannen, D. 1979. Individual and social differences in language use. In C. Fillmore, D. Kempler, and W.S.-Y. Wang, eds., *Individual Differences in Language Ability and Language Behavior*. New York: Academic Press. 305–325.

Hamilton, H. 1994. *Conversations with an Alzheimer's Patient*. Cambridge: Cambridge University Press.

Irigaray, L. 1973. *Le langage de dements*. The Hague: Mouton.

Kempler, D. 1984. Syntactic and symbolic abilities in Alzheimer's disease. Unpublished Ph.D. dissertation.

McKhann, G., Drachman, M., Folstein, M.F., Katzman, R., Price, D., and Stadlan, E.M. 1984. Clinical diagnosis of Alzheimer's disease: Report of the NINCDS-ADRDA work group under the auspices of the Department of Health and Human Services task force on Alzheimer's Disease. *Neurology* 34, 939–944.

Obler, L. 1981. Review of *Le langage des dements*, by L. Irigaray. *Brain and Language* 12, 375–386.

Reisberg, B., Ferris, S.H., and Crook, T. 1982. Signs, symbols, and course of age-associated cognitive decline. In S. Corkin, K.L. Davis, J.H. Growdin, E. Usdin, and R.J. Wurtman, eds., *Aging: Vol. 19. Alzheimer's Disease: A Report of Progress in Research*. New York: Academic Press.

Rommetveit, R. 1974. *On Message Structure: A Framework for the Study of Language and Communication*. London: Wiley.

Sabat, S.R. 1991. Facilitating conversation via indirect repair: A case study of Alzheimer's disease. *The Georgetown Journal of Languages and Linguistics* 2, 284–296.

Sabat, S.R. 1994. Excess disability and malignant social psychology: A cases study of Alzheimer's disease. *Journal of Community and Applied Social Psychology* 4, 157–166.

Sabat, S.R., and Harre, R. 1992. The construction and deconstruction of self in Alzheimer's disease. *Ageing and Society* 12, 443–461.

Sabat, S.R., and Harre, R. 1994. The Alzheimer's disease sufferer as a semiotic subject. *Philosophy, Psychiatry, Psychology*, 1, 145–160.

Shuttleworth, E.C., and Huber, S.J. 1988. The naming disorder of dementia of Alzheimer's type. *Brain and Language* 34, 222–234.

Identity in Old Age

Part Three
Identity in Old Age

CHAPTER 7

Evaluation in the Bereavement Narratives of Elderly Irish American Widowers[1]

Anne R. Bower

INTRODUCTION

Widowhood is one of the pre-eminent events of old age in the United States. The 1980 U.S. Census reports that, of the 10 million American men aged sixty-five and older, 1.4 million (14%) are widowers. Widowhood brings with it major social and psychological transitions in later life (Littlewood, 1992; Lund, 1989; Parkes and Weiss, 1983; George, 1980; Lopata, 1973; Berardo, 1970) and significantly challenges the widower's adaptive ability (Luborsky and Rubinstein, 1990, 1987) by altering his social role and social identity. The emotions related to the loss of a long-term spouse and other affective states must be weathered and overcome (Brabant, Forsyth, and Melancon, 1992; Campbell and Silverman, 1987). As Parkes and Weiss (1983) note:

> The death of a spouse invalidates a multitude of assumptions about the world that, up to that time, have been taken for granted. These affect almost every area of mental functioning: habits of thought which have built up over the years of interaction, plans and routines that involved the other person, hopes or wishes that can no longer be realized. (70)

A spouse's death is a key event in the life of the elderly man.

The topic I will take up in this chapter is the manner in which elderly Irish American widowers talk about their personal feelings and inner state at the time of their wife's death. Or, to be more accurate, I should say the manner in which they do not talk about such things, since the central characteristic of their discourse about their wife's passing is the apparent lack of expressed emotion. Few of the speakers communicate their emotional reactions to the events they report. Those who do, communicate that feeling so indirectly that only inference and speculation will permit an interpretation of the emotion that the speaker might have felt. The few speakers who do reveal their feelings overtly do so in textually disruptive ways, for example, by postposing statements of affect related to the bereavement into other topical areas or by segmenting emotional statements between sequences of detailed talk which are seemingly irrelevant to the events of the specific narrative.

Instead of emotional statements or descriptions of their inner state, these elderly Irish American widowers present facts. Their discourse on this topic constitutes factual accounts of the events of the day their wife died, factual exchanges between participants in the events, factual testimonies from medical authorities. Evaluative statements that report the emotional contours of the experience as they experienced it are typically factual in content and tend to offer evaluation of other facts rather than personal feelings. This focus on fact, the containment of affect, or the exclusion of emotional statements altogether creates an overall impression of dry, often unconnected, discourse which makes the listener work hard to follow the discourse, and at the end, leaves the listener wondering to what extent or how deeply the speaker was touched by the loss of his wife. This is an interesting phenomenon for a number of reasons, among which is the insight it offers into how language is utilized and manipulated to convey or suppress information about personal experience and inner state.

However, bereavement narrative also has a profound relevance for the wider field of gerontological linguistics. Review of these elderly widowers' stories about their bereavement offers an opportunity to reconsider the analytic perspectives that we invoke in our efforts to understand the speech of elderly people. At present, for example, one important band of research offers a coherent, overarching theory about the linguistic and communicative capabilities of elderly speakers. This paradigm, referred to here as biomedical or developmental, routinely characterizes the linguistic capabilities of older speakers in such negative terms as "reduced," "deteriorating," "declining," or "compromised." It concludes that elderly speakers' "inferior" linguistic performance, compared to younger adults, is attributable to normal deterioration of cognitive function related to old age. These gloomy findings are based on language data gathered under experimental or clinical research conditions. It relies on linguistic data that is elicited from standardized batteries of structured, highly artificial, verbal, reading, and written tasks designed to measure the linguistic acuity of the test-takers. The results of such testing is purported to reflect the linguistic capabilities of older speakers.

Within this paradigm, narrative discourse has drawn considerable attention, since it is considered to embody the complex interaction between linguistic, communicative, and cognitive processes to a greater extent than any other type of connected discourse (Ulatowska and Chapman, 1991). However, as with other linguistic and communicative units, elders' narrative discourse (as collected within test situations) is typically found to be significantly reduced or even lacking in complexity, content, and structure. From this perspective, the abbreviated event structures of the death narratives that we shall examine are likely to be construed as deficient. Similarly, the absence of the evaluative component is likely to be regarded not simply as an absence but as a lack and one which may be attributed to the cognitive decline typical in old age.

While sociolinguists are increasingly concerned with the vernacular speech of the elderly (e.g. Labov and Auger, 1991), the personal narratives of older speakers have only begun to be addressed. Most sociolinguistic analysis of personal narrative has been preoccupied with its effectiveness or dramatic adequacy. Oral narratives are described as effective, dramatic, or vivid, and these characteristics are widely regarded as conveyed through the evaluative components of the narrative (Johnstone, 1990; Tannen, 1989; Polanyi, 1979, 1985). Since the evaluative sections of these older widowers' narratives are typically reduced or absent, they are likely to be regarded by sociolinguists as ineffective or poorly told. Inadvertently, this feature of sociolinguistic narrative analysis supports the biomedical/developmental paradigm's deficit analysis.

In this chapter, I would like to propose an alternative analysis, one that is based on sociolinguistic principles and that takes into account the speech community's cultural parameters for speaking. The interpretation I propose is that the structural contours of the elderly widowers' bereavement narratives do not reflect cognitive and linguistic decline on the part of the speakers, nor do they represent poor storytelling. Rather, they represent an expressive speech style characteristic of the Irish American community. Further, this speech style is directly tied to Irish American cultural values and beliefs that govern talk about personal emotion. Despite the fact that both native Irish and American Irish cultures value talk highly, they are cultures that constrain disclosure of interior experience. Inner state is carefully shielded from view and revealed only guardedly in discourse.

Cultural anthropology and linguistic ethnography have demonstrated that speech community norms profoundly influence what members may or may not say, and how what may be said must be said (Hymes, 1972; Irvine, 1979; Schiffrin, 1984; Ochs, 1988). There is substantial literature on the extent and ways in which culture and oral narrative interact, and it has become widely accepted in cultural anthropology and linguistic ethnography that the language and structure of the narrative will also reflect the speech community's preferred or permissible forms for reported personal experience and indeed, will influence the individual's very perception of that experience (Price, 1987; Holland and Quinn, 1987; Basso, 1984; Rosaldo, 1986).

Although comparatively little systematic investigation of the speaking styles and roles adopted by the elderly in speech communities has been forthcoming to date (but for exceptions, see Coupland, Coupland, and Giles 1991; Williams, 1990), it seems unlikely that elderly speakers would relinquish their participation in their speech communities simply because they have aged. Consequently, it is reasonable to assume that the content of personal experience narratives will reflect the values, attitudes, and judgments of the social group of which the elderly narrator is a member. Further, the language and structure of the narrative will also reflect the speech community's preferred or permissible forms for reporting personal experience.

In the discussion to follow, I will argue that speaking about bereavement is a culturally delineated behavior and that the use of affective language to describe a traumatic experience is likely to be culturally determined (Schweder, 1991; Hill and Irvine, 1993). Further, I will argue that the use of elderly speakers' vernacular narratives about topics of deep, personal meaning can provide a picture of their linguistic and communicative abilities that differs dramatically from those formulated on the bases of language data elicited in clinical or experimental settings. Analysis of personal narratives used in this study offers an opportunity to examine healthy older speakers' language as it occurs in a speech situation that is similar to the one in which they might ordinarily engage, speaking on a topic of the most compelling relevance. As such, it represents a valuable, necessary contrast to the current biomedical/developmental approach which draws its data from standardized assessment batteries administered in experimental or clinical settings.

After a brief description of the narrators and context of talk, the sociolinguistic model for narrative analysis will be reviewed and illustrated with sample narratives from the data. The technical, linguistic means for evaluating the events that are presented in the narrative will be discussed. Specific evaluative strategies that convey the narrator's inner state will be examined in light of culturally defined values and attitudes surrounding the expression of emotion. The final section will discuss these findings in terms of their implications for the study of elderly speakers' language and for achieving a more realistic perspective on the linguistic and communicative capabilities of the elderly.

NARRATORS, CONTEXT, AND TOPIC

Narrators. The speakers represented in this study are 14 men between the ages of seventy-five and eighty-four years. At the time of the interviews during which the data were collected, these speakers were assessed by the original research team (Rubinstein, 1985) to be in good physical condition, not depressed, and not cognitively impaired. Speakers' health and morale were assessed using the short version of the Philadelphia Geriatric Center Multilevel Assessment Instrument (Lawton, Moss, Fulcome, and Kleban, 1982) and a version of Antonucci's (n.d.) social network instrument was used to assess current social network involvement. Thus, the language we will be exposed to in this study is that of healthy, alert men in an age range often characterized as "old" or "very old."

These respondents identify themselves as first- and second-generation Irish Americans, with both parents of Irish ancestry. They are native Philadelphians, with education, occupation, and income levels indicative of upper working and lower-middle class social economic status. A variety of questions based on Dashefsky and Shapiro's (1974) behavior trait approach was used to assess speakers' degree of ethnic saturation.

They are widowers whose long-term spouses died two to six years prior to the interview. All but two of the speakers describe themselves as having "gotten back to normal" after the death of their partners.

Context. The narratives in question derive from the second phase of extended, in-depth, qualitative interviews that covered a range of topics about the individual's life history, the circumstances surrounding the death of his spouse, the death itself, post-funeral life, and life-reorganization after bereavement. The interviews were typically three to five hours long and were conducted over a period of two to three days. The aim of the interview was to get as much detailed personal information as possible about the individual's bereavement experience in order to understand the role of ethnicity in life re-organization after bereavement.

For most respondents, the actual discussion of the wife's death took place on the second day of a three-day interview, after some familiarity and rapport with the interviewer had been established via discussion of the speaker's life history. The interviews were conducted in the respondent's home by a male interviewer, 30 to 40 years younger than the respondent. Only the interviewer and the respondent were present at the time of the interview. The interview itself was open-ended by design, with a set of questions accessible to the interviewer to guide the discussion and ensure topical comparability, but the respondent was permitted to control the length of the answers he offered to the questions he was asked.

Topic. In all, 12 of the 14 respondents offered a total of 34 narratives about some aspect of their bereavement experience. About half of the narratives focus on the circumstances leading up to and surrounding the death itself. The remainder address life after bereavement, for example, successful efforts in self-sufficiency in the new life without a spouse, encounters with new friends, or specific incidents from the speaker's early married life with his spouse.

This discussion will focus on responses to the question about how the spouse died. This question was always asked in the same form:

"Can you tell me a little bit about the circumstances leading up to your wife's death? Was she ill for a long while, or was it a sudden sort of thing?"

Nine of the 12 respondents answered this query with a narrative account of the death. Three speakers reported their wife's death in non-narrative discourse, typically with a single sentence answer that conveyed the death date, the cause of death, or that generally characterized the circumstances surrounding the death. For example:

"She was sick for mostly one and a half—or maybe two years. She died June 22, 1980."

"It was very gradual."

"She had a heart condition, as I said, for several years before she actually died. And-uh-she was—she'd get around pretty good. And-uh-then gradually, near the end of her life—why, she was—it was a struggle, you know."

While personal narrative represents only one of several options available to the speaker in presenting this important event (Riessman, 1990; Schatzman and Strauss, 1955), this discussion will examine the nine narrative accounts offered by these respondents. Typical narrative responses to this question were:

Example 1: Kilcullen

a) Well, it was Easter Sunday night, two years ago in 1984.
b) And—uh—after we come home from church
c) and—uh—she wasn't feelin' too good that day
d) and that night—she lapsed into unconsciousness

(Did she go to church?)

No.
Not—she didn't——.

(You say "We went to church." It was you and—?)

Well, my daughter and her family and myself, we went to church.
And my son-in-law stayed there.
And then, when we came back—uh—we—uh——.
She—she—she wasn't feeling good that day at all, and—uh—that night, she lapsed into unconsciousness.
e) And my oldest daughter was there with her
f) And she called down to me,
   she said "You better come up.
   I don't think-don't-don't think——.
   Things don't look good at all."
g) And that time, she was sort of laborin', breathin', laborin' and breathin'.

h)   So——.

(This was what? Like 8 o'clock at night?)

Yeah.
i)   We tried to get a hold of the doctor.
j)   Of course, it was Easter Sunday night.
k)   It was pretty hard to get a hold of the doctor.
l)   But—uh—he came.
m)   And—uh—then—and then, she died.
n)   He said
       there was nothin' we could—
       that we could do.

Example 2: Medd

a)   She wasn't terribly ill 'til she dropped dead on April the 23rd, 1980.
b)   She would holler for me.
c)   She did have a couple of falls,
d)   but she would always call—at night, or anything.
e)   She would call me
       if she had difficulty or pain or anything.

(Yeah, for example, if she went to the bathroom is that what you're saying?)

That's right.
f)   She went to the bathroom.
g)   It was 4:15 in the morning.
h)   And I heard her fall.
i)   And I knew
       that it was somethin' terrible
       because—she didn't call me.

(Uh-hunh)

j)   So—uh—Denise was here then.
k)   And Denise—I called for emergency service right away,
       and the police, and the first aid ambulance.
l)   They gave her artificial respiration,
m)   but when she got to the hospital,
       she was dead.

Example 3: O'Brien

a) And—uh—then one Friday morning, it was
b) Uh—I normally came home
c) and did my report writing on Fridays.
d) And—uh—so she knew
    I didn't have to get up early
e) So she slept in the boys' room, in Andy's bed,
    because he was away at college.
g) And-uh-the other kids woke up at seven o'clock.
h) And—uh—Jimmy said "Come on, Mother!
    It's time to go to—go to school.
    We got to get up."
i) And he went in and took a shower.
j) And when he came out,
    she was still in bed.
k) And he said "Mother! Come on! Come on!"
l) And he shook her,
m) and she didn't move.
n) And then he said to my boy Jack,
    who was—I guess Jack was in premed at LaSalle, then,
o) eh—he said—uh—"Hey, Jack!
    Somethin's wrong with Mother!"
p) So he jumped over,
q) and he—he saw.
r) And he started to give her—artificial respiration
    and stuff like that.
s) And I—and then I heard the kids scream,
t) and I run in the room,
    'cause she had let me sleep by myself, you know.
u) And I ran in the room,
v) and he said to me "Dad, she's gone."
    And he said "She's cold.
    She's been gone at least four hours."

(God.)

w) So that's the way she went.

ORAL NARRATIVE OF PERSONAL EXPERIENCE: THE SOCIOLINGUISTIC PERSPECTIVE

While there is considerable debate about the structural organization of personal narrative, there is general agreement about its nature and purpose. Personal narrative is widely regarded as one verbal means by which speakers utilize both the resources of their grammar and their cultures to present their individual experience of reality (Labov and Waletsky, 1967; Watson, 1973; Goodwin, 1990; Linde, 1993). Two key components are also generally recognized as constituents of narrative, namely, an event or action component and an evaluative component.

The analytic model that will serve for this discussion is a sociolinguistic one developed in the now classic study of oral narrative by Labov and Waletsky in 1967, further amplified by Labov in 1972 and 1982, and applied by a wide variety of analysts for their various purposes (Wachs, 1988; Johnstone, 1990; van Dijk, 1984). Within this paradigm, the action or event component of narrative is referred to as referential (Labov and Waletsky, 1967; Labov, 1972). The referential component of the narrative (i.e., its action or event structure) is realized in a temporally ordered sequence of clauses, the order of which is inferred to reflect the order of the events as they actually occurred. Altering the order of the sequence of clauses effects a change in the inferred chronology of the events reported (Labov and Waletsky, 1967; Labov, 1972).

The evaluative component of the narrative is regarded as the counterpoint to the referential component. It is best conceptualized as an independent dimension of narrative (van Dijk, 1984) by which the speaker reveals a complex of individual reactions to and assessments of the events he reports in the narrative. The evaluative function is realized at several levels within the narrative and can assume a variety of structural or syntactic shapes.

The referential and evaluative components of the narrative confer a distinctive formal structure on the narrative, which is often referred to as "linear", "chronological" (Gee, 1986) or "plotted" (Hudson et al., 1992). Since the structural properties of narrative are of primary importance to the argument to follow, it will be useful to review them briefly here. A five-part overall structure organizes the narrative in terms of its temporal and evaluative components. The five parts are the abstract, orientation, complication action sequence, evaluation, and coda.

Narrative's temporal sequence and the overall structure are illustrated below with a story from Maguire, who reports the accident that he believes precipitated the eventual death of his wife. Following Labovian convention, the narrative is presented as a sequence of independent clauses, each lettered. Dependent clauses, and other syntactic material are accorded separate, indented, and unlettered lines.

Example 4: Maguire

(During the time before her death, what went on? Did she die suddenly? Was there an illness?)

    Yes.
a) Now, this is what happened.
b) It was in May.
c) It was '78—in May.
d) She was slee-layin' down, upstairs.
e) And she got up.
f) As she was comin' down the stairs,
    she tripped
g) and fell.
h) And she broke her ankle.
i) So, I took her to the hospital.
j) And she was in the hospital about a week.
k) And they had to put pins in her, stuff like that there.
l) It was a pretty bad break.
m) And-uh-that stuck her—[in a cast].
n) That was from May—June, July, August.
o) All these months she had a cast on her.
p) It was for a long—maybe six weeks, eight weeks.
q) And I took her [to the doctor's]
r) and then her cast came off.
s) But from the time she broke her ankle,
t) she couldn't walk up and down the stairs.
u) So I set a cot up downstairs for her.
v) So that's where she slept, on this cot.

Abstract: The abstract may or may not be present and is represented by one or two clauses that summarize the narrative's point.

a) Now, this is what happened.

Orientation: The orientation section is a sequence of clauses that situates the main action by explaining the background issues and circumstances that lead up to the event reported in the complication.

b)   It was in May.
c)   It was '78—in May.
d)   She was slee—layin' down, upstairs.

Complication: The complication (or complicating action) is the sequence of temporally ordered clauses that report the main sequence of action. Their order cannot be reversed without changing the meaning of the events encoded in the temporal sequence.

e)   And she got up.
f)   As she was comin' down the stairs,
     she tripped
g)   and fell.
h)   And she broke her ankle.
i)   So, I took her to the hospital.

Evaluation: The evaluative component of narrative is a complex phenomenon which can assume a variety of shapes. One structural configuration that conveys evaluative material is a series of clauses which may appear at any point throughout the narrative. When this cluster appears following the complication, as it does in here in Maguire's narrative, it suspends the action before the moment of resolution.

j)   And she was in the hospital about a week.
k)   And they had to put pins in her, stuff like that there.
l)   It was a pretty bad break.

Resolution: A resolution clause (or clauses), as the name suggests, closes the action by providing a resolution to the action that was reported in the complication.

m)   And-uh-that stuck her—[in a cast].
n)   That was from May—June, July, August.
o)   All these months she had a cast on her.
p)   It was for a long—maybe six weeks, eight weeks.
q)   And I took her [to the doctor's]
r)   and then her cast came off.

Coda: Finally, a coda (which, like the abstract, may or may not be present) returns the action to the moment of speaking and functions to close the narrative turn at talk.

s)   But from the time she broke her ankle,
t)   she couldn't walk up and down the stairs.
u)   So I set a cot up downstairs for her.
v)   So that's where she slept, on this cot.

THE WIDOWERS' NARRATIVE STRUCTURE

The complicating action conveys the narrative's central sequence of actions. In the death narratives, the central event is the wife's death and the events that surround it. The death narratives of these Irish widowers reveal two distinctive structural profiles of the complicating action section: a contracted complication and an expanded complication. The contracted complication predominates in these data and will be shown to represent a characteristic development of the temporal sequence of events in the narrative. It should be noted that there is nothing sacrosanct about the descriptive terms selected for the present analysis. The reader is free to find other more suitable words: contracted complication might be also be described as terse, economical, concatenated, or summary. Expanded complications might be further described as extended, unabridged, or patulous.

Contracted Complications. Contracted complications are constituted by short sequences of temporally ordered narrative clauses that report a single portion of the event. This type of complication is referred to here as *contracted* because it is short. It focuses on what are presumably the key events for the narrator as he recounts the circumstances surrounding his wife's death. Contracted complications do not include some actions and occurrences that are related to the death although the narrator is likely to have participated in them. Examples 5 and 6 below from Medd's and Hannan's narratives illustrate the contracted complication. Complicating action clauses are in bold print.

Example 5: Medd

e)   She would call me
     if she had difficulty or pain
     or anything.

f) **She went to the bathroom.**
g) It was 4:15 in the morning.
h) **And I heard her fall.**
i) And I knew
    that it was somethin' terrible
    because—she didn't call me.

(Uh-hunh)

j) So—uh—Denise was here then.
k) **And Denise—I called for emergency service right away,**
    and the police, and the first aid ambulance.
m) **They gave her artificial respiration,**
n) **but when she got to the hospital,**
    she was dead.

(I see.)

Example 6: Hannan

c) And it was close to Christmas.
d) So she said "Well,"
    she says "I'm not goin' into the hospital anyhow."
    She says "You can put me in it if you want to,"
    she says, "But I'm not goin' nowhere."
e) **So I come home here,**
f) **And—uh—Barbara come home from work soon afterwards.**
g) **And I wanted to help her with the supper.**
h) **She says "No."**
    She says "The two of you get outside,
    and I'll get the supper" she says.
i) **She died at—nine o'clock that night.**

In Example 5, Medd focuses on a single part of the action
surrounding the moment of death, namely his awareness that something
was wrong, his call to the paramedics, and their failed attempt to
resuscitate his wife. He omits the discovery of his wife in the bathroom
and how his daughter Denise became involved in the action. He does
not report these actions, neither does he tell about his wife's state nor
what Denise did. In his narrative, the action sequence moves from not
hearing his wife's call, to his telephone call to the emergency team, and

from their efforts to her death. In Hannan's narrative, the action is even more concatenated. He tells us that his wife insisted on making dinner herself the night she died. The action sequence moves from his family's ordinary dinner time routine to her death.

Expanded Complications. In contrast, expanded complications enumerate actions rather than collapse them. Relative to contracted complications, they display longer action sequences which are composed of multiple location and participant changes. Example 7 from O'Brien's narrative illustrates the expanded complication. Complicating action clauses are in bold print.

Example 7: O'Brien:

e) So she slept in the boys' room, in Andy's bed,
    because he was away at college.
f) **And-uh-the other kids woke up at seven o'clock.**
g) **And-uh-Jimmy said "Come on, Mother!**
    It's time to go to—go to school.
    We gotta get up."
h) **And he went in and took a shower.**
i) **And when he came out,**
    she was still in bed.
j) **And he said "Mother! Come on! Come on!"**
k) **And he shook her,**
l) **and she didn't move.**
m) **And then he said to my boy Jack,**
    who was—I guess Jack was in premed at LaSalle then,
n) **eh-he said-uh-"Hey, Jack!**
    Somethin's wrong with Mother!"
o) **So he jumped over,**
p) **and he-he saw.**
q) **And he started to give her-artificial respiration**
    and stuff like that.
r) **And I-and then I heard the kids scream,**
s) **and I run in the room,**
    'cause she had let me sleep by myself, you know.
t) **And I ran in the room,**
u) **and he said to me "Dad, she's gone."**
    And he said "She's cold.
    She's been gone at least four hours."

(God.)

v)   So that's the way she went.

The contrast between expanded and contracted complications is thrown into sharp relief by comparing Medd's or Hannan's summary complications to O'Brien's expanded complication. As O'Brien moves from point to point in his children's discovery of their dead mother, and then to his own discovery, this expanded sequence offers as much information as Medd's and Hannan's offer little. Interestingly, O'Brien can only have known the events reported in clauses (f-q) because his sons told him. However, these events are incorporated in the narrative as if O'Brien were an eyewitness to them.

Profile of the Complication. The apparent preference for a contracted presentation of this melancholy event represents a key characteristic of Irish American narrative. The wife's death is reported in the complications of all the narratives, irrespective of the complication's degree of expansion. However, the contracted complication is the dominant structure for presenting the moment of the death in seven of the nine death narratives. Only two of the nine narratives offer an expanded complication.

This is how events are presented, and the evaluative patterns present in the narrative must be considered against the backdrop of this manner of presenting event structures. The evaluative structures encountered in the death narratives represent a second key characteristic of these speakers' narration.

TALKING ABOUT EMOTION: EVALUATIVE STRUCTURES

The personal emotions and reactions surrounding the moments of a spouse's death are an integral aspect of the experience. The subjective nature of this experience suggests that we should look for linguistic evidence of it in the evaluative function of the narrative, i.e., in those narrative components that tell what the reported events mean to the narrator. Yet, as mentioned earlier, a key feature of the Irish widowers' death narratives is the minimalist or absent commentary on the narrator's emotional reaction to the events he is recounting. This absence of emotional statement is visible in the structure of the narrative.

In his discussion of evaluation in oral narrative, Labov (1972) distinguishes between internal and external types of evaluation. Internal evaluation results from clause-internal permutations and complexity in the syntax of clauses that departs from the straightforward, simple structure of narrative clause syntax. External evaluation is structural. It is realized at the overall organizational level of the narrative via the distribution of evaluative clauses throughout the narrative sequence. While a narrative's point is constructed through both internal and external evaluation, in my view, they represent distinctive mechanisms that merit individual consideration before their joint operation can be addressed. Consequently, the present discussion will focus on patterns of external evaluation within these elders' death narratives. Irish American narrative is characterized by several distinct handlings of evaluation.

The Distribution of Evaluative Segments. Within the Labovian paradigm, evaluation in narrative is carried out by clauses that are not temporally ordered with regard to each other. Evaluative clauses appear throughout the temporal sequence of actions, and narrative analysts have identified a variety of placement and distribution patterns (Bower, 1996; Tannen, 1989; Polanyi, 1985; Labov, 1972). Several of these are apparent in the death narratives.

A particularly common pattern in narrative evaluation is the distribution of free evaluative clauses throughout the complication, either as free-standing evaluative clauses or as dependent clauses subordinated to a narrative clause. Kilcullen's narrative (Example 8 below) and Medd's narrative (Example 9 below) illustrate this evaluative clause configuration. The evaluative clauses are in bold print, and spaces between lines indicate separate structural components of the narrative.

Example 8: Kilcullen

a)   Well, it was Easter Sunday night, two years ago in 1984.
b)   And-uh-after we come home from church,
c)   and-uh-she wasn't feelin' too good that day,
d)   and that night—she lapsed into unconsciousness.
e)   And my oldest daughter was there with her.

f)   And she called down to me,
     she said "You better come up.
     I don't think-don't-don't think——.
     Things don't look good at all."

g) **And that time, she was sort of laborin', breathin', laborin' and breathin'.**

h) So——we tried to get a hold of the doctor.

i) **Of course, it was Easter Sunday night.**

j) **It was pretty hard to get a hold of the doctor.**

k) But-uh-he came.

l) **And-uh-then—and then, she died.**

m) He said there was nothin' we could—
    that we could do.

The complication is bounded by clauses (f-l) in Kilcullen's narrative. The complicating action clauses are (f, h, k, l), which are interspersed by evaluative clauses (g, i, j) and punctuated by evaluative clause (m). The evaluative clauses provide orienting information about the physical condition of Kilcullen's wife, an explanation for the difficulty in getting a physician, and finally the physician's authoritative statement about what could or could not have been done.

Similarly, in Medd's narrative (Example 9 below), evaluative clauses (g, i, j) intersperse with the temporally ordered narrative clauses in the complicating action section (clauses f-n).

Example 9: Medd

a) She wasn't terrible ill
    'til she dropped dead on April 23, 1980.

b) She would holler for me.

c) She did have a couple of falls.

d) But she would always call—at night or anything.

e) She would call me
    if she had difficulty or pain or anything.

f) She went to the bathroom.

g) **It was 4:15 in the morning.**

h) And I heard her fall.

i) **And I knew
    that it was somethin' terrible
    because she didn't call me.**

j) **So-uh-Denise was here then.**

k) and Denise—I called for the emergency service right away, and the police, and the first aid ambulance.
l) By the time they got her to the hospital—they gave her artificial respiration.
m) but when she got to the hospital,
    she was dead.

(I see.)

In Medd's narrative, the complicating action section, clauses (f, h, k, l, m) report the sequence of temporally ordered events, but this sequence is interspersed with evaluative clauses (g, i, j). The content of these evaluative clauses provides orienting information about time and place. Clause (i) reveals the narrator's interpretation of the meaning of the call that did not come.

A second identifiable external pattern involves the clustering of evaluative clauses in a discrete section after the last clause of the temporally ordered sequence of events but before the resolutive clauses. Often described as a "suspension" of the narrative at the "high-point" of the action, this cluster pattern is widely regarded as heightening the dramatic impact of the reported action and as reflecting the speaker's perception of the importance of the event that precedes or follows the cluster. (Labov, 1972; Peterson and McCabe, 1983; Linde, 1993).

Thus, for example in Maguire's narrative (Example 10 below), a cluster of seven evaluative clauses (j-p) suspends the complicating action sequence (clauses e-i) and separates the complication from the resolution (clauses q-r).

Example 10: Maguire

c) It was '78—in May.
d) She was slee—layin' down, upstairs

e) And she got up.
f) As she was comin' down the stairs, she tripped
g) and fell,
h) and she broke her ankle.
i) So, I took her to the hospital.

j) **And she was in the hospital about a week.**
k) **And they had to put pins her, stuff life that there.**

l)   **It was a pretty bad break.**
m)   **And-uh-that stuck her—[in a cast].**
n)   **That was from May, June, July, August,**
o)   **all these months she had a cast on her.**
p)   **It was for a long—maybe six weeks, eight weeks.**

q)   And I took her [to the doctor's],
r)   and then her cast came off.

The number and content of the evaluative clauses (j-p) emphasize the importance of the break (reported in narrative clause h) by mentioning the length of hospital stay, the treatment required as an indication of the complexity of the break, the length of time his wife wore the cast, and a direct statement about the fracture itself, "It was a pretty bad break."

Single clauses also suspend the complication as in Hotchkiss' narrative below.

Example 11: Hotchkiss

a)   We had this neighbor
     who we was always jokin' with about the Phillies always losin',
     my son and me and this neighbor.

b)   And—uh—my son and I had been over [to visit her in the hospital]
     on a Sunday night.
c)   And we left her about quarter of ten.
d)   And she wasn't good then.

e)   But—uh—we got home.
f)   And—[pause]—an hour later, why, this neighbor came over,
g)   and my son came over.
h)   And he said—uh—"We lost. [Pause] We lost."
i)   I said "Aawwwhh, the damn Phillies!
     They're always losin'!"
j)   And they repeated again: "We lost her."
k)   I heard the "her"

l)   **I hadn't heard that.**

m) She was gone.

n) **So—[pause]—that—she had—she had 78 years of age, 57 years married, and—dying—in the same month**

o) **It's really hard.**

In this narrative, evaluative clause (l) briefly suspends the complicating action at (k) before resuming at the resolution clause (m). Clauses (n,o) are evaluative clauses that illustrate yet another important location at which evaluative clauses cluster, namely after the resolution clause. In this position, they can function as a coda, as they do here.

Factual Content of the Evaluative Segments. Irish American narratives are unremarkable with respect to the dispersed, clustered, and suspension patterns described above. Dispersed and clustered distributions are apparent in half the death narratives. What is distinctive about these narratives, however, is the semantic content of the evaluative clauses. While the structural placement of these clauses with respect to the narrative clauses indicates their importance to the narrator, the actual content focuses not on emotional state but on factual information pertinent to the evaluated complication.

For example, in Kilcullen's narrative (Example 8), evaluative clauses (i-j) interrupt the complicating sequence to focus on the difficulty of getting a physician on a holiday weekend. The clauses do not address the narrator's emotional state nor that of any one of his family members. The evaluative focus of clause (m) is not on the emotion of the moment but on the medical authority's assessment of the adequacy and appropriateness of the actions taken to assist the spouse in extremis. Similarly, the evaluative clauses of Medd's narrative (Example 9) focus on details of time and participant, although the call that did not come from his wife is subordinated to his prescient knowledge that her silence was an indication that something was wrong. Maguire's lengthy evaluative segment (clauses j-p in Example 10) focuses on the severity of the bone fracture that eventually caused his wife's death but does not allude to his or his wife's personal reaction to the break. Finally, Hotchkiss' misunderstanding of what his son and neighbor are telling him as they announce his wife's death to him is evaluated only by a factual statement about his acoustic perceptions (Example 11).

Thus far, two structural and semantic patterns of evaluation can be isolated in these death narratives. In half the narratives from these Irish

American speakers, the narratives demonstrate typical patterns of distributed or clustered evaluative clauses. The content of the evaluative clauses and segments does not focus on inner states of the narrator or any of the participants but rather on facts about participants, locations, diagnoses, and medical procedures. If, following the conventional analysis of narrative evaluation, we contend that the placement and content of evaluative clauses reflects what is important to speakers, then we must conclude that for these narrators at least, the emotional turmoil caused by a death is less important than the factual, logistical aspects surrounding the death.

The Absence of an Evaluative Segment. While half of the death narratives do exhibit distributed or cluster evaluative clauses, the other half do not. For half of the Irish widowers' narratives, no external evaluative structure of any type is present. For these narratives, the overall structure is represented by abstract, orientation, complication, and coda, and the distributed or clustered evaluative clauses that were apparent in the previous narrative examples are markedly absent. Hannan's narrative (Example 12 below) and O'Brien's narrative (Example 13 below) offer examples of narratives with no external evaluation section. Again, spaces between clauses indicate separate narrative segments.

Example 12: Hannan

a)   That afternoon, I had her to the doctor.
b)   And he said
        he'd put her in the hospital.
c)   And it was close to Christmas.
d)   So she said "Well,"
        she says "I'm not goin' into the hospital anyhow."
        She says "You can put me in it if you want to,"
        she says "but I'm not goin' in it."

e)   So, I come home here,
f)   and Barbara came home from work soon afterwards.
g)   And I wanted to help her with the supper.
h)   She says "No."
        She says "The two of you get outside,
        and I'll get the supper" she says.

i) She died at—nine o'clock that night.

(She made supper that night, too?)

Yes.

The complication closes with the quotative clauses of (h) and the resolution clause (i) ends the narrative. Given the preceding discussion about the likely structural locations for evaluative clauses, a predictable location for the clause or cluster of clauses that might report Hannan's emotion, inner state, or even factual commentary (considering these narrators' predisposition toward factual comment) would be between clauses (h) and (i). Another predictable location for such clusters is after the resolution clause (j), where Hannan could reveal the overall meaning of this event, as Hotchkiss did (Example 11) when he eulogized his wife in the last evaluative clauses of his narrative (n,o). However, Hannan does not offer such evaluation in his narrative.

Similarly, in O'Brien's narrative, with two exceptions, no discrete evaluation sections are present. Example 13 picks up with clause (e):

Example 13: O'Brien

e) So she slept in the boys' room, in Andy's bed,
    because he was away at college.

g) And-uh-the other kids woke up at seven o'clock.
h) And-uh-Jimmy said "Come on, Mother!
    It's time to go to—go to school.
    We gotta get up."
i) And he went in and took a shower.
j) And when he came out,
    she was still in bed.
k) And he said "Mother! Come on! Come on!"
l) And he shook her,
m) and she didn't move.
n) And then he said to my boy Jack,
    who was—I guess Jack was in premed at LaSalle then,
o) eh—he said—uh—"Hey, Jack!
    Somethin's wrong with Mother!"
p) So he jumped over,
q) and he-he saw.

r)   And he started to give her-artificial respiration
     and stuff like that.
s)   And I-and then I heard the kids scream,
t)   and I run in the room,
     'cause she had let me sleep by myself, you know.
u)   And I ran in the room,
v)   and he said to me "Dad, she's gone."
     And he said "She's cold.
     She's been gone at least four hours."

(God.)

w)   So that's the way she went.

In O'Brien's expanded complication, the evaluative component is only minimally present. No cluster of evaluative clauses suspends the complication at a likely position, such as (u) or (v), nor does a cluster of evaluative clauses appear after the resolution clause (w) which ends the narrative. O'Brien goes on after (w) to tell another narrative about his wife's funeral with no further interaction with the interviewer.

The evaluative material that *is* present appears in two non-narrative clauses that are subordinated to a main, narrative clause of the complication in clause (n) and (t). It is the only material in the complication that does not directly relate to the action sequence as it is unfolding and the non-temporal status of this information is neatly conveyed by the subordination. The content of these clauses establishes them as embedded orientations, that is, orienting clauses that appear in the complication (Labov, 1972). Clause (n) appears as ancillary information that is important to the speaker in establishing his son's authority to correctly identify death and (t) reiterates O'Brien's explanation for his wife's absence from their bedroom. The content of these clauses indicates neither the narrator's nor his sons' emotional reactions to the unfolding events.

The Absent Emotional Component. The absence of such external evaluative structures means that the effect of the death on the narrator as presented in the narrative remains largely uninterpreted for the analyst or the listener. The narrator provides no direct statements about the meaning of the event for him or his reaction to those events. Our interpretation about how the speaker felt is based on inferences that we, as analysts and listeners, make based in a variety of other sources, for example internal evaluative material, our own experiences, expectations, and ethnographic knowledge of the narrator's speech community.

The factual orientation of an evaluative segment or its absence altogether assumes a heightened significance when placed against the contracted complication's economical presentation of action (see Medd's, Hannan's or Kilcullen's accounts for examples). In such cases, both the events and the meaning of the death are reported in its tersest form. The focus on fact and the containment of affect or interpretive meaning results in a dry, seemingly disconnected narrative.

Although we are dealing with a relatively small corpus of narratives (nine narratives from eight speakers), the absence of an evaluation section in four of the narratives and the fact- rather than emotion-oriented content of the evaluative clauses in three of the others are provocative. Admittedly, generalizing from a small number of narratives must be carried out with caution, but the proportion of unevaluated narratives is suggestive of an expressive style in personal narrative that precludes the articulation of much personal feeling. This view is supported by the next data which illustrate the disruption in the narrative structure caused by the articulation of personal emotion.

THE PRESENCE OF AN EVALUATIVE SEGMENT

Thus far, the topic has been the absence or minimal presence of emotional statements in Irish-American narratives. This section examines how emotional statements are presented in narrative and the narrative structures that convey them.

In two of the death narratives, the narrators talk about their personal emotions and reactions in the moments surrounding their spouse's death. In doing so, however, the identity and contours of the emotional expression are obscured in various ways. This is the third key feature of these death narratives, namely, that when emotion is recounted, its force obscures or diffuses the event structure of the complicating action. Two examples from the data will illustrate this process of diffusion.

Maguire's narrative (from which Example 14 is excerpted) is a long narrative (clause a-u3) which offers an expanded complication section (i-h3) telling how his wife's physical condition moved in a few hours from headache to back pain to respiratory difficulty and finally to cardiac compromise. The complication is suspended in its progress by a cluster of evaluative clauses (r2-u2). The example below picks up halfway through the complication. Evaluative clauses are in bold print and a space separates narrative segments.

Example 14: Maguire

o2) And so Denise told her, she said "Mom,
      we're goin' to take you down to the hospital
      where the doctors can really check you—
      give you a check-up."

p2) So she said "All right."

q2) So we were tryin' to get her things ready.

r2) **And—and—it's—that's the one thing
      I still regret today,**

s2) **'Cause, see, things you—you don't know stuff,
      see, at the time.**

t2) **But she probably knew.**

u2) **And I didn't know that, see, at the time.**

v2) She said to me "Sit with me.
      Hold me."

w2) And I said "I can't!"
      I said "'Cause I'm helpin' Denise," you know,
      "get your stuff ready."

x2) **I didn't know.**

y2) Then the first thing you know,
      she just laid back.

z2) And when [Denise] saw that, you know,
      she said "This could be something really serious."

a3) She tried to work on her heart, you know, breath in her mouth, and
      stuff like that, you know.

b3) And she grabbed the phone

c3) and called the rescue.

d3) And we called a priest.

e3) She said "You better call the priest too, Dad."

f3) I said "What are you thinkin'?"
      I said "She ain't dyin'!"

g3) She said "You never can tell.
      It looks bad."

(Yeah.)

h3) But, [snaps fingers] that's how fast it happened.

While the structural outlines of the evaluative segment (r2-u2) are clear cut, the semantic content is elusive. Its evaluative force is powerful, but the extraction of meaning relies on inference and is obscured by the clause level semantics.

Structurally, clauses (r2-u2) and (x2) are easily identified as serving a straightforward evaluative function in that they suspend the action of the temporal sequence of events to focus on the actions in clauses (v2-w2). As discussed earlier, they represent what is often called the "classic" suspension of the narrative at a central (or "high") point of action. The linguistic profile of the clauses themselves further identify their evaluative function since the syntactic embedding in clauses (r2, s2) is typical of evaluative clauses (Labov, 1972). The repetition of content in clauses (s2, u2, and x2: " . . . didn't know . . . ") serves a broader discourse function of coherence and emphasis (Tannen, 1989).

In contrast to its simple structural identity, the clause level semantics of this evaluative segment obscures its meaning. For example, while the structure of the evaluative section signals the importance of the content of the following clauses, the semantics of the four evaluative clauses offers no hint as to what the importance may be. The forward reference of the demonstrative pronoun "that" (r2, u2) and the unspecified referent of "things" and "stuff" (r2, s2) point to the fact that what is to come causes Maguire regret to contemplate, but does not tell what it is. Similarly, the object of the verb "know," which would tell what "that" is, is not articulated (s2, t2, u2). Each of these cataphoric referents points to clauses (v2) and (w2) as the key to understanding what is to be regretted, but in these two clauses Maguire simply describes Mrs. Maguire's request and his refusal. The evaluative clause (x2) reiterates that Maguire did not know but does not reveal the object of his ignorance.

A sequence of inferences is required to grasp a likely meaning. One interpretation may be summarized as follows: At the time of narration, Maguire has come to interpret his wife's request to "Sit with me. Hold me." as her last request to him. At the time about which he is narrating, Maguire was ignorant of the import of this request, although he believes that his wife may have known that her death was impending and understood that this was her last moment to to be near to him. To this day, while he understands that some things cannot be known in advance, his lack of prescience in this regard troubles him.

This interpretation is purely speculation, of course. Maguire does not explicitly state that this was his wife's last request to him and the narrative action itself is straightforward. A literal interpretation of the complication tells us only that Mrs. Maguire asked her husband to sit and hold her (v2) while Maguire and his daughter were getting her ready to go to the hospital (q2). He refused because he was busy getting her ready to go (w2). After that, Mrs. Maguire's condition worsened (y2-a3). The rescue squad was called (b3-c3), the priest was called (d3-g3), and Mrs. Maguire died (h3). However, for the evaluative section to be meaningful, that is, for there to be something for Maguire not to have known and then later to have come to know and then to regret, the interpretation of Mrs. Maguire's request as a dying request must be in place. Indeed, the only way to make sense of the internal mini-debate in clauses (s2), (t2) and (u2) about who knew what, who did not, and what is possible to know hinges upon an interpretation of the unspoken object as Mrs. Maguire's impending death and her request subsequently as her dying request.

The semantic complexity of these four clauses supports this sequence of inferences via a counterbalance of multiple contexts (Bauman, 1986) or "storyworlds" (Young, 1987; Polanyi, 1985) in which the narrative is situated. There are two temporal frames in the narrative: the time of the action and the time of narration. There are three individual perspectives on the action articulated: Maguire's understanding of his wife's request at the time of the action, his wife's (attributed) understanding of the true nature of her request, and Maguire's latter-day understanding of the request. Finally, a continuum of inner feeling that extends from the past into the present is articulated: there were several aspects of his wife's death that Maguire regretted. These have been resolved with the passage of years with the exception of his perduring regret that he did not understand her "last request."

Thus, while the structure of this evaluative segment signals the importance of the information that is to come, the clause level semantics diffuses its emotional impact by obscuring the identity of the cause for regret. Maguire does reveal something of his inner state surrounding a crucial moment in his wife's death, but the identity and impact of the feeling he reports about are obscured and diffused in the clause level language. When distilled, the complex of temporal perspectives, point-of-view, and emotional continuum revealed in these clauses powerfully suggests Maguire's emotional turmoil over his perceived failure to anticipate the true nature of his wife's request.

However, the affective force of the evaluation may derive from its structural position rather than its content, since a reading of the request as a "last request" reveals itself only with examination and explanation and depends heavily on the sequence of inference outlined here.

A second example of a present evaluation comes from Carroll's death narrative (Example 15), which offers the baldest statements about inner feelings of any encountered in the discussion thus far. This narrative also offers the most contracted complicating action segment in the data, so contracted that it is difficult to follow and requires considerable expansion. The complication segment of this narrative is only four clauses in length (f, g, r, t) but the tiers of evaluation that separate the complicating action clauses are full of feeling. Evaluative clauses are in bold print, and line spaces separate narrative segments.

Example 15: Carroll

a) And that night, my sister was the one.

b) She didn't want——.
c) "Catherine's dyin'."
d) I don't know how she knew.
e) I was sleepin',

f) and she woke me.
g) "Harry, Catherine's dyin'."

h) **Aaaaaaah—I was so glad.**
i) **I wouldn't know**
    she was goin' to die.
j) **But-uh-you *talk* about death!**
k) **I heard it—and nurses are deathly afraid of death,**
    nurses in hospitals!
l) **But I'm a great believer in this is—**
    this world is only a try-out.
m) **This is not our home.**
n) **I'm a firm believer in the——.**
o) **This is a precursor.**
p) **And when Catherine died,**
    I was so glad for her sake
    that she died at that time.

q) **It came very—*oh*, thank God.**

r) And-uh-she-Maureen's goin' "Catherine just died."
s) **She knew just to look at her.**

t) So, I called the cops.

The brevity of this complication segment requires that we infer (because Carroll does not explicate it) that during the night, his sister Maureen, who has experience attending the dying, has recognized Catherine Carroll's impending death (a-d). She comes to Carroll's bedside to wake him and leads him into his wife's bedroom (e-g). While they attend her, Catherine takes her last breath and dies (r). Carroll calls the police (t).

The narrative action is suspended in the classic pattern at Maureen's announcement of Mrs. Carroll's impending death (g) by an extended cluster of evaluative clauses (h-q). The linguistic profile of the clauses themselves further identify their evaluative function since the syntactic embedding in clauses (i, l, p) is typical of evaluative clauses.

This evaluation is the most emotion laden of any of the Irish American widowers' narratives in these data. It articulates Carroll's emotions and places them in the context of his philosophical belief. The emotion Carroll reports is strikingly contiguous with the moment of death. He reveals his gladness, perhaps gratitude, at being present at his wife's death bed (h-i) and then again his gladness, perhaps gratitude, for her peaceful death (p-q). He also talks about the fear of death (j-k) and, by inference, his own lack of fear, placing his wife's death in his broader understanding of another life after this one (l-m). This evaluation is accomplished through a sequence of four topic changes, which, when examined on their own, are cogent and coherent: Carroll's gladness (although the reason for his gladness is obscured by the semantic content of the clauses), professionals' reaction to death, the afterlife, and feelings about his wife's death.

Yet, despite the topical coherence and balance of these evaluative clauses when considered outside the structural context, the length of the sequence overwhelms an event structure which is already minimal and which relies heavily for meaning on expansion and inference. The evaluative segment separates the narrative's two key events (b) ". . . Catherine is dying" and (r) "Catherine just died", and evaluates the second event so heavily, that the continuity of the event structure is reduced, even decimated. Consequently, while the emotional component is clearly present, its structural realization overwhelms and submerges the very actions to which it has to give meaning.

Discussion. While the majority of the Irish American widowers appear to prefer to leave emotional statements out of their narratives, when they do express an emotional aspect of their experience, that expression obscures the very events of the death that they evaluate. In Maguire's narrative, veiled reference obscures the cause for regret: we are left to infer what it is about his wife's request he regrets. In Carroll's narrative, the evaluative content is clear but so developed that the temporal sequence is overwhelmed: we are left to reconstruct what sequence of events it is he evaluates. In this respect, the presence of an evaluative component operates in exactly the same manner as an absent or fact-centered evaluation. In either case, referential and evaluative components of the narrative do not work in synchrony to reveal the meaning of the death for the narrator. In either case, the death and its meaning are addressed in an expressive manner that is guarded, veiled, or obscured.

CONCLUSIONS AND IMPLICATIONS

While the corpus of data is slender, in my view, it adequately supports a characterization of these widowers' death narratives. Four identifiable patterns are revealed, which, taken together, point toward a distinctive expressive style. First, these narratives are characterized by short, terse, complicating action sequences in which only parts of (what must be presumed to be) the whole event are revealed. Second, the narratives' evaluative components report factual information about medical assessments, emergency transportation logistics, or health conditions at the time of the death rather than information about the emotional or inner state of those involved in this important event. Third, in many instances, there is no (external) evaluative component present at all. The actions of the event stand without interpretation. Finally, when emotional content is introduced into the evaluative segments of the narrative, it obscures the event structure or completely overwhelms it.

The need to account for the distinctive profile of this narrative style offers an important opportunity to examine the assumptions upon which the explanation rests. The literature on narrative articulates several interpretative perspectives from which potential explanations may be drawn. These include the cognitive deficiency perspective, the performance deficit perspective, and the inner state perspective. A fourth perspective, namely ethnicity, will be advanced at the conclusion of this section. Each perspective's interpretation of these elderly widowers' narrative capabilities hinges on what the structural configurations of their narratives are felt to represent.

The Cognitive Deficiency Explanation Linguists working within the biomedical/developmental paradigm tend to regard and evaluate narrative structure in terms of its perceived structural completeness. From this perspective, evaluative material and referential material are both required for a narrative to be regarded as complete or well formed. As a result, (perceived) gaps in the narrative action sequence, the probability that some events which occurred are not reported in the narrative, and the absence of evaluative material are all likely to be taken as important evidence of reduced cognitive ability among elderly narrators (Ulatowska and Chapman, 1991; Ripich, 1991).

Among developmentalists who study the personal narratives of elderly (and child) narrators, it is not uncommon to encounter descriptions of narrative complications that reveal a sharp bias toward length and perceived completeness. For example, narratives which offer the "contracted" complications we have been considering in the preceding discussion are typically referred to as "fragments of experience" (Bokus, 1992), as "underdeveloped" (Pratt and Robins, 1991), "inadequate" (Ripich, 1991) or "impoverished" (Peterson and McCabe, 1983). More specifically, the brevity of the contracted complications such as Medd's (Example 5) or Hannan's (Example 6) risks being construed as evidence for the elderly narrator's inability to adequately produce an action sequence due to cognitive deficiency (Ripich, 1991; Ulatowska and Chapman, 1991). In contrast, narratives with expanded sequences such as O'Brien's (Example 7) are positively described by developmentalists as "well-ordered sequences" or "complete" (Peterson and McCabe, 1983), although the absence of an evaluative component may be suspect. Elders who produce these lengthier, seemingly more complete, complications are less likely to be classified as impaired. The tone of these characterizations suggests a judgmental predisposition in favor of a perceived level of narrative completeness. Such a predisposition can be dangerous, since it requires that criteria for completeness be established and raises the vexing question of whose criteria should be employed in defining a complete narrative.

A biomedical/developmental interpretation of these elderly narrators' capabilities is not encouraging and might be paraphrased in the following way: these elderly speakers can only produce narratives of the simplest chronological sequences in the simplest of syntax. The majority of the narratives are minimalist productions, composed of short utterances, typically sequences of main clauses. Such syntax reflects the elders' declining ability to initiate and produce syntactically complex or elaborate sentences (Emery, 1986; Kemper, 1988). The absence of important narrative structures, specifically evaluation, indicates that they cannot properly evaluate or convey the meaning of the events they recount (North et al., 1986; Walker, 1988). In a few of the death narratives, the referential and evaluative material is apparent enough to qualify the story for the status of structural completeness, e.g., Maguire (Example 14) and Carroll (Example 15). However, their chronological integrity and meaning is badly obscured by thematically irrelevant or tangential material (Obler and Albert, 1980; Gold and Andres, 1988). Further, compensatory strategies undertaken to conceal self-perceived deficits in narrative ability (Hutchinson and Jensen, 1980) lead these speakers to self-initiated interjections, "fillers" and athematic talk (Johnstone, 1990) that creates the impression of verbose rambling.

Thus, the distinctive structural contours of the death narratives that typically concatenate referential material and reduce or eliminate evaluative material are interpreted as structural deficiency. This deficiency is, in turn, attributed to the "normal" loss of linguistic and communicative function with aging, at best, or, at worst, as indicative of cognitive deficit or impairment due to disease.

The Performance Deficit Explanation. Narrative analysts from many perspectives adopt the view that personal narrative is a performance. As such, its structure works to convey not only the personal meaning of the events reported in the narrative but also to legitimate the very narrative turn at talk itself. In this context, the presence or absence of evaluative material becomes a performance issue: does the narrative convey the meaning of the reported events to the listener, and how effectively does the narrator accomplish this? Is the narrative "worth" telling (Linde, 1993) or is the listener left asking "So what?" (Labov, 1972). When the evaluative material in narrative is regarded as so closely tied to the reason for and legitimacy of its telling, it is not surprising that the absence of evaluative material will be construed as a stripping away of both meaning and *raison d'etre*. As in the biomedical/developmental paradigm, a judgmental note is sounded. For example, in their original analysis of oral narrative, Labov and Waletsky (1967) suggested that oral narrative without evaluation is "aberrant." Subsequent narrative analyses have echoed this viewpoint (Linde, 1993; Polanyi, 1985; Tannen, 1989; Robinson, 1981). It should be noted that proponents of the deficit explanation can find support for their view of decline in this performance oriented approach to oral narrative by arguing that sociolinguists (and other discourse analysts) have also linked effective narration to structural completeness.

Consequently, a performance orientation can lead to a negative assessment of these narratives on the grounds that they are largely devoid of external evaluative structures and that their focus on the factual aspects of the event reveals little or nothing about the personal, emotional impact of the death. If it is the narrator's responsibility to make the meaning of events clear to the listener via the evaluative material, then these are not successful narratives.

Interestingly, while the personal meaning of the events reported may be regarded as unsuccessfully communicated in these narratives, the legitimacy of the narrative turn at talk is not likely to be in question. The "so what?" question may be forestalled by the overarching importance of death as a topic. Death commands attention in modern American culture, and talk about the events and actions surrounding it is so compelling under most circumstances, that even the most poorly told narrative cannot dim its intrinsic interest.

The Inner State Explanation. Another explanation for the absent (external) evaluative component proceeds from the view that narrative expression of emotion is linked to emotional experience. The assumption here is that a narrator's inner state is reflected in some aspects of the narrative structure. For example, in their study of children's narratives about a significant death (parent, friend, or pet), Menig-Peterson amd McCabe (1977) noted a pattern of absent evaluation very similar to that isolated in the widowers' narratives. Menig-Peterson and McCabe described these narratives as "devoid" of almost all evaluation and characterized them as heavily "chronological." They interpreted the absence of evaluation as an indication of the child narrators' difficulty in coping with the emotions generated by the death of the loved one. For them, the absence of evaluation does not indicate a cognitive or performance deficit on the part of the narrator but rather represents the presence of suppressed emotion. Similarly, Rubinstein's (1995) analysis of middle-aged daughters' narratives about the death of their elderly mother clearly associates length and depth of narrative with the level of care-giving involvement. Daughters who were very active caregivers for their mothers in the last year before death tended to offer lengthy, multidimensional and emotional "explications" of their mothers' death. In contrast, daughters who provided little or no care in the last year of mother's life produced shorter, chronologically simple "accounts" of the death.

If emotional experience can indeed be tracked through the narrative structure, then several conflicting explanations for the distinctive structure of the elderly widowers' narratives can be suggested. For example, on the one hand, it might be argued that the concatenated and overtly unevaluated presentation of a wife's death variously reflects the narrator's difficulty in coping with the emotions generated by the loss, a lack of resolution about the death, or an unfinished integration of the death into his own biography. On the other hand, it might be argued that a terse, unemotional narrative reflects a man emotionally uninvolved with his wife or one who does not perceive her death as a great loss. It might be argued still further, that recalling the death is so overwhelming an emotional experience that the narrator's control over the sociolinguistic skills that produce effective, dramatic narrative recedes or is lost in the face of his memories of the event. While such explanations are purely speculative (within the scope of this study), the value of this approach is that it links variation in narrative structure to inner state rather than to deficiency in cognitive or performative skills.

The Ethnicity Explanation. A fourth explanation regards the distinctive profile of these narratives as reflective of an ethnic speech style. Accruing evidence from sociological and anthropological studies of dying, death, and bereavement suggests that ethnicity rather than age, gender, or social class, has the most profound influence in shaping individuals' understanding of and approach to death (Counts and Counts, 1991; Walsh and McGoldrick, 1991; Williams, 1990; Palgi and Abramovitch, 1984; Huntington and Metcalfe, 1979; Kalish and Reynolds, 1976; Rosenblatt, Walsh, and Jackson, 1976). Ethnicity has been demonstrated to dramatically shape individuals' reaction to the bereavement experience, specifically in providing important guidelines for perceptions about what constitutes proper and appropriate inner emotional states as well as for the outward expression of emotions relative to the loss (Luborsky and Rubinstein, 1990). Consequently, the concatenated and unevaluated presentation of both the objective and affective aspects of a wife's death may be taken to reflect an Irish American expressive style when speaking about significant, personal issues.

This conclusion is based on our examination of the structural contours of one type of speech event, namely, the personal narrative, but similar observations have been made by psychologists, sociologists and anthropologists about the verbal behavior in other speech situations of both Irish Americans and native-born Irish. For example, McGoldrick's (1982) description of Irish American families in family therapy clearly delineates a pattern of response that reflects what we have encountered in these narratives. McGoldrick describes her Irish American clients as typically "silent" and "inexpressive" in therapy; not, she writes, because they are resistant to therapy but from an inability to articulate their feelings. She observes a "reticence to share information with personal content" and reports that while these clients offer brief, factual descriptions of family interactions, they do not readily elaborate on their feelings about what they have experienced. In a cross-cultural study of mourning, McGoldrick also notes that Irish American and native-born Irish are alike in responding to "any statement of feelings as if it were an overstatement." Similarly, Zborowski (1969) associates an unemotional speech style with the Irish American respondents in his cross-cultural comparison of reactions to pain. He describes these respondents' difficulty in expressing their experience of pain as a "reluctance" verging on an "inability" to articulate their feelings.

Observations of native-born Irish verbal behavior support the view developed here of a conservative approach to the expression of emotion. Scheper-Hughes' (1979) study of West Kerry village life reports a marked predisposition toward "reserved" social behavior, especially among men, in which general sociability is emphasized to the exclusion of intimate friendships with one or two individuals. Glassie makes a similar observation in his discussion about the oral folk traditions of an Ulster village (1982). He notes that stories and personal narratives that emphasize general, impersonal topics are highly valued and strongly preferred to narratives that report personal reactions and experience.

In the death narratives, the preference for contracted event structure, the marked absence of overt expressive statements about personal feeling or inner state, the focus on factual reports, and the diffusing strategies as a means of drawing attention away from personal emotion when it is expressed, all represent narrative strategies for presenting personal emotional experience that are consistent with the analyses of Irish American verbal behavior outlined above. In my view, the structure of these narratives strongly suggests a contained approach to the linguistic expression of personal experience that is consistent with the speech attitudes and values of this American ethnic group. The death narratives are produced in accordance with Irish American beliefs about the proper linguistic expression of emotional topics and, as such, conform to the standards for verbal behavior that are valued by the socio-cultural group of which the speakers are members. On these grounds, interpretations of the distinctive structural profile of the death narratives as either indicative of old-age-related cognitive decline or as ineffective story-telling is rejected. The inner state explanation for the emotionally terse character of these narratives is appealing and perhaps not unrelated to the ethnicity explanation. However, the individual's inner state that produces such an absence can only be speculated about since the narrators are certainly not telling us. Because it is speculative, the inner state explanation is on considerably shakier ground than an explanation that regards the absence of an overtly articulated emotional component as a reflection of cultural values that govern expressivity in narratives about emotional topics, namely, the ethnicity explanation.

In conclusion, the view of these narratives as illustrative of a particular ethnic expressive style, in this case Irish American, has relevance for current research on the interaction of aging and language. The interpretations we arrive at based on the structural configurations of elders' narratives have extraordinary implications for our overall view of elderly speakers' linguistic and communicative capabilities. It suggests that evaluations of both healthy and impaired elders' speech be rooted in an understanding of the informal, contextualized, and situated discourse practices of the group to which they belong, taking into full account what sociolinguistic parameters and constraints their ethnicity places upon what may be spoken about and how it may be expressed. It recommends ethnographically sound analyses of the verbal repertoire of the speech community of which the speakers being studied are members before making determinations about cognitive or performative capabilities.

NOTE

1. The research described in this chapter was conducted as part of a project entitled "Ethnicity and Life Reorganization by Elderly Widowers" (Robert Rubinstein and Mark Luborsky, primary investigators). Support of this project by Grant AGO5204 from the National Institute of Aging is gratefully acknowledged. The primary investigators' permission to use these ethnographic data for sociolinguistic purposes is also acknowledged with gratitude. All of the names used in this discussion are pseudonyms, and some details have been altered to to preserve respondents' anonymity.

REFERENCES

Antonucci, T. Unpublished manuscript. Personal characteristics, social support and social behavior.

Basso, K. 1984. Stalking with stories: names, places and moral narrative among the Western Apache." In *Text, Play and Story: The Reconstruction of Self and Society*. E. Bruner, ed. *1983 Proceedings of the American Ethnological Society*. Washington, D.C.: American Ethnological Society.

Bauman, R. 1986. *Story, Performance, and Event: Contextual Studies of Oral Narrative*. Cambridge: Cambridge University Press.

Berardo, F. 1970. Survivorship and social isolation: The case of the aged widower. *Family Co-ordinator* 19: 11–25.

Bokus, B. 1992. Peer co-narration: changes in structure of pre-schoolers participation. *Journal of Narrative and Life History* 2 (3).

Bower, A. 1996. Deliberate action constructs: reference and evaluation in narrative. In *Toward a Social Science of Language: A Festschrift for William Labov*. G. Guy, J. Baugh, and D. Schiffrin, eds. Cambridge: Cambridge University Press.

Brabant, S., Forsyth, C., and Melancon, C. 1992. Grieving men: thoughts, feelings and behaviors following deaths of wives. In *Hospice Journal* 8(4): 33–47.

Campbell, S., and Silverman, P. 1987. *Widower*. New York: Prentice Hall.

Counts, D. and Counts, D. 1991. *Coping with the Final Tragedy: Cultural Variation in Dying and Grieving*. Amityville, New York: Baywood Publishing Co.

Coupland, N., Coupland J., and Giles H. 1991. *Language, Society and the Elderly*. Oxford: Blackwell Publishers.

Dashefsky, A., and Shapiro, H. 1974. *Ethnic Identification Among American Jews*. Lexington, Massachusetts: Lexington Books.

Emery, O. 1986. Linguistic decrement in normal aging. *Language and Communication* 6 (1–2): 47–64.

Gee, J. 1986. Units in the production of narrative discourse. *Discourse Processes* 9: 391–422.

George, L. 1980. *Role Transitions in Later Life.* Belmont, California: Wadsworth.

Glassie, H. 1982. *Passing the Time in Ballymenone.* Philadelphia: University of Pennsylvania Press.

Gold, D., and Andres, D. 1988. Measurement and correlates of verbosity in elderly people. *Journal of Gerontology* 43 (2): 27–33.

Goodwin, M. 1990. *He-Said-She-Said: Talk as Social Organization among Black Children.* Bloomington: University of Indiana Press.

Hill, J., and Irvine, J. 1993. *Responsibility and Evidence in Oral Discourse.* Cambridge: Cambridge University Press.

Holland, D., and Quinn, N. 1987. *Cultural Models in Language and Thought.* New York: Cambridge University Press.

Hudson, J., Gebelt, J., Haviland, J., and Bentivegra, C. 1992. Emotion and narrative structure in young children's personal accounts. *Journal of Narrative and Life History* 2(2) 129–150.

Huntington, R., and Metcalfe, P. 1979. *Celebrations of Death: The Anthropology of Mortuary Ritual.* Cambridge: Cambridge University Press.

Hutchinson, J., and Jensen, M. 1980. A pragmatic evaluation of discourse in normal and senile elderly in a nursing home. In *Language and Communication in the Elderly.* L. Obler, and M. Albert, eds. Lexington, Massachusetts: Lexington Books.

Hymes, D. 1972. Models of interaction of language and social life. In *Directions in Sociolinguistics.* J. Gumperz, and D. Hymes, eds. New York: Holt, Rinehart, Winston.

Irvine, J. 1979. Formality and informality in communicative events. *American Anthropologist* 81: 773–90.

Johnstone, B. 1990. *Stories, Community and Place: Narratives from Middle America.* Bloomington: Indiana University Press.

Kalish, R., and Reynolds, D. 1976. *Death and Ethnicity: A Psychocultural Study.* Los Angeles: University of Southern California Press.

Kemper, S. 1988. Geriatric psycholinguistics: syntactic limitations of oral and written language. In *Language, Memory and Aging.* L. Light and D. Burke, eds. New York: Cambridge University Press.

Labov, W. 1972. The transformation of experience in narrative syntax. In *Language in the Inner City: Studies in the Black English Vernacular.* Philadelphia: University of Pennsylvania Press. 354–396.

Labov, W. 1982. Speech actions and reactions in personal narrative. In *Analyzing Discourse: Text and Talk.* Georgetown University Round Table on Language and Linguistics. Deborah Tannen, ed. Washington DC: Georgetown University Press.

Labov, W. and Auger, J. 1991. The effects of normal aging on discourse: a sociolinguistic perspective. In *Narrative Discourse in Neurologically Impaired and Normal Aging Adults.* Hiram Brownell and Yves Joanette, eds. San Diego: Singular Publishing Group, Inc.

Labov, W. and Waletsky, J. 1967. Narrative analysis: oral versions of personal experience. In *Essays on the Visual and Verbal Arts.* June Helm, ed. Seattle: University of Washington Press. 12–44.

Lawton, P.; Moss, M.; Fulcome, M., and Kleban, M. 1982. A research and service oriented multilevel assessment instrument. *Journal of Gerontology* 37:91–99.

Linde, C. 1993. *Life Stories: The Creation of Coherence.* New York: Oxford University Press.

Littlewood, J. 1992. *Aspects of Grief: Bereavement in Later Adult Life.* London: Tavistock/Routledge.

Lopata, H. 1973. *Widowhood in an American City.* Cambridge, Massachusetts: Schenkman.

Luborksy, M., and Rubinstein, R. 1987. Ethnicity and lifetimes: self-concepts and situational concepts of ethnic identity in late life. In *Ethnicity and Aging: New Perspectives.* D. Gelfand and C. Barresi, eds. New York: Springer.

———. 1990. Ethnic identity and bereavement in later life: the case of elderly widowers. In *Aging, Culture, and Society.* J. Sokolovsky, ed. Brooklyn: Bergin and Garvey.

Lund, D. 1989. *Older Bereaved Spouses.* New York: Hemisphere Press.

McCabe, A., and Peterson, C. 1991. *Developing Narrative Structure.* Hillsdale: Lawrence Erlbaum Associates.

McGoldrick, M. 1982. Irish families. In *Ethnicity and Family Therapy.* McGoldrick, M., Pearce, J., and Giordano, J., eds. New York: Guilford Press. 310–339.

———, Almeida, R., Hines, P., Garcia-Preto, N., Rosen, E., and Lee, E. 1991. Mourning in different cultures. In *Living Beyond Loss: Death in the Family.* F. Walsh, and M. McGoldrick, eds. New York: Norton. 176–206.

Menig-Peterson, C., and McCabe, A. 1977. Children talk about death. *Omega* 8(4): 305–317.

North, A., Ulatowska, H., and Bell, H. 1986. Discourse performance in older adults. *International Journal of Aging and Human Development* 23(4): 267–289.

Obler, L., and Albert, M. 1980. *Language and Communication in the Elderly.* Lexington, Massachusetts: D.C. Heath.

Ochs, E. 1988. *Culture and Language Development.* New York: Cambridge University Press.

Palgi, P., and Abramovitch, H. 1984. Death: a cross-cultural perspective. In *Annual Review of Anthropology* (13). Bernard Siegel, Alan Beals, and Stephen Tyler, eds. Palo Alto, California: Annual Reviews Inc. 385–417.

Parkes, C., and Weiss, R. 1983. *Recovery from Bereavement.* New York: Basic Books.

Peterson, C., and McCabe, A. 1983. *Developmental Psycholinguistics: Three Ways of Looking at a Child's Narrative.* New York: Plenum.

Polanyi, L. 1979. So what's the point? *Semiotica* 25 (3–4): 207–241.

——— 1981. What stories can tell us about their tellers' world. *Poetics Today* 2: 97–112.

———1985. *Telling the American Story: A Structural and Cultural Analysis of Conversational Storytelling.* Cambridge: M.I.T. Press.

Pratt, M., and Robins, S. 1991. 'That's the way it was:' age differences in the structure and quality of adult personal narratives. *Discourse Processes* 14.

Price, L. 1987. Ecuadorian illness stories. In *Cultural Models in Language and Thought.* D. Holland, and N. Quinn, eds. New York: Cambridge University Press.

Riessman, C. 1990. *Divorce Talk: Women and Men Make Sense of Personal Relationships.* New Brunswick, New Jersey: Rutgers University Press.

Ripich, D. 1991. Differential diagnosis and assessment. In *Dementia and Communication.* R. Lubinski, ed. Philadelphia: Decker.

Robinson, J. 1981. Personal narratives reconsidered. *Journal of American Folklore* 94: 58–85.

Rosaldo, R. 1986. Ilongot hunting as story and experience. In *The Anthropology of Experience.* V. Turner, and E. Bruner, eds. Urbana: University of Illinois Press.

Rosenblatt, P., Walsh R., and Jackson, D. 1976. *Grief and Mourning in a Cross-Cultural Perspective.* New Haven: HRF Press.

Rubinstein, R. 1995. Narratives of elder parental death: a structural and cultural analysis. *Medical Anthropology Quarterly* 9(2): 258–277.

———. 1985. Ethnicity and life reorganization by elderly widowers. National Institute on Aging Grant #AGO5204.

Schatzman, L., and Strauss, A. 1955. Social class and modes of communication. *American Journal of Sociology* 60(4): 329–338.

Scheper-Hughes, N. 1979. *Saints, Scholars and Schizophrenics: Mental Illness in Rural Ireland.* Berkeley: University of California Press.

Schiffrin, D. 1984. Jewish argument as sociability. *Language in Society* 13: 311–335.

Schweder, R. 1991. *Thinking Through Cultures: Expeditions in Cultural Psychology.* Cambridge, Massachusetts: Harvard University Press.

Tannen, D. 1989. *Talking Voices: Repetition, Dialogue and Imagery in Conversational Discourse.* Cambridge: Cambridge University Press.

Ulatowska, H. 1985. *The Aging Brain: Communication in the Elderly.* San Diego: College Hill Press.

———, and Chapman, S. 1991. Discourse studies. In *Dementia and Communication.* R. Lubinski, ed. Philadelphia: B. Decker.

van Dijk, T. 1984. *Prejudice in Discourse: An Analysis of Ethnic Prejudice in Cognition and Communication.* Philadelphia: John Benjamins.

Wachs, E. 1988. *Crime Victim Stories.* Bloomington: Indiana University Press.

Walker, V. 1988. Linguistic analyses of the discourse narratives of young and aged Women." In *Folia Phoniatrica* 40:58–64.

Walsh, F., and McGoldrick, M. 1991. *Living Beyond Loss: Death in the Family.* New York: Norton.

Watson, K-A. 1973. A rhetorical and sociolinguistic analysis of narrative." *American Anthropologist.* 75. 243–64.

Williams, R. 1990. *A Protestant Legacy: Attitudes Toward Death and Illness among Elderly Aberdonians.* Oxford: Clarendon Press.

Young, K. 1987. *Taleworlds and Storyrealms.* (Martinus Nijhoff Philosphy Library 16) Dordrecht: Martinus Nijhoff.

Zborowski, M. 1969. *People in Pain.* San Francisco: Jossey-Bass Inc.

CHAPTER 8

Ageing, Ageism and Anti-Ageism
Moral Stance in Geriatric Medical Discourse

Nikolas Coupland
Justine Coupland

INTRODUCTION

The notion of "ageism" is becoming increasingly familiar, both in everyday usage and in academic and professional contexts.[1] This shift in what we can think of as contemporary discourses of ageing and the lifespan reflects the West's late awakening to moral and political considerations centring on older people. But attributions that social practices (including forms of talk), socio-structural arrangements, or social policies are "ageist" do not seem to be based on entirely consistent moral and political assumptions. Some inconsistency of this sort may be normative for public accounts of discrimination and disadvantage. The wide diversity of circumstances, of needs and opportunities, and not least of ages, among so-called "elderly people" makes it inappropriate to appeal to "ageism" as an undifferentiated and grandiose moral assessment. Ageism in a variety of forms is certainly rife, but this assessment clearly does not relate to a uniform and circumscribed set of moral criteria which apply across all social contexts. On the other hand, there is an urgent need to recognise the many arenas and processes of prejudice and disadvantage that do threaten the self-esteem and quality of life of many older people. And discourses that witness and promote awareness of "ageism" are potentially very powerful agents of social policy formation and of social change.

We do not set out to provide "correct" or even "adequate" formulations of the concept of ageism—and certainly not a single formulation. Rather, in this chapter we consider how the everyday talk of older people can itself be taken to reproduce ageist assumptions (in this case, about health-in-ageing) and how such talk can become a focus for anti-ageist conversational work by others (in this case, in what is said by doctors in medical consultations). We feel there is a need to investigate the relationship between ageist discourse (the forms of talk and ways of meaning to which the ascription "ageist" is locally applied) and discourses of ageism (the forms of talk and ways of meaning that negotiate rights, obligations, and opportunities in the context of an attribution of ageist practice). In approaching discourse and ageism in this way, we loosen the obligation upon researchers to evidence and to defend their own moral judgements about the desirability or problem status of specific linguistic or other behaviours. We shift research attention onto how individuals and groups themselves represent and respond to moral and political evaluations in specific cases. Discursive accounts of ageism can then be seen as attempts at social influence and change at the micro level.

In the chapter, we first consider some current public accounts of ageism. Important as they are, we want to suggest that they contain certain internal contradictions. There are multiple routes to the attribution of ageism, even to the extent that what are considered anti-ageist practices may themselves endorse some arguably ageist assumptions. Then, we examine some formulations of ageism that have surfaced in different literatures, in our own earlier work on intergenerational talk, and in some recent and challenging critical theory perspectives on ageing and late life. In the second half of the chapter, we show how these perspectives can help us understand both ageist discourse and discourse about ageism in conversational data from a geriatric outpatients clinic.

AGEISM AS DISENFRANCHISEMENT

An academic and social policy discourse of ageism is becoming more common in the UK, although it seems to be more firmly established in the USA. It asserts, convincingly, that ageism in diverse formations is prevalent and even structurally enmeshed in society. This analysis can be traced back to Butler's (1969, also 1975) seminal discussion of societal ageism, elaborated by Levin and Levin (1980), and carried on, for example, through contemporary publications by the UK Centre for

Policy on Ageing (e.g. Norman, 1987) and Age Concern England (e.g. McEwen, 1990; see also Tyler, 1986).

A recent instance is Scrutton (1990), writing on behalf of Age Concern England:

> Where the assumptions made about old age are negative they lead to ageism, which treats older people not as individuals but as a homogeneous group which can be discriminated against. Ageism creates and fosters prejudices about the nature and experience of old age. These usually project unpleasant images of older people which subtly undermine their personal value and worth. Commonly held ideas restrict the social role and status of older people, structure their expectations of themselves, prevent them achieving their potential and deny them equal opportunities. (p.13)

In this account, ageism is defined as the overlapping processes of deindividuation, devaluation, and, above all, disenfranchisement. Ageism is a force which denies older people access to levels of respect and opportunity which are the right of all individuals. In the context of presumed universal human rights, ageism parallels sexism, racism, and classism. Accounts of ageism commonly recognise this parallelism but also that there are some unique considerations. Scrutton continues:

> First, older people do not form an exclusive group, but one of which every individual will eventually become a member. . . . Second, the discrimination which emanates from ageism can appear to result from the natural process of biological ageing rather than social creation. It is important to emphasise that the concept of ageism does not deny the ageing process, but rather seeks to distinguish between—on the one hand—ageing as a process of physiological decline and—on the other—the social phenomenon which forms the basis of the disadvantage and oppression of older people. Any consideration of ageism has to be clear about the difference. (p.14)

There are many difficulties in setting ageism in direct comparison with other recognised 'isms," although the two familiar caveats in the second quoted passage may well explain the relatively limited currency of the ageism attribution until recently. In the West we have been prepared to tolerate discrimination against, in a sense, our ageing selves more readily than against some more obviously delimitable and disenfranchised outgroup. Strong perceived intergroup boundaries (cf. Giles and Coupland, 1991) are necessary for the mobilisation of a political discourse of discrimination. But it may also be the case that people have actually believed that different thresholds of deservingness legitimately exist across the lifespan. 'Evidence' supporting this view may be that the body, its health and activity, and older people's perceived contribution to and involvement in society all arguably decline with advancing old age. If these are common beliefs, a discourse of ageism first has to assert that principles of social equality are in fact applicable to old age before it evaluates how they have been compromised.

Statements like those of Scrutton do set a crucial moral and political agenda for "ageing" Western societies as we move from a three-plus to a four-plus generational family format and as the social group we have thought of as "post-retirement" swells to half the adult population. (This last sentence itself contributes to what Turner [1982] and Featherstone [1982] call the demographic discourse of ageing, which is already very strongly represented in political life and in the mass media. Construing elderly people as an unexpected population mass draining "our" health resources has huge potential as an ageist formation in its own right.) A coherent discourse of ageism, such as Scrutton's, will presumably help to build some wider awareness of ageism—as concept and as social practice—within the political consciousness. The current lack of such an awareness is noteworthy in many unrelated contexts. For example, as we have argued previously (see Coupland, Coupland, and Giles, 1991, for an overview), academic research in the language sciences can itself be shown to be ageist in its assumptions about lifespan development. Language research has predominantly treated ageing, if at all, in terms of speakers' decrementing faculties. Social science as a whole has paid highly selective attention to social issues and populations and has often overrepresented young adults as all adults in survey research. In the (UK) media, it is not uncommon to find rather blatant pejorative references to old age and the elderly—of the sort that tend to be tabooed in liberal democracies that have achieved at least a threshold awareness of the prejudiced and discriminatory bases of such practices.

But having access to the concept of "ageism" does not itself outlaw ageist practices. Sex-based discrimination in many domains of life is clearly able to survive untouched by there being ubiquitous everyday references to sexism. And as van Dijk has convincingly shown (e.g.,

1992), racism referred to and denied is integrally part of racist discourse. We simply observe that, on the whole, the West (and again particularly, we think, the UK) has not arrived even at the point where ageism is regularly agendaised—in whatever way and with whatever focus.

In terms of disenfranchisement, there are blatantly age-discriminatory social practices to be identified. Institutional arrangements for fixed retirement ages and the absence of legislation banning age-specific job-advertisements (Laczko and Phillipson, 1990) are clear instances of structural ageism. As an extreme case of devaluation, abuse of elderly residents in long-stay care, inferior health-care provision and delivery are even more obviously so (Adelman, Greene, and Charon, 1987; Henwood, 1990). In such instances, convincing cases can be made on comparative grounds. Where it is demonstrably true that individuals are being debarred from security, dignity, services or careers by virtue of age alone, relative to other age groups, universalistic principles of human rights and equality of opportunity are indeed the appropriate point of reference. The social arrangements that permit, endorse, or encourage discriminatory processes can be identified as emanating from power structures with vested interests; an instance is the withholding of resources from older people in the interests of other (younger) favoured social groups (see the detailed discussion in Levin and Levin, 1980). The facts of ageism of this sort are incontrovertible and campaigning initiatives can and should be directed against discriminatory practices of this sort.

AGEISM AND ANTI-AGEISM

But, in the context of our analysis of language research on ageing (Coupland and Coupland, 1990), we also identified a critical tradition that we labelled "anti-ageism." Most obviously within the social sciences and the social services, but also to be found in the negotiation of everyday intergenerational relations generally, an ideology exists which is principally sustained by the recognition, at some modest level, that there is social injustice towards the elderly. Its overt politics are to resist this injustice (whether or not fixed by the label "ageism"). For example, we find paradigms of critical commentary and research which set out to demonstrate the fact that, the extents to which and the circumstances under which, older people are the objects of social prejudice and discrimination. Much research into social stereotyping of the elderly is anti-ageist in this sense. Studies that demonstrate how some older people are spoken to in simplified and/or "babytalk" registers (e.g. Caporael and Culbertson, 1986, and for that matter our own studies of accommodation in talk across the generations—see below). In everyday talk, we very often find a sympathetic and defensive orientation to older people—as topics of talk or as addressees (Henwood, Giles, Coupland, and Coupland, 1993).

And resisting ageism, as we argued above, is what societies must be committed to. But there is a problem of setting boundaries to discourses of anti-ageism, so as to distinguish them from ageist ideologies themselves. Because clearly enough, within the anti-ageist tradition, there is a seductive if simplistic morality of protecting the weak and oppressed minority. In the very act of exposing prejudiced or discriminatory orientations to old people, there is a risk of contributing to society's perception of the elderly as necessarily vulnerable and oppressed. In everyday conversation between the generations there are many indications of we have called "over-accommodation"—the tendency to use overbearing and often patronising styles of talk to older people, generally stemming from nurturing and (over)protective intents (Coupland et al., 1988; Hamilton, 1994; Ryan, Bourhis and Knops, 1991). What we have called "under-accommodation" is the subjective assessment that talk to the old can, at the other extreme, be dismissive and insufficiently attentive, solicitous, or respectful, as for example in the case of the "deflecting" strategies that nurses use in their talk to long-stay residents (Grainger, Atkinson, and Coupland, 1990).

Parallelling this distinction, Scrutton (1990) refers to "patronising ageism" (p.12) as existing alongside another "more pernicious form of ageism . . . that arises from neglect, and from discounting the needs of older people" (p.13). Our social institutions have to chart the same difficult course as conversationalists do—between under- and over-accommodative orientations. Despite its positive orientation, anti-ageism risks problematising the circumstances of the elderly and smothering them in misplaced concern. Anti-ageism recreates ageism when it draws from the same inventory of prejudiced assumptions about the old, for example, as necessarily having lower autonomy and higher vulnerability. Not surprisingly, these competing discourses of ageism can lead to highly confused policies and practices. One instance we have considered in detail is the overt ideology of "over-accommodation avoidance" (Atkinson and Coupland, 1988) that is paradoxically interconnected with actual over-accommodative talk in the training of home care assistants in the UK.

AGEISM AS UNIVERSALISM AND REPRESSION

But another contradiction surfaces here too. If there are risks attached to singling out older people as especially disenfranchised, so too there are risks in assuming that old age has no distinctive characteristics. It is very clearly one version of anti-ageism to assume and assert that elderly people should not be differentiated from the category of all adults, and this is the general thrust of Scrutton's first quoted paragraph (above). On the other hand, this same ideology can easily fail to acknowledge the ways in which many older people's circumstances are genuinely distinct from the young adult norm, e.g., in terms of economic and health-related limitations. This is why Scrutton is at pains to "emphasise that the concept of ageism does not deny the ageing process" (see the second quoted paragraph, above).

In fact, some recent critical theoretical writings have isolated denial of ageing as the cornerstone of contemporary social ageism in the West. Perhaps the richest contemporary perspective is Woodward's (1991) interpretation in *Aging and Its Discontents*. Working in the post-Freudian psychoanalytic traditions and building her accounts primarily around literary representations, Woodward argues that the dominant contemporary Western response to old age and ageing is repression. Working outwards from personal anecdotes about the unwatchability of elderly nude forms, she argues that the repression of old age is in part a Freudian legacy, since "Freud repressed the subject of aging in his construction of a powerful discourse of subjectivity and generational relations so firmly anchored in infancy and early childhood" (p.9). This is a tradition that predisposes us to "reproduce dark if not tragic portraits of aging" (p.10) which she shows are commonplace as literary representations. This is one facet of the supposed pathology of "gerontophobia," as discussed by Bunzel (1972) and Levin and Levin (1980). (We say "supposed" because it is at least possible that pathologising fear and hatred of ageing and the elderly is one ageist strategy for legitimising discrimination.)

Cole's (1986) historical contextualisation of ageism connects well to Woodward's ideas about contemporary repressive responses. Cole contrasts a pre-industrial and essentially religious mythology of old age, which was able to infuse spiritual meaning into late life, with a secularised and far more materialistic conception. The nineteenth century generated a dualistic vision of old age, still prevalent, which contrasted decay and dependency with health, virtue, and self-reliance (p.123). Effectively, Cole argues, this was the birth of the modern myth that old age is intrinsically no different from youth, except in its supposedly deviant (frail and decremental) forms. The consequence is the denial and hence repression of old age, largely in that we no longer perceive old age to have a legitimate place as a distinct period of lifespan occupancy with its own spiritual agenda.

In fostering the alternative myth of a normatively healthy and "youthful" old age, and very largely as part of an anti-ageist ideology, it seems therefore that we are cutting away old age's "natural" or at least established territory, creating an ideological vacuum in which older people must strive to exist. As Cole also argues, we thereby actively construct the "deviant" cases of ill health and frailty as marginal, and certainly as less acceptable. Elderly frailty, if we can extend Woodward's idea, is unwatchable in this more profound sense. The analysis has much in common with Guggenbuhl-Craig's treatise on the "pitfalls of the health/wholeness archetype" (1980, p.21). In a human environment where (Guggenbuhl-Craig says) we need to accept ill health and infirmity as the normal condition; if we assert and assume that good health and vitality in old age are not only viable but normative, we store up dissatisfactions and prejudices for ourselves and our ageing identities.

It is again consistent with societal repression of ageing that the condition of old age itself should be fraught with uncertainties and contradictions. And Hagestad (1985) has independently argued that the social role of, for example, grandparenting is a highly ambiguous one nowadays—integral or peripheral to "the family"?; a time of opportunity or constraint?; and so on. Featherstone and Hepworth (1990) generally support the contention that postmodernity is "producing a reversal in those processes of industrialisation and modernisation which brought about the institutionalisation of life stages . . . (the prescription of, for example, rules concerning childhood and development, schooling, careers, marriage, retirement)" (p.144). They cite Meyrowitz's (1984) claims that in contemporary Western society children are becoming more adult-like and adults more childlike.

One of their examples is that styles of dress are far less prescriptively considered age-appropriate nowadays—60-year-olds wearing tennis shoes and jeans, for instance. Is clothing on the verge of becoming uni-age as it has, in some contexts, become uni-sex? Featherstone and Hepworth themselves note that post-retirement casual dressing tends to be restricted to the affluent, urban middle classes, and it may this far be a specifically "young-old" phenomenon. Still, this speculative view that such changes may be indications of a postmodern blurring of age-related social roles deserves empirical attention. A society that represses old age leaves us casting around, in later life, for warrantable social identities and accounts of our own place and purpose. These ideas may help us understand some of the origins of low levels of life satisfaction and, in extreme cases, of mental health in old age.

These ideas present an agenda for discourse analytic research that has only recently been embarked upon. Our own previous accounts of patterns of intergenerational talk are, nevertheless, in some specific respects indicative of repression. Woodward's anecdotal experience is as follows:

> It is my experience that when people do speak personally about their own experience of old age or their own fears of aging and death, especially when they are old, the common response of others is to reject what they say. Nervous anxiety is masked by a denial of another's subjectivity in a way that appears to be reassuring but is in reality silencing and repressive. (Woodward, 1991, p.3)

In our own empirical work, we have found that young adults' responses to elderly troubles telling can quite often indicate discomfort with this mode of talk. Silence and minimal back-channelling are common, and they occasionally "lighten" the key of these conversations by strategically "looking on the bright side" of an otherwise worrying or unhappy circumstance (Coupland et al., 1988). An alternative strategy is shifting topic to elicit a different, more positive aspect of the elderly person's life circumstances. If we interpret these responses as young conversationalists not allowing troubles tellers to present troubles in fully elaborated ways, they do constitute a form of repression. But a more common strategy is for troubles-tellers themselves to do this lightening work. One instance from the cited study (p.234) is an elderly woman who discloses: "I can't walk far because (.) I'm full of arthritis (laughs).. but er (.) oh wh what else (.) can we expect . . . we're lucky that we've got the day centre to go to."[2] There are possibilities here for an analysis in terms of elderly self-repression (which is also appropriate in the medical consultation data we shall consider shortly). Again, the study we referred to above where nurses systematically deflect the troubles that their elderly patients report to them represents the denial of elderly experiences of problems and discomfort.

Similarly, young adults' responses to disclosures of age by older people ("I was seventy-eight last February") do very commonly involve expressions of surprise and denials (Coupland, Coupland, and Giles, 1989). Henwood, Giles, Coupland, and Coupland (1993) show how young people discussing audio-recorded instances of elderly troubles talk either overtly or covertly discredit the speakers' motives for telling problems and recast these disclosures as discountable elderly conversational routines. So, on balance, the interactional evidence from our own studies does support the repression model, and theorising ageism as repression would seem to be one valuable organising principle for diverse future discourse analytic studies.

One implication is that what we might be tempted to gloss as "negative" (infirm, problematised) representations of old age, say in the media, may at one level be socially productive as well as potentially damaging. Viewing later life across its full range—old age as healthy but also infirm, potentially a time of fulfilment but for many a time of deprivation and anxiety—may at least succeed in challenging our arguably naive postmodern assumptions that old age can and perhaps should be "youth with grey hair." It is important to assume that there is a dialectic to be entered into about how we should interpret the moral utility/reprehensibility of such images. Foregrounding the genuinely predictable limitations and worries associated with old age (physical frailty, bereavement and loss, sometimes economic stresses) is often taken as a central case of ageist practice. But to portray elderly frailty and the rest may also be salutary as a discourse counteracting simplistic, benign assumptions about the intrinsic positivity of old age (vis. overt anti-ageism), just as validating the achievable satisfactions and benefits of late life can counteract doom-and-gloom ageist assumptions about necessary decrement. What is clear is that social texts do not construct themselves as ageist or otherwise simply through the positivity/negativity of the images of old age they portray (although this has been a dominant assumption—see Atkins, Jenkins, and Perkins, 1990; Cassata and Irwin, 1989; Davis and Kubey, 1981). Texts establish a dialogue, often critical, with an ideology of ageing that obtains in their own local contexts.[3]

GERIATRIC MEDICINE AND THE DATA CONTEXT

Medical consultations involving elderly patients provide one context for analysing discourses about ageism in more specific terms. To the extent that so-called "geriatric" medicine is practised as a distinct medical domain, we can expect its practitioners to subscribe to ideologies that reflect its distinctiveness and, at least in more "progressive" institutional contexts, its inherent value.

In the UK, it is recognised that geriatrics is being re-born out of a particularly troubled and undistinguished past (Anderson, 1991; see also the discussion in Coupland and Coupland, 1994). Geriatrics originally had close associations with the Poor Law and it is only in the last 50 years that certain fundamental arguments—e.g., that old age is not a disease and that bed-rest without reason is dangerous—have been unequivocally accepted. Swift (1991) adds that the notion that "old patients are not acute" and that waiting lists for services are acceptable has bedevilled care of the elderly for decades. Swift also documents how a radical reappraisal of the bases and goals of geriatric medicine is currently under way, based on a rich and differentiated modern system of patient assessment. Within this, emphasis will necessarily fall on medical professionals' communication skills and sensitivities as an integral part of care delivery. In its public, reflective, published accounts of its own ideals, modern geriatrics therefore commits itself to an anti-ageist ideology, geared to counteracting an earlier set of clearly ageist assumptions and policies.

The data for this study were collected at a Geriatric Outpatients Clinic at a major hospital in South Wales over six weeks of participant observation, interviewing, and audio- and video-recording. The study was designed on ethnographic lines, to involve multiple intersecting levels of analysis, centring on audio-tape-recording of interactions between staff and patients during clinic hours but supplemented with open-ended interviewing of all participants. We focus here on audio-recordings of the doctor-patient consultations themselves and associated observers' notes. There are 102 interactions involving 98 patients and 8 doctors (6 males and 2 female) ranging in status from junior housemen through registrars and consultants to very senior staff. Patients were aged between 62 and 97. Their presence in the clinic to some extent simply reflects their age: the existence of the Geriatrics Unit means that older patients in the Health Authority region are referred here for care and treatment. Hence, the Clinic staff deal with a wide variety of more and less routine ailments, though there is a predictable predominance of age-related medical conditions represented, from minor to acute.

Each doctor who participated in the study agreed to have a micro-recorder running on his/her desk and a researcher present during the entire consultation. The observer sat in full view of doctor and patient but towards the back of the consulting room. S/he made written notes of contextual information and non-verbal behaviours particular to each consultation as it progressed and took no direct part in the interaction other than minimal responses if spoken to by another participant. Doctors asked patients' permission to record the consultations for research purposes soon after they entered the consultation room. (In addition, patients had in all cases been alerted when they entered the clinic to the fact that recordings were being made at the clinic on that particular day.) In all but one case this permission was readily granted. Micro-recorders were placed in open view on the desk between the doctor and patient. To ensure protection of confidentiality and patients' privacy under any special circumstances that arose, doctors were given discretionary rights to stop the recording if they felt that the procedure at any point constituted too great an intrusion. This option was taken up on two occasions, when one patient became ill and the other extremely upset during the consultation. These interactions were of course excluded from the data set. All details of these procedures were fully endorsed by the relevant Medical Ethics Committees of the Local Health Authority in advance of the recording sessions.

Large sections of the recorded data have been transcribed using a modified version of the conventions we describe in Coupland, Coupland, and Giles, 1991. Our transcriptions are produced with varying degrees of delicacy depending on the analytic questions being addressed. But in all cases, interpretive commentaries derive from repeated listenings to the recordings themselves, supported by the observational notes and post-interaction interviews. That is, we use transcriptions as one of several analytic resources rather than as objects of analysis in their own right.

The Clinic is a very progressive centre for geriatric medicine in the UK and several senior doctors associated with it are at the forefront of modern geriatric medical theory. We feel that these data give us an opportunity to observe some of the most positively motivated contemporary UK practice in geriatrics. The clinic very clearly allies itself with the anti-ageist ideal, as our interviews with all doctors who participated in the observational phases of the work confirmed. A senior doctor at the clinic comments on elderly patients' damaging orientations to their own health in the following terms:

> old people often don't seek help and they don't see it often as sickness, they see it as part of getting old and they accept it . . . they don't see that this is something you tell a doctor and the result is that they don't actually seek advice . . . this is a problem . . . often they [geriatric patients] don't see there's anything that they can successfully do or it will have benefits. . . .

The work of the clinic, beyond addressing patients' clinical and socio-environmental problems, is therefore anticipated to include ideological work in opposition to such predictable formulations of health-in-ageing brought forward by patients themselves. In the views of at least certain professionals, clinical consultations are established in advance as potential arenas for conflictual discourses of ageism and anti-ageism. And these issues are in fact central to the geriatric enterprise, because elderly patients' understandings of their own health-in-ageing are crucial to their self esteem, life satisfaction, and health.

SELF-DISENFRANCHISING DISCOURSE

Contemporary discourses of age and health can easily be seen as a legacy of the same fundamentally ageist assumptions that suppressed basic health care provision for older people for so long. The general agenda for our own work (Coupland, Coupland, and Giles, 1991; Coupland, Coupland, and Grainger, 1991; Coupland and Nussbaum, 1993) has been to show how the uncertainties of lifespan identity are very frequently reflected in lay and medical conversations between people of different ages. One recurring feature in earlier data is how, for very many older people and for younger people interacting with them, discursive representations of age are systematically enmeshed with considerations of health-identity. For example, ill-health or its denial establishes a preference for disclosing age (in expressions of the type "I'm eighty-five, what can I expect?"; or "I'm doing well for eighty-five"). Examples from elderly people's responses to a "How are you?" elicitation in interviews that we conducted about experiences of health (see Coupland, Coupland, and Robinson, 1992) are:

erm (.) not too bad (.) no (.) not on top of the world but none of us are
are we (.) no (.) but when you come to eighty-three years of age you
can't expect ((to be like)) a spring chicken can you? as well as can be
expected (.) I'll be ninety on the seventh of August if all goes well (.)
I'm quite well actually (.) considering I'm seventy-five

As in the first two of these instances, disclosing age can act as an
account for a general or specific health problem. Conversely (as in the
third example), one can claim credit for being in relatively good health
"despite" one's advancing age. Health and age thereby become tokens
in a rather ritualised series of lay exchanges across the lifespan but
particularly (our data suggest) in the talk of older speakers. The
ideologies of ageing that are reproduced in such talk are potentially
very damaging ones and an obstacle to professionals who are trying to
enact an explicitly anti-ageist ideology of geriatric medicine. Such
statements endorse a view of ageing as an unremitting decremental
process with expectable stages of decline in physical and emotional
well-being linked to chronological ageing (see Coupland and Coupland,
1993).

In the Outpatients data, elderly patients' self-disenfranchising
discourse takes several forms. It includes comments about individuals
being "too old to change" (unhealthy lifestyles) and about lowered
expectations for own health and well-being generally. The central and
most frequent case, however, is references to own-health-in-ageing
which invoke, in one way or another, the stereotype of ineluctable age-
graded health degeneration. The following extracts are illustrative.

Extract 1

Doctor A (male); Patient 09 (male, aged 71)

Dr A :   we've been seeing you here because of a thrombosis you had
           in the right calf
           [   ]
P09:   that's right yes yes
Dr A: ah (.) and you had that (.) about two or three months ago?
                                                                    [
P09:   yes
Dr A: have you had any further problems?
P09:   nothing at all no pain nothing at all
Dr A: have you got any complaints at the moment?

                                    [
P09:   (breathes in loudly)
        (thoughtfully) um (3.0) well (1.0) I don't feel (1.0) er how can
        I put it? (.) (louder and faster) well at seventy-one you you you
        you everything seems important doesn't it so I think I'm
        alright yes yes ((you can write it down I'm alright))
                                    [
Dr A: (slight laugh) OK (.) who's at
        home (.) Mr Cameron?

Extract 2

Doctor A (male); Patient 10 (female, aged 88)
After the physical examination, patient and doctor have been talking
about P10's recent hospital stay

P10:   everything was done for me I was well looked after (.) you
        can't expect much at eighty-eight can you? (chuckles at
        length) still I see some of them are flying across the world at
        ninety (.) true (laughs)
                        [
Dr A: that's r that's right
                        [   ]
P10:   (laughs)
        (more seriously) so I don't know (.) (coughs) as long as I can
        get this breathing (.) better (.) bit easier you see
Dr A: yeah

Extract 3

Doctor C (female); Patient 71 (male, aged 81)

Dr C: right (.) er right (.) now (.) any problem? (.) anything I can?
P71:   problem?
Dr C: mm (.) anything I can't erm (.) anything that (.) erm
P71:   oh about myself you mean?
Dr C: yes yes
P71:   well (.) er (.) I get tired (.) rather quickly but I course I (.) I'm
        not getting younger am I I mean
Dr C: well nobody gets younger but (.) that's not the reason that you
        should get tired
P71:   well I'm hoping it is (laughs briefly)

Dr C:
                           [
                           (laughs)

Extract 4

Doctor G (female); Patient 83 (female, age 77)
The patient has reported bouts of dizziness and repeated falls

Dr G: how long have you had blood pressure trouble for?
P83:   ooh! many years (The doctor examines the patient's sprained
          ankle and takes her blood pressure)
Dr G: just sit you up a minute (.) there we are (.)
          now let's just listen to your heart could you just open your
          blouse (5.0)
P083:   (sighs) (2.0) it's old age this is nothing else (2.0)
Dr G: you may well be right
PO83:   nothing else at all

Extract 5

Doctor G (female); Patient 74 (male, age 73)

Dr G: all right (.) so what I'd like to know is what have you been
          doing since you've been at home
P74:   well er
Dr G: good bad?
P74:   good I (.) I get out of breath (.) more easily than I used to
Dr G: right
P74:   but er (1.0) well that's old age
wife: (laughs slightly)
Dr G: but you've noticed that more in the last five weeks since
          you've been at home?
P74:   I think so yes

Extract 6

Doctor F (male); Patient 51 (female, age 83) accompanied by her
granddaughter (GD)

GD: she dosen't eat an awful lot a sandwich a day
Dr F: yeah
          [
P51:   mm?

GD: you don't eat an awful lot
P51:   oh well I mean as you get older your appetite
                                              [
GD: she throws her dinner away and
         has a sandwich
P51:   isn't the same ((funny how)) people think I've
                          [   ]
Dr F: are you losing weight? . . .
Dr F: do you get short of breath at all?
P51:   not that no not really no I have slowed up (.) this last few
         weeks but I course that's my age ((that's what I)) think you
         know
Dr F: yeah
P051:   yeah

Extract 7

Doctor E (male); Patient 113 (female, age 83)
The doctor is finishing a physical examination of the patient

Dr E: where my hand is is it? oh dear (.) oh alright then
                                    [   ]   [   ]
P113:   yeah   yeah
Dr E: there we are then (.) good (.) OK (.) you know you're not bad
         though (.) you're really very good=
                              [   ]
P113   no!
P113:   =well for eight eighty-three I'm not bad am I?
Dr E: you're jolly good
P113:   yeah that's it (laughs)

In the first extract, the patient does not apply the stereotype
unequivocally to himself and appears to struggle to formulate his
response to the doctor's question about any complaints at the
moment—for example, "er how can I put it?" He has given a positive
report about lack of further symptoms following a thrombosis, although
his health-in-age formulation ("well at seventy-one you you you you
everything seems important doesn't it") obliquely qualifies the
positivity of his earlier report. There is a suggestion here that there are
many reportable symptoms which he might attribute to his age and so
deems not worth reporting to the doctor.

In each of the other extracts, the patient makes a more explicit claim about the relationship of health to age: "you can't expect much at eighty-eight, can you?" (extract 2); "I get tired (.) rather quickly but I course I (.) I'm not getting younger am I I mean" (extract 3); "(sighs) (2.0) it's old age this is nothing else (2.0)" (extract 4); "I get out of breath (.) more easily than I used to . . . but er (1.0) well that's old age" (extract 5); "oh well I mean as you get older your appetite isn't the same" (extract 6); and "well for eight eighty-three I'm not bad am I?" (extract 7). The last of these articulates a positive relationship between how the patient feels she "is" and her age (what we have previously called the disjunctive formulation of age-health identity—see Coupland, Coupland, and Giles, 1991). In each of the other cases, the patient takes age to function as an account for some undesirable or problematic circumstance—lowered expectations for medical care, tiredness, dizziness and falls, breathlessness, and loss of appetite.

These instances confirm our findings from studies of discourse in lay settings (see Coupland, Coupland, and Giles, 1991). But in a geriatric medical setting, attributing health problems to age is hearable not only as self-handicapping and defeatist but also as a challenge to the goals of the medical enterprise itself. Nevertheless, a closer examination of the organisation of individual instances repays attention. Note, for example, how patient 10's "can't expect much" comment is followed by laughter. Also, she goes on to challenge the stereotype she has just endorsed when she implicitly compares her own circumstances to those of others who are "flying across the world at ninety (.) true." She thus acknowledges that the stereotype of poor health-in-ageing is not invariable, and the light-hearted key offers a possible interpretation of her ageist claim as not being sincerely held. The patient's expressed wish to alleviate her breathing problem (which follows in the extract) itself implies that, even if you can't expect much, she herself does nevertheless hope for some improvement in the specific medical regard of her breathing.

Extract 3 follows a series of exchanges where the patient has been stressing how well he feels generally. This is why the doctor's questions in her first two turns of the extract are so open-ended, and why the patient's first two turns show he takes some time to orient to a problems format. When the patient tells that he gets "tired (.) rather quickly," it is in a general context of being reportedly very well. So in this instance, it is specifically a very slight ailment that is being characterised and attributed to not getting younger. Laughter again follows (though see below). The "it's old age this is nothing else" formulation in extract 4 apparently reflects a far more fundamental concern, relating to the patient's earlier comment about having had blood pressure trouble for many years. On the other hand, patients 74 and 51 (in extracts 5 and 6) are referring to being out of breath and slowing up as relatively minor problems in the context of discussing more significant health concerns. They offer ageing as an account for these minor reported conditions, specifically without implying it accounts for their whole range of symptoms. The patient's partner in extract 5 again mitigates the patient's ageist remark with laughter.

Clearly, then, patients vary in the scope of their age-attributions. Some present ageing as coterminous with all their medical problems; other patients allow it to be inferred that they selectively allocate some symptoms to ageing (and predictably the less determinate and less obviously remediable ones) and others to medical domains. They also command discursive devices (humour and the scheduling of contrary claims) to project self-disenfranchising remarks as light-hearted or at least to ambiguate the degree of sincerity with which they are held.

DILEMMAS OF ANTI-AGEISM

Other traditions of research have established that older patients tend to be in various ways less involved in their own medical care than are younger patients. For example, Haug (1981), Strull, Lo, and Charles (1984), and Beisecker (1988) showed that older patients indicate less desire to make or assist in making medical decisions than younger patients. Haug and Lavin (1981) suggested there are two conflicting models of doctor-elderly patient roles: physician authority and patient consumerism (see also Betz and O'Connell, 1983). They argued that the two competing models "apply differentially, depending on the characteristics of the actors, their orientation to power and dependence, and the circumstances under which they meet" (p. 222); also that it is predominantly younger people who are more predisposed to adopt the consumerist orientation, to be sceptical of professionals' authority and to be convinced of their own rights to make health care decisions. Relatedly, Haug and Ory (1987, pp. 24–25) overviewed research into cancer patients' predispositions to being told their prognoses, where people over sixty were significantly less likely to prefer either hearing details of their conditions or participating in decisions about their care.

Taken together, these studies indicate that older patients have relatively low expectations of the extent to which the medical services can improve their lives, and low aspirations towards understanding and being personally involved in decisions about their own health. If doctors want to instantiate their anti-ageist ideology in the texts of their consultations with patients, they need to convey that patients themselves do have a part to play in taking responsibility for the maintenance of their good health and well-being. Doctors may need to argue that better health is achievable despite advancing age. It follows that they may need to resist or even refute elderly patients' self-disenfranchising statements.

But refutations in general, and particularly refutations of claims made about speakers' own areas of control and experience, are tricky conversational acts. In the terms of Brown and Levinson (1987), they constitute threats to both speaking parties' face. They intrude on patients' private domains (their negative face). They threaten patients' knowledge base, perceived competence, and personal awareness (their positive face), also risking doctors' own projections of themselves as likeable individuals (doctors' positive face). Doctors' understandings of their professional roles and their ideological commitments are the forces that may mobilise them, in individual instances, to override local considerations of face-threat (cf. Coupland, Grainger, and Coupland, 1988).

A wide range of response-alternatives is evident in the consultation data. In extract 1, the doctor laughs slightly after the patient reaches his formulation of how he is, which may be more particularly a response to the patient's presuming to prescribe what the doctor should write in the medical notes. In any event, the doctor does not make any more explicit comment and moves on to a question about the patient's life at home. In extract 2, the doctor expresses agreement ("that's r that's right"), but does this directly after the patient's alternative version of how elderly lives can be rich and active. In extract 4, the doctor gives explicit, positively support to the contention that the patient's problems are due to old age and nothing else; he says, "you may well be right." In extract 6, doctor F makes no comment in response to the patient's remark about losing appetite as you get older but later acquiesces to the patient's suggestion that her slowing up should be attributed to her age (he offers "yeah"). In extract 7, doctor E appears to agree with the patient's claim that she is not bad for eighty-three, although his emphasized endorsement ("you're jolly good") does not explicitly confirm that he believes she is good specifically "for her age."

Why might doctors acquiesce to ageist self-disenfranchising remarks or offer bland non-committal responses? The degree of face-threat entailed, shortage of time, and a ubiquitous preference for agreement in conversation are certainly relevant considerations. When patients themselves ambiguate their ageist claims (through humour or denials, as we noticed above), doctors will probably be wary of responding in too heavily health-ideological terms. The very predictability and ritualisation of the health-age association in older people's self-presentations may lead doctors too to produce conventionalised responses (see Coupland, Robinson, and Coupland, 1994).

But there are several occasions when doctors in the data do explicitly work to counter patients' formulations of their own health. A minor instance is in extract 5. After the patient produces "but er (1.0) well that's old age," and his spouse laughs, the doctor probes about the specific circumstances of the breathlessness in her next question. When the patient, in responding, notes that he has in fact noticed the problem more in the last five weeks, this functions as an implicit counter to the ageist claim. Towards the end of extract 3, we see doctor C formulating a very explicit anti-ageist claim: "well nobody gets any younger but (.) that's not the reason that you should get tired." She is prepared to challenge the conventionalised appeal to old age as an account for tiredness. As we noted earlier, in this case the doctor may feel that there is pre-existing evidence for the likely success of this interventionist strategy, because the patient has already reported his generally positive health experiences.

Extract 8 is part of a sustained debate between a doctor and a patient about the appropriate health-horizons for older people. We include a relatively long portion of the transcribed text to illustrate the degree of elaboration that can occasionally be found in the negotiation of health and age in the Outpatients data.

Extract 8

Doctor F (male); Patient 08 (female, age 77)

The sequence occurs well into the consultation after the question/answer diagnosis, a lengthy series of exchanges between the doctor and the patient's daughter (while the patient talks to the nurse in the examination cubicle) about the patient's smoking and drinking problems and recent weight loss, and the doctor's physical examination of the patient. The patient has just been helped to dress by the nurse and has returned to sit in the main consulting room.

Dr F: I've told your daughter (clears throat) not to buy you any
          drinks (.) not to give you any cigarettes either (4.0)
P08:   (quietly, ironically) what a nice man you are!
Dr F: (amused) hm!
P08:   that you think that somebody at seventy seven
Dr F: mm
          [
P08:   can (breathes) give up smoking when she's smoked since she
          was fifteen
Dr F: well that is the reason that you have to give up
P08:   yes well ye
               [
Dr F: because you have smoked for so long (1.0)
P08:   but also really
                  [
Dr F: I think it is time you gave up (1.0)
          (clears throat)
P08:   (clears throat) I think it's also a reason why you won't be able
          to give it up=
Dr F: =(indignantly and loudly) who said you won't be able to
                              [   ]
P08:   because
P08:   (a little indignantly) don't you think I've tried
          in the past years?
              [
Dr F: o::h I you may have tried you may have tried Mrs. Casey on
          your own (.) but not with me (4.0) I have not been un I have
          not been unsuccessful in the past
P08:   very good
Dr F: and so we should still be we should be able to stop you
          smoking this time
P08:   (haughtily) and how do you suggest
                                  [
Dr F: do you want to stop smoking for
          a start?

P08: er no I don't want to stop it's the only pleasure I have
                                              [

Dr F: you don't want

P08: I don't go out at all (1.0)

Dr F: what s (.) w w what sort of pleasure does that give you?

P08: (1.0.) er (.) well I don't know I expect it's just that I've always been used to it and if I haven't got one

Dr F: mm

P08: I go berserk (1.0)

Dr F: mm

P08: you know

Dr F: how (.) er realistically (.) how many do you think (.) will keep you (.) without going berserk (.) ten? ten a day?

(they negotiate how she will try to control her cravings for smoking . . .)

P08: oh one twenty a day (.) if I'm having (.) er just two little puffs just now and again (.) I'll have I'll have over half of them left!

Dr F: well that would be good (.) I do want to see that happen (4.0)

P08: I'm a bit old now to to give it up
      [

Dr F: (loudly, emphatically) no you're not! you see (.) what is happening is your lungs are are disappearing fast (.) you're getting
                                 [

P08:   my my lungs have
already disappeared I've had TB
   [

Dr F: no! you're getting (.) well the TB hasn't done too much damage (.) as as much damage as your smoking is doing (2.0)

(they go on to negotiate a time and place for P08 to be admitted to hospital)

Dr F begins his post-examination discourse with the patient in a highly confrontational manner. He presents her with a *fait accompli* decision about her future drinking and smoking without reference to the patient's own responsibility for these issues. He assumes control, mediated via the daughter's actions ("I've told your daughter"). Dr F's bald statement about the imposed regime may well have been intended to shock, and this doctor uses this strategy elsewhere in the data. The patient replies with an ironic remark that is unusually direct and face-threatening for medical interaction in general (and for the present corpus); she then begins to argue her point of view.

In the developing argument, both speakers have recourse to length-of-time arguments, which they use in different ways to suit their own ends. The patient's appeal to the doctor raises two overlapping considerations: her age (seventy-seven), and how long she has already been smoking (since she was fifteen). The related implications are that old people cannot be expected to change their ways (somebody at seventy-seven), and that habitual smokers (possibly of whatever age) cannot be expected to quit through the strength of their addiction. These themes reverberate through the whole of the conversation.

The doctor makes various attempts to counter these arguments, invoking length of time as "the reason that you have to give up," "because you have smoked for so long." When he says, "I think it is time you gave up," he subverts both the "too old" and the "too addicted" implications. His own version implies the need to revert to a "normal" (non-smoking) lifestyle for reasons to do with future health status. The patient counters by reinstating the length of addiction claim: "I think it's also a reason why you [she means herself] won't be able to give it up." And the doctor then refutes her inability. His own perspective asserts the importance of individual influences (his own participation ["not with me"], and particular attempts to give up smoking ["this time"]) in opposition to the patient's remarks about the generalised past ("in the past years"). The doctor projects this time as just another time in a sequence, rather than a time (of old age) when it will be harder than others to give up a (lifelong) habit.

Having been checked in the temporal debate, the patient raises a new age-related consideration: smoking is "the only pleasure I have." This statement invokes a pleasureless old age. Doctor F challenges her account of what is pleasurable ("what sort of pleasure does that give you?") which moves the patient back to earlier claims about habituality ("I expect it's just that I've always been used to it") and addiction ("I go berserk").

The doctor makes clear headway in persuading her to cut down but the patient then produces a defeatist, age-self-handicapping formulation: "I'm a bit old now to to give it up." In proclaiming herself too old, and having already raised the "only pleasure I have" argument just before, the patient is suggesting she has achieved a life stage that puts her beyond the responsibilities and demands that apply to younger patients. Her age is offered as a criterion that should afford her refuge of the sort suggested by Greer when she describes the post-menopausal woman: "after a lifetime of pleasing others, she was about to please herself" (Greer, 1991, p.36). Greer argues that this transition is liberating. But, in the context of the extract 8 consultation, Dr F takes it to be disempowering and dangerous. It is at this point that he makes his most vociferous contributions, including the loud, emphatic denial "no you're not!" His attempt to shock the patient further with frighteningly explicit images of degeneration ("your lungs are are disappearing fast") arguably backfires, in that the patient can take this as evidence that it is indeed too late. Therefore the doctor needs to retract this threat and to imply that there is indeed a future of possible improved health: "no! you're getting (.) well the TB hasn't done too much damage."

Predictably enough, the argument is not clearly concluded. After the transcribed extract ends, the patient effectively withdraws from the consultation. When an X-ray procedure is suggested, she says,"don't do any more today now I've had enough." In itself this is an appeal to be allowed one of the supposed luxuries of growing older, "a right to resist being rushed" (Greer 1991, p.143). The patient continues to protest about the doctor's suggested no-drinking regimen, appealing to her life-long drinking, and then to her own death; she says: "I may as well drink the little bit I'm left my life left mightn't I?"

OVERVIEW

We have seen that doctors in the corpus do challenge the age-health association that is commonly available to elderly people, in lay or medical contexts, as a way of organising their discourse about their own health statuses and symptoms, but that they do not do this either consistently or wholly successfully. When they do embark on discursive attempts to construct alternative versions of health-in-ageing, these are consistent with public statements about the ideology of the "new" geriatrics. From the standpoint of geriatric medical professionals, interventionist attempts are motivated by their concern that elderly patients have unnecessarily low aspirations for their own health. They see patients perpetuating ageist ideologies which restrict their access to possibly improved health. Their own strategies are by that account anti-ageist. The data that we have examined do indeed go some way to supporting the findings of quantitative studies that have foregrounded some older patients' low aspirations and non-consumerist orientations to medicine (and, of course, that doctors find this position a matter of professional concern).

We commented at the beginning of this chapter that we do not see it as our own role to legislate on the "correct" interpretation of "ageist" and "anti-ageist" practices. Having said this, we do suspect that many will find the dominant professional version of rights and responsibilities here a convincing one. Medicine is presumably expected to maximise opportunities for health promotion and to intervene to counteract social processes that promote unhealthy lifestyles. The issues that underlie this debate, opportunities and responsibilities for good health, have been central to medical ethics from Hypocrates onwards.

But at the level of situated talk—the level at which ethical arguments and medical ideologies have to be implemented—it is not always obvious how to attribute the designations "ageist" or "anti-ageist." Firstly, when ideologies need to be articulated as social actions (and most obviously as conversational acts), they can only have force as positions in local arguments. In the last and longest extract we considered, the patient shifted her ideological ground from one turn to another, invoking her own age, her long-standing addiction, and her pleasureless life, eclectically and contingent upon how she saw the argument to be balanced from moment to moment. Correspondingly, a committed doctor acted to reduce her unhealthy habits by asserting his own control, by projecting the patient's potential control, by holding up the threat of physical damage already caused but also by denying that damage already done was irreversible. In this instance, at least, local, sequential considerations seem to have imposed very significant constraints on the implementation of any one "pure" ideological position.

But beyond this, it is clear that in the text of these consultations, participants can conjure quite radically different ideologies of health-in-ageing. Again in the last extract, the patient was able to reference the far-from-idiosyncratic belief that old age should be a time of liberation from earlier constraints and conformity to norms—even normative regimens for good health. A discourse of the universalist version of ageism was constructed, allowing the patient momentarily to imply that the doctor's prescription to stop smoking was a curtailment of her rights to a pleasurable activity as an older person. From that point of view, the argument between doctor and patient was transformed, again momentarily, into a debate about ageism itself: should geriatric medicine after all be asserting the supposedly universal truth of health promotion—at the expense of ephemeral but no doubt genuine satisfactions? And if the answer is affirmative, at what point in the life course or in the health course should these priorities be modified?

At several points in the data, doctors themselves come to endorse positions that the dominant ideology considers ageist. We suggested earlier that there are many local factors that conspire to make this all but inevitable. But when doctor G in the fourth extract agrees with her patient that the patient's problems are attributable to old age and nothing else, she voices support for the Cole/Woodward stance—that old age does predictably bring physical limitations and problems for many older people, and that it is arguably "ageist" (in the sense of universalist ageism) to deny this. So, in extract 3, there is a striking resonance to the patient's brief response to Dr C's insistence that "nobody gets younger but (.) that's not the reason that you should get tired." He simply comments, "well I'm hoping it is."

As we age, we inevitably modify our subjective assessments of what we can and should age-appropriately be able to achieve. This may be in relation to physical abilities, styles of dress and self-presentation, or for that matter modes and roles of talk (Coupland and Nussbaum, 1993). This ongoing process of self-reassessment includes aspects of self-handicapping, although the social psychological literature dealing with this phenomenon (e.g. Jones and Berglas, 1978) has always been clear about its potential benefits as well as its risks. To set our health horizons as low as many prevalent social stereotypes of late life presume appropriate is indeed to disenfranchise ourselves, with possibly disastrous consequences. But the latitude to interpret a certain set of health experiences as "the result of old age" may be a source of reassurance for some people, a formulation that allows us to believe there is no immediately threatening or more acute health problem to be overcome. If health in later life is as much a matter of good morale as a matter of bio-medical integrity, the potential health impact of a whole array of self-accounts should be closely examined rather than dismissed out of hand. What discourse analysis offers this debate, and the broader one about ageism and anti-ageism, is the ability to develop highly contextualised readings of how moral imperatives impinge on the negotiated realities of older people's lives.

NOTES

1. An earlier version of this chapter was presented at the 1992 Workshop on Discourse, Institutions, and the Elderly at the Uppsala conference on Discourse and the Professions and published in the Proceedings of that Workshop (as Coupland and Coupland, 1993). The revised text is reproduced here with the kind permission of Professor Jay Gubrium and JAI Press. We are grateful to Mike Hepworth, Jake Harwood, Angie Williams, and Heidi Hamilton for very helpful comments on earlier drafts of the chapter.

2. Following the usage of Gail Jefferson, in this and subsequent examples the symbol (.) indicates an untimed pause.

3. It is from this position that we would want to modify Harwood and Giles' (1992) conclusion that the American television show *The Golden Girls* juxtaposes humour and age-marking in "problematic" ways. The fact that the show often focuses on "negative" and stereotypical features of old age and the fact that elderliness is undeniably a source of humour there seem to us to establish rather healthy oppositions to several potentially ageist assumptions which are made elsewhere in the media: that old age is uniform (the four principal characters of *The Golden Girls* are remarkably diverse on many dimensions, as Harwood and Giles point out); that advanced old age entails slow-wittedness (the oldest character has the sharpest and most acerbic wit); that retirement in the Sun Belt is either depressingly predictable and staid or wholly absolved from personal and social worries; and that old age is an inherently serious matter. Perhaps principally the show resists the ideology that represses old age as unwatchable in many of its diverse attributes.

REFERENCES

Adelman, R., Greene, M.G., and Charon, R. 1987. The physician-elderly patient-companion triad in the medical encounter: The development of a conceptual framework and research agenda. *The Gerontologist* 27 (6): 729–734.

Anderson, Sir Ferguson. 1991. An historical overview of geriatric medicine: Definitions and aims. In M. S. J. Pathy, ed. *Principles and Practice of Geriatric Medicine*, 2nd Edition. London: Wiley. 1435–1442.

Atkins, T. V., Jenkins, M. C., and Perkins, M. H. 1990. Portrayal of persons in television commercials age 50 and over. *Psychology, a Journal of Human Behavior* 27: 30–37.

Atkinson, K., and Coupland, N. 1988. Accommodation as ideology. *Language and Communication* 8 (3/4): 321–328.

Beisecker, A.L. 1988. Aging and the desire for information and input in medical decisions: Patient consumerism in medical encounters. *The Geronotologist* 28: 330–335.

Betz, M., and O'Connell, L. 1983. Changing doctor-patient relationships and the rise in concern for accountability. *Social Problems* 31 (1): 84–95.

Brown, P., and Levinson, S. 1987. *Politeness: Some Universals in Language Usage*. Cambridge: Cambridge University Press.

Bunzel, J.H. 1972. Note on the history of a concept: gerontophobia. *The Gerontologist* 12: 116–203.

Butler, R.N. 1969. Age-ism: another form of bigotry. *The Gerontologist* 9: 243–246.

Butler, R. N. 1975. *Why Survive? Being Old in America*. New York: Harper and Row.

Caporael, L., and Culbertson, G.H. 1986. Verbal response modes of baby talk and other speech at institutions for the aged. *Language and Communication* 6 (1/2): 99–112.

Cassata, M., and Irwin, B. 1989. Going for the gold: Prime time's sexy seniors have turned around their age group's TV image. *Media and Values*, 45: 12–14.

Cole, T. R. 1986. The 'enlightened' view of ageing: Victorian morality in a new key. In T. R. Cole and S. A. Gadow, eds. *What Does It Mean to Grow Old?: Reflections from the Humanities*. Durham: Duke University Press. 117–130.

Coupland, J., and Coupland, N. 1994. "Old age doesn't come alone": discursive representations of health-in-ageing in geriatric medicine. *International Journal of Aging and Human Development* 39 (1): 81–95.

Coupland, J., Coupland, N., and Grainger, K. 1991. Intergenerational discourse: Contextual versions of ageing and elderliness. *Ageing and Society* 11: 189–208.

Coupland, J., Coupland, N., and Robinson, J. D. 1992. "How are you?": Negotiating phatic communion. *Language in Society* 21: 207-230.

Coupland, J., Robinson, J., and Coupland, N. 1994. Frame negotiation in doctor-elderly patient consultations. *Discourse and Society* 5 (1): 89–124.

Coupland, N., and Coupland, J. 1990. Language and later life: The diachrony and decrement predicament. In H. Giles and P. Robinson, eds. *Handbook of Language and Social Psychology*. Chichester: Wiley. 451–468.

Coupland, N., and Coupland, J. 1993. Discourses of ageism and anti-ageism. *Journal of Aging Studies* 7 (3): 279–301.

Coupland, N., Coupland, J., and Giles, H. 1989. Telling age in later life: Identity and face implications. *Text* 9 (2): 129–151.

Coupland, N., Coupland, J., and Giles, H. 1991. *Language, Society, and the Elderly: Discourse, Identity and Ageing*. Oxford: Basil Blackwell.

Coupland, N., Coupland, J., Giles, H. Henwood, K., and Wiemann, J. 1988. Accommodating the elderly: Invoking and extending a theory. *Language in Society* 17 (1): 1–42.

Coupland, N., Grainger, K., and Coupland, J. 1988. (Review article) Politeness in context: Intergenerational issues. Review of P. Brown and S.C. Levinson. 1987. *Politeness: Some Universals in Language Usage.* Cambridge: Cambridge University Press. *Language in Society* 17 (2): 253–262.

Coupland, N., and Nussbaum, J., eds. 1993. *Discourse and Lifespan Identity.* Newbury Park: Sage.

Davis, R. H., and Kubey, R. W. 1981. Growing old on television and with television. In D. Pearl, L. Bouthilet, and J. Lazar, eds. *Television and Behavior: Ten Years of Scientific Progress and Implications for the Eighties* (Vol. 2). Rockville, Maryland: National Institute of Mental Health. 201–208.

Featherstone, M. 1982. The body in consumer culture. *Theory, Culture and Society* 1: 18–33.

Featherstone, M., and Hepworth, M. 1990. Ageing and old age: Reflections on the postmodern life course. In B. Bytheway, T. Keil, P. Allatt and A. Bryman, eds. *Becoming and Being Old: Sociological Approaches to Later Life*. London: Sage. 133–157.

Giles, H., and Coupland, N. 1991. *Language: Contexts and Consequences.* London: Open University Press.

Grainger, K., Atkinson, K., and Coupland, N. 1990. Responding to the elderly: Troubles talk in the caring context. In H. Giles, N. Coupland, and J. Wiemann, eds. *Communication, Health and the Elderly* (Proceedings of Fulbright International Colloquium 1988), Manchester: Manchester University Press. 192–212.

Greer, G. 1991. *The Change: Woman, Ageing and the Menopause.* London: Hamish Hamilton.

Guggenbuhl-Craig, A. 1980. *Eros on Crutches: On the Nature of the Psychopath*. Dallas, Texas: Spring.

Hagestad, G. O. 1985. Continuity and connectedness. In V. L. Bengston, and J. F. Robertson, eds. *Grandparenthood.* Beverly Hills: Sage. 31–48.

Hamilton, H. 1994. *Conversations with an Alzheimer's Patient*. Cambridge: Cambridge University Press.

Harwood, J., and Giles, H. 1992. "Don't make me laugh." Age representations in a humorous context. *Discourse and Society* 3 (4): 403–436.

Haug. M. ed. 1981. *Elderly Patients and Their Doctors*. New York: Springer.

Haug, M.R., and Lavin, B. 1981. Practitioner or patient—Who's in charge. *Journal of Health and Social Behavior* 22: 212–229.

Haug, M.R., and Ory, M.G. 1987. Issues in elderly patient-provider interactions. *Research on Ageing* 9 (1): 3–44.

Henwood, K., Giles, H., Coupland, J., and Coupland, N. 1993. Stereotyping and affect in discourse: Interpreting the meaning of elderly painful self-disclosure. In D. Mackie and D. Hamilton, eds. *Affect, Cognition, and Stereotying: Interactive Processes in Group Perception*. New York: Academic Press. 269–296.

Henwood, M. 1990. No sense of urgency: Age discrimination in health care. In E. McEwen, ed. *Age: The Unrecognised Discrimination*. London: Age Concern England. 43–57.

Jones, E.E., and Berglas, S. 1978. Control of attributions about the self through self-handicapping strategies: The appeal of alcohol and the role of underachievement. *Personality and Social Psychology Bulletin*, 4: 200–206.

Laczko, F., and Phillipson, C. 1990. Defending the right to work: Age discrimination in employment. In E. McEwen, ed. *Age: The Unrecognised Discrimination*. London: Age Concern England. 84–96.

Levin, J., and Levin, W.C. 1980. *Ageism: Prejudice and Discrimination Against the Elderly*. Belmont CA.: Wadsworth.

McEwen, E., ed. 1990. *Age: The Unrecognised Discrimination*. London: Age Concern England.

Meyrowitz, J. 1984. The adult child and the childlike adult. *Daedalus* 113 (3): 19–48.

Norman, A. 1987. Aspects of ageism: A discussion paper. London: Centre for Policy on Ageing.

Ryan, E. B., Bourhis, R. Y., and Knops, U. 1991. Evaluative perceptions of patronizing speech addressed to elders. *Psychology and Aging* 6: 442–450.

Scrutton, J. 1990. Ageism: The foundation of age discrimination. In E. McEwen, ed. *Age: The Unrecognised Discrimination*. London: Age Concern England. 12–27.

Strull, W.M., Lo, J., and Charles, G. 1984. Do patients want to participate in medical decision-making. *Journal of the American Medical Association* 252: 2990–2994.

Swift, C. G. 1991. The problem-orientated approach to geriatric medicine. In M. S. J. Pathy, ed. *Principles and Practice of Geriatric Medicine*, 2nd Edition. London: Wiley. 299–312.

Turner, B.S. 1982. The discourse of diet. *Theory, Culture and Society* 1 (1): 23–32.

Tyler, W. 1986. Structural ageism as a phenomenon in British society. *Journal of Educational Gerontology* 1 (2): 38–46.

van Dijk, T. 1992. Discourse and the denial of racism. *Discourse and Society* 3 (1): 87–118.

Woodward, K. 1991. *Aging and Its Discontents: Freud and Other Fictions.* Bloomington: Indiana University Press.

CHAPTER 9

When and How Old Age Is Relevant in Discourse of the Elderly

A Case Study of Georgia O'Keeffe

Elif Tolga Rosenfeld

INTRODUCTION

Research on the discourse of the elderly often tends to focus on either the discourse of the elderly who are cognitively impaired or on discourse produced in contexts in which old age is at issue. For example, studies focus on intergenerational talk and talk within care-giving institutions. In both types of talk, age difference is often viewed as causing a problem in communication. While these studies contribute to our knowledge of the problems faced by the elderly in communicating, there is still relatively little research which focuses on elderly discourse in which 'problems' do not seem to arise. The implicit assumption is that discourse of the elderly in which there is no obvious problem nor obvious avoidance of a problem is the same as the discourse of younger people. Thus, while these studies often seek to avoid viewing aging as a process of decrement, they support a decrement perspective by primarily focusing on problematic discourse specific to the elderly segment of the population.

In analyzing the discourse of Georgia O'Keeffe, as presented in the 1977 WNET–13 movie *Georgia O'Keeffe*, produced by Perry Miller Adato, a movie celebrating O'Keeffe's 90th birthday, I have found that although there are no apparent breakdowns in communication, her discourse, nonetheless, is distinctly that of an elderly woman. Specifically analyzing prosodic, discourse, and paralinguistic features of her discourse, I have found linguistic evidence to support the claim that her old age is but one characteristic of her identity. Further, this characteristic varies in the extent to which it is relevant and whether it is positively or negatively valued within the different identities she presents through her discourse.

In my analysis of O'Keeffe's discourse, I focus on her register use from an interactional sociolinguistic perspective, drawing on the work of Goffman (1981) and Tannen and Wallat (1983). Similar to the work of Tannen and Wallat, I identify the different registers (speech styles) O'Keeffe uses and identify shifts in the activity being engaged in at the time of talk, what Goffman (1981) identifies as shifts in "footings." That is, I identify the activity O'Keeffe is engaged in at the time of talk for each register. I then identify the different roles of O'Keeffe reflected in the talk within each register. Having identified the registers as well as the footings and roles associated with each, I then analyze the discourse to determine whether or not age is relevant as part of her role and, further, whether it is considered negative or positive. I have identified four footings which correspond with four different registers (or speech styles), which, in turn, reflect four different roles (or identities) that O'Keeffe presents through her discourse.

In what follows I present my analysis of O'Keeffe's discourse, discussing background literature focusing on the issue of 'age' as a variable in social science, previous work concerning discourse and aging, and the interactional sociolinguistic approach taken in the analysis which follows; the data; and my analysis of the data, identifying the different registers used by O'Keeffe, and analyzing the relevance of age based on these registers. Ultimately I argue that being elderly has a different qualitative and quantitative impact on O'Keeffe's role in the interaction depending on the context of the particular moment of interaction. Being elderly can be salient or not, and it can be valued positively or negatively. Thus, my analysis supports the claim that the diversity found in the elderly as a group can also be found within a single elderly person.

OLD AGE

Research on the elderly population has led to the realization that "age" is itself a vague term, indicating both chronological and social age. Eckert (1984:219) suggests that the label "age" does not adequately describe age as an independent variable in any research in which age differences are compared to behavior differences. She claims age can and should be broken down into two categories, chronological age and social age, arguing that "insofar as individuals' linguistic behavior is part of a strategy associated with social roles, it is the roles that each individual plays that correlate with linguistic variation" (1984:224). Thus, in researching social old age, Eckert (*ibid.*, 230) claims that one is discovering sociolinguistic behaviors which "might not correlate with linguistic differences" between the chronologically old and young, "but rather the roles and linguistic needs associated with" old age as a life stage.

Although Eckert is specifically addressing sociolinguistic variation studies of sound change, this distinction seems relevant for any linguistic study of the discourse of the elderly. Thus, in my analysis, although O'Keeffe is chronologically eighty-nine years old, I consider this to be only a rough indicator of the social roles that might be reflected in her discourse.

Research on the elderly population also shows that there may be an important difference between the way the elderly view their lives and the way the rest of society does. Eckert (1984:229) notes that the "elderly, being the farthest from the experience of young and middle-aged researchers, comprise the age group that is most subject to stereotyping in linguistics as well as other research." Thus, as researchers we are not within the group we are describing and our descriptions run the risk of being outsiders' descriptions rather than descriptions of how aging is experienced by the elderly themselves.

In analyzing child behavior, adult researchers face a similar problem. One difference, however, is that, although at the time of research they are not within the group, they once were. Further, childhood is thought of as a positive stage in the life span, in which one develops into an adult. Old age, however, is something which has not been experienced *yet* and which is generally viewed in American society as a time of decrement. Sankar, for example, cites a Harris poll in claiming that:

> Americans believe that the main causes of the disabilities associated with old age is age itself. For Americans old age is seen as a kind of disease, a terminal illness that uniformly begins in the sixties. (1984:251)

Thus, our "own anxieties about the inevitability of death are associated with old age as a disease—a disease whose only outcome is ultimately death" (*ibid.*, 262). The belief that the process of decrement begins due to chronological old age is also supported, as Sankar (*ibid.*, 261) points out, by social legislation which has fixed sixty-five as a marker of old age. Further, as Ward (1984:228) notes, in modern societies the aged receive a low status due to our work ethic as well as intellectual and moral segregation of the old and young.

The belief that the aging process is an inevitable process of decrement is often reflected not only in the public at large but also in the work of gerontology. Ward (1984) discusses the conflict between outsiders' and insiders' views of old age as a paradox in the gerontological literature. That is, while it is found that old age has a marginal and stigmatized status in our society, it is also found that this status does not seem to significantly affect the daily lives and self-evaluation of the elderly themselves (1984:227).

Ward (*ibid.*: 230) claims that "our models and methods still lead us to expect that age will have a central significance and to look for its effects in our research of the elderly." That is, an outsider's view of old age as a negative and salient characteristic of elderly people influences our research. He urges us to "strive to understand lives *as they are lived*," in other words, to gain an insider's perspective (*ibid.*, 230).

It is important to note that while the decrement paradigm for research is clearly a faulty one, the extreme opposite to this, an anti-ageist paradigm, is equally faulty. To claim that any research supporting the idea of decrement is ageist is clearly misguided since there is obvious decrement with aging. Thus, in agreement with Coupland and Coupland (1990), I suggest that one should not select either of these outsiders' research perspectives but rather seek to understand decrement as *part* of the aging process.

Ward ultimately suggests that age is a social fact which represents one characteristic of the many possessed by an elderly individual. Thus, as researchers we must seek to identify the contexts in which age is relevant. Further, one must discover how, in these contexts, age is valued. Rather than assuming that whenever age is salient it will be negatively valued, Ward (1984:230) claims that "under some conditions being old may be both salient and positive, as when later life is linked with such favorable qualities as wisdom."

There are at least two research methods which might lead to an insiders' understanding of the elderly. One, which has traditionally been used by anthropologists, is to use an ingroup informant. For example, Sankar (1984:259) notes that although doctors seem to have difficulties in distinguishing illness due to specific diseases from illness due to old age, her elderly informants "could be clear and concise concerning the distinction between their complaints due to old age and those due to illness." Thus, the physical condition of the elderly is viewed differently by the doctors and the elderly.

A second method for gaining an insiders' perspective on the experience of aging is discourse analysis. Although an outsiders' analysis of discourse of the elderly is equally possible, an insiders' perspective can be gained by grounding one's analysis on the discourse itself as much as possible and at the same time being aware of researcher bias. In my analysis of the O'Keeffe data, I analyze the discourse which reflects how O'Keeffe, herself, manages her identity as an elderly woman.

DISCOURSE AND AGING

While my analysis is based primarily upon an application of an interactional sociolinguistic approach to register use, it also draws upon two specific findings in the literature on language and aging as well. First, Coupland and Coupland (1990:454), reviewing the literature, refer to the work of Ramig (1986) in which it has been shown by matched guise tasks that the elderly voice is "regularly discriminable from younger voices," to the extent that subjects were able to correctly identify the elderly voice based on single prolonged vowels. Ramig (1986) claims that the regular change in voice is due to degenerative changes in the larynx. Coupland and Coupland (454) further claim that "voice quality . . . has the potential to act as a social marker of elderly speech." Thus, in my analysis of O'Keeffe's discourse, although I identify subtle shifts in her register, her voice is always clearly identifiable as that of an elderly woman.

Second, Coupland, Coupland, Giles, and Henwood (1988) study the functions of disclosing chronological age in discourse of the elderly. They identify disjunctive disclosing of chronological age as instances when telling one's old age reflects either "favorable self evaluation" or "perceived incongruence between chronological age and contextual age" (1988:137). The O'Keeffe film was made to celebrate O'Keeffe's 90th birthday. Although she does not disclose her chronological age in the discourse, there are instances in the discourse when a disjunctive sense of O'Keeffe's age is clearly expressed.

Previous research on discourse and aging includes the development of communication accommodation theory (cf. Giles et al., 1987; Coupland et al., 1990, Giles et al., 1991) which allows researchers to analyze the way in which the elderly communicate with others from an interactive perspective. Communication accommodation is defined by Shadden (1988:35) as referring to "modifications in speech style designed to expedite the transmission of a message and to signal willingness to engage in communication interactions." Thus, breakdowns in intergenerational talk have been identified as being due to problems in accommodation strategies, where, for example, either the elderly or the younger participants over- or underaccommodate each other's speech style. One example of accommodation is the use of baby talk (BT) by younger interlocutors with elderly people. It can be a case of overaccommodation, when perceived as demeaning by the elderly individual. Caporeal (1981), however, has shown that not using baby talk can be seen as underaccommodation in some contexts, in which BT is perceived as nurturing, and thus, when care-takers do not use it they are perceived as not being nurturing.

While I take an interactional approach to the analysis of O'Keeffe's discourse, the analysis does not focus on the intergenerational aspect of the interaction. Understanding how O'Keeffe and her interlocutors accommodate to one another is not a central concern. Rather than applying communication accommodation theory (CAT) and focusing on the general research question "how do people manage interactions when one of the participants is elderly?", the general research question for the current analysis is "to what extent is age relevant at all, and how is it valued, by the elderly themselves?"

Using the term "register," I take an interactional sociolinguistic approach, focusing on the relative (qualitative) variation in the use of certain prosodic, discourse, and paralinguistic features of O'Keeffe's talk in my analysis of the data. The five prosodic features are as follows: (1) pitch or relative differences in (overall) pitch; (2) tempo or the rate of speech production; (3) intonational range or the extent to which contrastive pitch is used (wider or narrower range); (4) function of intonation or whether contrastive pitch is functioning primarily grammatically (e.g., to distinguish between questions and statements), emphatically (to emphasis a single word), or to express emotion (e.g., surprise) (cf. Crystal: 1969)[1]; (5) loudness for emphasis. Further, I identify quoted dialogue as a discourse feature. Quoted dialogue is commonly thought of as reported speech. In this study, quoted dialogue includes not only reports of what has been uttered in the past but also the representation of previous thoughts that were not necessarily uttered. Finally, I identify laughter as a paralinguistic feature of the discourse.

O'Keeffe's use of these features varies throughout the discourse. Identifying distinct registers is not a matter of a discrete "use" or "absence of use" of the features but rather the different degrees of use within each register. I identify the registers based on the distinctive (relative) use of certain features with each register.

AN INTERACTIONAL SOCIOLINGUISTIC APPROACH

The analysis of the O'Keeffe data draws on Goffman's (1981) concept of footing. Goffman (1981:126) identifies as changes in footing cases in which the tone of discourse changes along with "an alteration in the social capacities in which the persons present claim to be active." He summarizes this phenomenon as follows:

1. Participant's alignment, or set, or stance, or posture, or projected self is somehow at issue.
2. The projection can be held across a strip of behavior that is shorter than a grammatical sentence or longer, so sentence grammar won't help us all that much, although it seem clear that a cognitive unit of some kind is involved, minimally, perhaps, a "phonemic clause." Prosodic, not syntactic, segments are implied.
3. A continuum must be considered, from gross changes in stance to the most subtle shifts in tone that can be perceived.
4. For speakers, code switching is usually involved or at least the sound markers that linguists study: pitch, volume, rhythm, stress, tonal quality.
5. The bracketing of a "higher level" phase or episode of interaction is commonly involved, the new footing having a liminal role, serving as a buffer between two more substantially sustained episodes.

Tannen and Wallat (1983:205) examine a pediatric interview, identifying the way in which the pediatrician, in communicating with the child, mother, and a video camera/crew (recording the interview for use in training students) is "addressing three audiences, each of which is involved in at least three 'frames' associated with distinct footings (Goffman 1979) marked by use of identifiable linguistic registers." My analysis of the data is similar to Tannen and Wallat's insofar as I identify four registers which are associated with four different footings. Thus the relationship between ways of speaking (register) and the social meaning reflected in and created by those ways of speaking (footing) is analyzed.

The term "frame," however, refers to "the definition of what is going on, without which no message could be interpreted" (Tannen and Wallat, 1983:207). Thus, the notion of frame involves the recognition by participants in the interaction of the frame (smooth communication) or the lack of such a joint understanding of what is going on in the interaction (problematic communication). In the current research, the data are excerpts from a movie which is clearly focused on O'Keeffe talking about herself, since it is an interview of her. The overall activity, or the frame, is "participating in an interview." While this does not mean that there is no further, subtler, shift in interactive frame throughout the interviewing, I do not analyze the frames in my data for two reasons.

First, the excerpts in the movie represent chunks of the discourse of the interview when, for the most part, O'Keeffe is dominant in the interaction. As a result, there is not enough evidence in the data to support theories concerning the reactions or participation of interlocutors other than O'Keeffe. Second, the goal of my analysis is to identify the way in which age is part of O'Keeffe's identity. Rather than focusing on people's reaction to how age is manifested in O'Keeffe's discourse, I wish to further understand how age is part of the identity O'Keeffe presents in her discourse.

It is possible to identify a hierarchy of levels of activities in the data. The higher level activity throughout the excerpts in the movie is "interviewing." Based upon my analysis of the different registers used in the data, I have identified four different footings, three of which are associated with the "interviewing" activity and one of which results in what Goffman (above) describes as a "bracketing" of the interviewing activity.

Goffman (1981:128) goes on to claim that "a change in footing implies a change in the alignment we take up to ourselves and the others present as expressed in the way we manage the production or reception of an utterance." Thus I also identify the different roles which correspond with the different footings.

The notion of role, as I use it here, is based on Goffman's (1981) analysis of the notion of speaker as "production format." The production format is made up of three elements. The animator is the person who produces the utterance; the author is the person who has determined what those utterances are to be; and the principal is the person "whose position is established by the words that are spoken, someone whose beliefs have been told, someone committed to what the words say" (*ibid.*: 144). He goes on to describe the principal suggesting that:

> one deals in this case not so much with body or mind as with a person active in some particular social identity or role, some special capacity as a member of a group, office, category, relationship, association, or whatever, some socially based source of self-identification. (*Ibid.*)

In my analysis I focus on the way in which the principal of O'Keeffe's production format changes, referring to the principal of her talk as her role. I have found that with each shift in register and footing, there is a corresponding shift in role. Further, in each role the value and relevance of age varies. That is, in the different roles her age seems to be either valued (negatively or positively) or not valued and seems to vary in the extent to which it is salient to her overall identity.[2]

THE DATA

The film, produced by Perry Miller Adato, for WNET–13 NY, celebrating Georgia O'Keeffe's 90th birthday was broadcast on WETA–23 DC in 1977. She was eighty-nine at the time of filming. The movie is a collection of excerpts of O'Keeffe talking with the interviewer and her assistant, Juan Hamilton, at her ranch in New Mexico. Interwoven with O'Keeffe's discourse are (1) images of her art work, (2) photographs of her, places she lived, and people involved in her life, (3) interviews with art critics, and (4) letters O'Keeffe wrote at earlier points in her life, read by a woman other than O'Keeffe. Thus, the film is, in a sense, a collage.

The movie celebrates O'Keeffe. One can assume that the excerpts from O'Keeffe's discourse which were included in the movie were

selected by the producers. It is important to remember, then, that there
may have been communication breakdowns during the interviews but
that these segments would obviously have been "edited out" of the final
film. As a result my analysis of O'Keeffe's discourse focuses on
understanding the discourse of an elderly woman which has been
favorably evaluated by the editors.

DATA ANALYSIS

In what follows I first identify four registers which O'Keeffe uses in the
data: reporting, narrating, teaching, and interacting registers. The
analysis focuses on her relative use of the following prosodic,
discourse, and paralinguistic features: pitch, tempo, intonational range,
function of intonation, loudness, quoted speech, and laughter. In
identifying the registers I also identify four different footings and four
different roles which correspond with these registers. Second, I analyze
the content of the discourse in each of these registers (and footings),
focusing on the references to O'Keeffe's age. This analysis contributes
to my identification of O'Keeffe's roles, allowing a determination of
whether old age is reflected in the discourse as a salient characteristic
of her identity in each role. Further, in those cases in which old age is
salient, the way in which it is valued is identified. That is, old age can
either be evaluated or not, and if evaluated it can be evaluated either
negatively or positively.

Four registers, four footings . . . four roles

In the following excerpt O'Keeffe shifts back and forth in her register
between reporting and narrating[3]. She is describing her paintings of
animal bones. She says:

| reporting | 1 | At first I painted the horses head. . . . |
| | 2 | And then I got this cow's head. |

narrating	3	And I had the cow's head painted against the blue
	4	and I thought
	5	"Well I have to do something else about that."

reporting	6	And that was at the time that
	7	the men were all talking about
	8	the great American . . . novel,
	9	the great American play,
	10	the great American . . .
	11	oh it was the great American everything.

narrating	12	And I thought they didn't know anything about America
	13	mo—a lot of them had never been across the Hudson.
	14	So I thought
	15	"I'll make my picture . . . a red white and blue (laughs)
	16	I'll make it an American painting
	17	for these people that don't go across the Hudson"

reporting	18	And this was my painting.
	19	I put a red stripe down either side . . .
	20	it entertained me
	21	but I don't think anybody else caught on to it
	22	for quite a while

In lines 1 and 2 O'Keeffe begins describing the paintings using a relatively flat intonation, emphasizing "horses" and "cow's" by using contrasting (higher) pitch and a louder voice and ending both lines with falling intonation. In line 3 there is a shift in register. Her voice has a subtle shift to a higher pitch than it has in lines 1 and 2. In line 3 she emphasizes the word "blue" by using a pitch which contrasts with her overall pitch more than the contrast in pitch when she utters "horse's' and "cow's' in lines 1 and 2. In fact, overall in lines 3–5 she uses a wider intonational range than she does in 1–2. Then, in line 5, "Well I'll have to do something else about that," O'Keeffe produces quoted discourse, reproducing her internal dialogue: she vocalizes her thoughts behind the painting.

In lines 1 and 2 O'Keeffe's speech is characterized by a relatively lower pitch and narrower intonational range, functioning to emphasis words or signal the end of the utterance with utterance-final falling intonation. I have labelled this register "reporting," based on the content of her talk. Here she is describing her art work itself, her artistic career: first she painted the horse's head, and then the cow's head. Thus, the footing, is "doing an interview on her artistic career." In this footing her role is that of an interviewee describing her career.

The register used in lines 3–5 I have labelled her "narrating" register[4]. This register is characterized by a relatively higher pitch, use of a relatively wider intonational range, and the use of quoted discourse. The content of her talk in this case is her personal experience in developing her painting. That is, in line 3 she refers to an original version of the painting of the cow's head and then communicates her decision to redo this painting by vocalizing her thoughts (at that time) in line 5, "Well I'll have to do something else about that." Here she is giving information about the personal life and experience behind the paintings described in lines 1 and 2. Thus, the footing is "telling personal stories about her art work." Her role in this footing is that of narrator of these personal anecdotes.

In line 6 there is a register shift back to "reporting." Her voice assumes a lower pitch, emphasizing the utterance-final "novel" and "play" (lines 7 and 8), indicating, with loudness as well as a slight rise in intonation, that the clauses are part of a list. In lines 1 and 2 O'Keeffe reports on her art work. In lines 6 through 11 she is describing the historical context in which these paintings were painted. Thus, the 'reporting' register is used to describe her career and to describe the historical context of her career.

In line 12, again there is a shift back to the "narrating" register. Her voice not only assumes a higher pitch, but again she uses a relatively wide intonational range. In line 12 her pitch gradually rises until "about," when it falls and then rises to a pitch relatively higher than the pitch preceding "about." Then, in pronouncing "America" she uses a lower pitch. In line 13 the intonational contour is similar to line 12, with a slight rising in pitch, culminating with the first syllable in "Hudson" being the highest pitch while the second syllable is uttered with a lower pitch. Unlike the reporting register, where changes in pitch are used only to emphasize certain words mark grammatical functions (such as the end of a sentence or an element in a list), in lines 12 and 13 the wider intonational range seems to express her amazement or disbelief that these people who were so concerned with America did not even know about America.

O'Keeffe also gives quoted discourse in lines 15–17, to describe her reasons for painting the cow's head the way she ultimately did, "I'll make my picture a red white and blue/ I'll make it an American painting/ for these people who don't go across the Hudson." Thus, again, the narrating register corresponds with talk about her personal experience behind the painting.

Finally, in lines 18–22, she switches back to the reporting register. She is describing the final version of the painting. Notice that in lines 20–22, although she is describing her views of the painting, she does not switch to the narrating register. I suggest that this is because she is not talking about her personal experience in producing the painting but, rather, is factually describing the way the painting was understood by the public. She claims in lines 21–22 that she does not think "anybody else caught on to it for quite a while," that is, people did not understand the significance of the color scheme, until later.

In excerpt 2 O'Keeffe talks about her artistic process on an abstract level. Here she uses the narrating register as well as two other registers, which I have labelled "teaching" and "interacting."

teaching	1	. . . I s— can see shapes.
	2	It's as if my mind creates shapes
	3	that I don't know about.

| interacting | 4 | I can't say it any other way (laughing) |

| teaching | 5 | that I get this shape in my head. |

| narrating | 6 | and sometimes I know what it comes from |
| | 7 | and sometimes I don't |

teaching	8	and I think . . . with myself . . .
	9	that there are few shapes
	10	that I have repeated

narrating	11	a number of times during my life
	12	and I haven't known I was repeating them
	13	until after I had done it.

Lines 1 through 3 are spoken with a slower tempo than the utterances spoken in the other three registers. She also articulates each word very clearly, to the extent that it seems as if her voice is putting emphasis on every word. In lines 1 through 3 O'Keeffe is describing the artistic process. I have labelled the register she uses her "teaching" register, since the characteristics of the register, slowness of speech and careful articulation, both function to make the discourse more easily understood. It is as if she is explaining to her audience something which may be difficult to understand. Thus, the register helps ease language comprehension. The footing when this register is used is "teaching the young what she has learned," while her role in this footing is that of a wise woman.

In line 4 O'Keeffe switches to what I have labelled her "interacting" register, that is, the register she uses when managing the social interaction at the time of speaking. In line 4, this register is reflected in her significantly faster rate of speech production, less careful articulation, and laughter. In line 4 O'Keeffe breaks from her description of her artistic process, to comment on this description. She recognizes that what she has said about visualizing shapes may not be easily comprehended by her interlocutor when she says "I can't say it any other way," laughing. While her description of her artistic process is not firmly grounded in the time and situation of talk, this utterance in line 4 is clearly more grounded in the immediate social context of talk. Thus, the footing here is "managing the social interaction at the time of talk." This footing represents a shift in activity (i.e., frame), from "doing an interview" to "interacting." Thus, it is a "bracketing" of the interview frame.

In the footings described as "doing an interview about an artist's career," "telling personal stories behind the art work," and "imparting wisdom," O'Keeffe's role (the principal of her talk) can be identified clearly as "interviewee," "storyteller," and "teacher." For the footing described as "managing the social situation at the time of interaction," however, O'Keeffe's role is not as clearly identifiable as one identity. Rather, since this footing involves interaction, her role is more clearly dependent on the immediate context of talk and her interlocutors' contributions. As a result O'Keeffe's interactive register seems to describe her everyday conversational style, (cf. Tannen, 1984).

Although the interacting register is used for longer segments at other points in the interview, it is important to recognize that a footing can be held momentarily as it is here. While this shift is clearly reflected as a register shift, it only lasts for one line in the transcript.

Again, the shift back to her teaching register in line 5 only lasts for one line. Although it is short, there is a clear shift in register. Her speech in line 5 is again relatively slow and she articulates each word carefully. Then in lines 6 and 7 she shifts to the narrating register. Although she does not use the fast speech of the "interacting" register, she is no longer using the slow rate of speech of the "teaching" register. This median rate of speech is characteristic of both the "reporting" and "narrating" register. What distinguishes lines 6 and 7 as narrating and not reporting is the higher pitch and the fact that she uses a wider intonational range.

In lines 8 and 9 the shift to the teaching register is again marked by a slower rate of speech production and careful articulation. Finally, in lines 11 through 14, O'Keeffe uses the narrating register.

The four registers, four footings, and four roles which represent the principal of O'Keeffe's discourse are summarized in Figure 1. While none of the features listed for each register are present in all four registers, there is some overlap between them. The features which distinguish the register from all other registers appear in bold. Note that the narrating register does not have a single distinctive feature, but the co-occurrence of the features of this register is unique.

When and how is old age salient?

Having identified these four registers as corresponding with four different footings and roles, the question remains: When and how is age relevant? That is, to what extent and how is O'Keeffe's identity as "old" associated with her role or identity reflected in the discourse? Analyzing the data in terms of the content of the discourse, I have identified the different ways in which "old age" seems to emerge in O'Keeffe's discourse. Each of these, again, corresponds with the different registers and footings.

When O'Keeffe is "doing an interview on her career as an artist," using the "reporting" register, her age does not seem to be very salient. Although she is talking about past events, her age does not emerge in the discourse. The only time her age does becomes relevant is when she is reporting on the historical context as in excerpt (1), which is reproduced here as excerpt (3). Here O'Keeffe is describing the cultural context which made her want to use a red, white, and blue theme in her painting of the cow's head:

(3)
1   And that was at the time the men were all talking about
2   the great American . . . novel,
3   the great American play,
4   the great American . . .
5   oh it was the great American everything.

Figure 1. Four Registers, Activities and Roles

Register	Characteristics of Register	Activity	Role
reporting	narrower intonational range; intonation used to signal grammatical relation or emphasis	doing an interview about her artistic career	interviewee
narrating	**wider intonational range; relatively higher pitch;** intonation used to signal grammatical relation or emphasis and to express emotion; laughter; quoted discourse	telling the personal stories behind her artwork	storyteller
teaching	**relatively slower rate of speech production; very clear articulation**	teaching the young what she has learned (imparting wisdom)	teacher
interacting	wider intonational range; intonation functions to signal grammatical relations and emphasis, or to express emotion; relatively higher pitch; **faster rate of speech;** laughter	managing the social situation at the time of interaction	participant in interaction (dependent on immediate context of talk)

In describing the spirit of America at the time she painted the picture, she is describing a time which the reporter and the public audience may not remember. She is describing something in the past which she experienced but which her younger audience did not. Thus, she has to describe a cultural context which her age allows her to have experienced. Here her "old age" does not seem to reflect either a particularly negative or positive value.

When O'Keeffe is "telling personal stories behind her art work" her age becomes more salient. In the following excerpt she describes what her daily painting schedule used to be when she would go out into the desert and paint in New Mexico:

(4)
1   I don't go out like that now
2   but I used to get right up in the morning
3   and start out and stay out all day.
4   I'd start off around seven
5   and not get back until around five.

In lines 1 and 2 O'Keeffe explicitly contrasts what she used to be able to do (physically) and what she can now do: "I *don't* go out like that *now*/ but I *used* to get right up in the morning." Since her ability to get up and "stay out all day" does not involve a particular physical ability but rather physical endurance, the contrast is between the physical vigor of youth and the frailty of age. Although age is more relevant here than in excerpt (3), the issue of her old age is still not central to the discourse. She goes on to talk about what she used to do when she painted in the desert. Thus, it seems that although her age is mentioned, her activities as an younger artist seem to be more salient than her age at the time of the discourse. It should be noted, however, that this subtle reference to physical weakness due to old age reflects the fact that old age is being negatively valued in this context.

Another way in which O'Keeffe's age becomes salient while she is "telling personal stories behind her art work," is in excerpt (2), repeated as excerpt (5):

(5)
1   and I think . . . with myself . . .
2   that there are few shapes
3   that I have repeated
4   a number of times during my life
5   and I haven't known I was repeating them
6   until after I had done it.

As mentioned previously, O'Keeffe uses the "teaching" register in lines 1–3 and then switches to the narrating register in lines 4–6. In lines 4–6 her old age is implied by the fact that she is describes a pattern over her lifetime. Thus, while her old age is not mentioned directly, the fact that she is looking back on her life with the hindsight of her age makes the fact of her old age salient. Further, whereas it was negatively valued in the previous excerpt as causing frailty, here it positively valued as it provides her with a lifetime of experience which she can look back on and use to understand her own artistic process more clearly. In summary, then, in the footing "telling personal stories" age is somewhat salient, but can be valued either positively *or* negatively.

When O'Keeffe is "imparting wisdom" her old age does not seem to be mentioned in the content of the discourse. For example, in the above excerpt, in lines 1–3, while using the teaching register, O'Keeffe does not mention her age. Although there is no direct reference to her age in the content of the discourse nor is it reflected in the features of her register, because of our stereotype of elderly wisdom, age is nonetheless salient to her identity as one who is imparting wisdom.[5]

Old age is clearly salient when O'Keeffe uses the 'interacting' register. For example, in the following excerpt Juan and O'Keeffe are in her studio, and Juan mentions O'Keeffe's health[6]:

(6)
1 Juan: Georgia you know everybody's not the way you are
2   they don't take care of themselves as well as you do
3 O'Keeffe: That's because they don't try to live to be a hundred

Although there is no explicit disclosing of chronological age, it seems clear that what Coupland, Coupland, and Giles (1989) identify as disjunctive age is the view of O'Keeffe's age presented here. Juan initiates the topic in lines 1 and 2 by claiming that O'Keeffe is not like everybody else in that she takes good care of herself. O'Keeffe responds, in line 3, "that's because they don't try to live to be a hundred." The discourse reflects an image of O'Keeffe as being in better health than most people due to the fact that she takes particularly good care of herself.

Another example of the disjunctive view of O'Keeffe's age which is made evident in the "interacting" register is the following. O'Keeffe is leaning on Juan's arms as they make their way across a rocky patch of ground in the desert:

(7)
1 O'Keeffe: Don't break your leg or anything like that Juan
2   It'd be awful hard for me (laughing) to carry you
3 Juan: Oh!
4   Well, you'd just have to work at it!
(O'Keeffe laughs)
5   Look over there there's no there's no

(O'Keeffe slips)
6   over there there's no stone
7   then we get into the good stuff

In lines 1–3 O'Keeffe jokes about her frailty, claiming that Juan should not hurt himself because she would not be able to carry him.[7] Juan responds to this in lines 3–4 by telling O'Keeffe she would "just have to work at it!" O'Keeffe positive response to this is made evident by her laughter. Then, while Juan is uttering lines 5–6, O'Keeffe slips on the rocks, but since she is leaning on Juan's arm, he manages to keep her standing and help her to regain her balance. There is no mention of the fact that she has slipped.

In the excerpt in which O'Keeffe is narrating the story of how she used to spend her days painting, analyzed above (4), the reference to her frailty due to old age is directly indicated. In the above excerpt, O'Keeffe makes reference to the same negatively valued characteristic of old age in a very indirect way: she sarcastically warns Juan to be careful and then mentions her frailty insofar as she would be unable to carry him. The idea of O'Keeffe's chronological age and social age being disjunctive was analyzed in the previous excerpt, in O'Keeffe's explanation that the reason is her efforts to try to live to be one hundred. Here, Juan expresses this same idea, that her disjunctive age is due to her efforts, when, in line 4 he says that she would just have to work at carrying him. The implication is that if she works at it she will be able to do it. That is, if she wishes to, she can overcome the negatively valued effects of old age.

Particularly interesting, however, is the fact that right after they joke about Juan hurting himself, she slips on the rocks. Neither Juan nor O'Keeffe draw any attention to this incident. Juan, in fact, seems to be diverting attention away from the incident by continuing his talk as if nothing had happened. Thus, while her old age was mentioned in talking about the past and contrasting what she could do then with her present frailty, the issue of her age seems more salient in this instance. It seems plausible that, when she is using the "interacting" register, the discourse and activity are firmly set in the present time and negatively valued effects of old age are very salient and very negative. Both Juan and O'Keeffe make efforts to avoid recognizing these effects explicitly although they are mentioned indirectly.

At other points in the discourse when O'Keeffe uses this "interacting" register, however, her age seems to be positively valued and salient. In the following excerpt, Juan and O'Keeffe are riding in a car.

(8)

1	Juan:	How do you like being one of the roots of Abstract American Art?
2	O'Keeffe:	Well, I must be one of the old roots.

Line 2 is the most direct reference O'Keeffe makes to her age. Whereas the salient characteristic of old age in the previous excerpt was her frailty, here her old age is positively valued: she is among the artists considered to have started an entire movement in American Art. Thus, here, she makes a more direct reference to her age within the present context in a positively valued way. In summary then, within the footing "managing the social interaction at the time of talk," age is very salient and can be valued either positively or negatively.

Figure 2 is an extension of the chart from Figure 1, incorporating the analysis of the saliency of old age and the evaluation of old age (as positive, negative, both positive and negative, or neither positive nor negative) to the previous chart which summarized the four registers, four footings, and four roles identified in O'Keeffe's discourse.

CONCLUSION

I have demonstrated that it is possible to identify subtle differences in O'Keeffe's register based on certain linguistic and paralinguistic features of her discourse. The use of these different registers can then be analyzed as corresponding with different footings: the registers are used when a certain type of activity is being engaged in. In turn, the roles of the speaker correspond with the different footings. In analyzing the content of the discourse it is then possible to determine where age is salient in the discourse and whether it is valued positively, negatively, both, or not at all. I have demonstrated that in my data the salience and value of old age vary depending on the specific role in which O'Keeffe is at the time of talk: it might not be salient, it may be salient but not valued, salient and negatively valued, salient and positively valued, or salient and both positively and negatively valued.

Figure 2. Registers, Activities, Roles: The Relevance and Evaluation of Old Age

	Characteristics of Register	Activity	Role	Relevance of Old Age	Evaluation of Old Age
r e p o r t i n g	narrower intonational range; intonation used to signal grammatical relation or emphasis	doing an interview about her artistic career	interviewee	not very relevant	neither positive nor negative
n a r r a t i n g	wider intonational range; relatively higher pitch; intonation used to signal grammatical relation or emphasis and to express emotion; laughter; quoted discourse	telling the personal stories behind her artwork	storyteller	somewhat relevant	negative or positive
t e a c h i n g	relatively slower rate of speech production; very clear articulation	teaching the young what she has learned (imparting wisdom)	teacher	relevant	positive
i n t e r a c t i n g	wider intonational range; intonation functions to signal grammatical relations and emphasis, or to express emotion; relatively higher pitch; faster rate of speech	managing the social situation at the time of interaction	participant in interaction (dependent on immediate context of talk)	very relevant	negative or positive

While many researchers recognize the heterogeneity of the elderly population as a whole as well as a diversity in the variety of behaviors a single elderly person may exhibit, the response is often to increase the number of subjects used in the study and thus be able to generalize about normative elderly behavior. In this case study of Georgia O'Keeffe's discourse, I have demonstrated that the diverse ways in which she speaks correspond with diverse ways in which old age is part of her identity. Age can be experienced in a variety of ways for each individual, and to try to eliminate this individual variation in research will ultimately inhibit researchers from understanding how the elderly experience old age in their everyday lives.

NOTES

1. I describe the function of intonation as *primarily* grammatical, emphatic, or attitudinal rather than *only* serving certain functions to indicate my agreement with Crystal's (1969:272) suggestion that when describing tonal contrasts one must speak of scales of contrastivity. He writes, ". . . it seems impossible to pronounce any utterance in such a way that it will be interpreted as carrying no attitude whatever—even the most 'objectively' pronounced utterances will be labelled 'cold,' 'unworried,' 'matter-of-fact,' 'precise,' etc." Thus, in distinguishing between different registers I identify in my data I describe the types of tonal contrast (grammatical, emphatic, or attitudinal) which are used "more" than others.

2. Applying Goffman's notion of footing, Tannen and Wallat (1983) identify three different footings in pediatric interviews. Each footing corresponds with a different register. In analyzing O'Keeffe's discourse I have found that she uses four different registers, which correspond with four different footings.

3. The transcription of the data follows the conventions which are further described in Tannen (1989:202–02). The discourse is divided into intonation units. Sentence final falling intonation is represented by a period (.); final rising intonation is represented by a question mark (?); pauses are represented by repeated periods (. . .), the number of which indicates roughly the length of pause.

4. The term "narrating" is being used as a general term, referring to the anecdotal nature of the talk uttered in this register. It is not being used to refer to the structural concept of narrative as presented in Labov (1972). The question naturally arises, however, as to what the relationship between the "narrating register" and the structural concept of narrative may be. Due to both

the scope of the present study as well as the amount of relevant data for further research on this issue, I have not explored this relationship.

5. While one might expect that her wisdom would be clearly connected with her old age, so that her old age would become positively valued and salient in the content of her discourse, this does not seem to be the case. It is interesting to note, however, that while the slowness and clarity of her teaching register can be interpreted as functioning to make what she is saying more easily comprehended, an alternate interpretation is possible. A slowing down of speech has been found to be typical of the aging voice. Although this is often accompanied by problems in articulation, it is possible that the linguistic characteristics of this teaching register signal two different identities. The clarity of articulation signals that she is teaching, while the slowness of a production signals that what she is teaching is the wisdom of old age.

6. Although Juan's age is not disclosed in the movie, it is clear that he is significantly younger than O'Keeffe.

7. In fact, due to O'Keeffe's size, one might argue that she never could have carried Juan. The idea of her carrying him now, thus can be seen as hyperbole. Used in this joking context, her disjunctive age is further emphasized.

REFERENCES

Caporeal, Linnda R. 1981. The paralanguage of caregiving: baby talk to the institutionalized aged. *Journal of Personality and Social Psychology*, 40: 876–884.

Coupland, Nikolas and Justine Coupland. 1990. Language and later life. In: H. Giles and P. Robinson, eds. *Handbook of Language and Social Psychology*. New York: John Wiley and Sons Ltd.

Coupland, Nikolas, Justine Coupland, and Howard Giles. 1989. Telling age in later life: identity and face implications. *Text*, 9: 129–151.

Coupland, Nikolas, Justine Coupland, Howard Giles, and Karen Henwood. 1988. Accommodating the elderly: invoking and extending a theory. *Language in Society*, 17: 1–41.

Coupland, Nikolas, Karen Henwood, Justine Coupland, and Howard Giles. 1990. Accommodating troubles-talk: The management of elderly self disclosure. In: Graham McGregor and R.S. White, eds. *Reception and Response: Hearer Creativity and the Analysis of Spoken and Written Texts*. London: Routledge.

Crystal, David. 1969. *Prosodic Systems and Intonation in English*. Cambridge: Cambridge University Press.

Eckert, Penelope. 1984. Age and linguistic change. In: D. Kertzer and J. Keith, eds. *Age and Anthropological Theory*. Ithaca: Cornell University Press.

Giles, Howard, Nikolas Coupland and Justine Coupland. 1991. Accommodation theory: communication, context, and consequence. In: Howard Giles, Justine Coupland and Nikolas Coupland, eds. *Contexts of Accommodation: Developments in Applied Sociolinguistics*, 1–68. Cambridge: Cambridge University Press.

Giles, Howard, Anthony Mulac, James J. Bradac, and Patricia Johnson. 1987. Speech accommodation theory: The first decade and beyond. In: Margaret L. McLaughlin, ed. *Communication Yearbook 10: An Annual Review Published for the International Communication Association*, 13–48. Newbury Park, California: Sage Publications.

Goffman, Erving. 1967. On face work. In: *Interaction Ritual*, 5–45. New York: Pantheon Books.

Goffman, E. 1979. Footing. *Semiotica* 25: 1–29.

Goffman, Erving. 1981. Footing. In: *Forms of Talk*, 124–159. Philadelphia: University of Pennsylvania Press.

Labov, William. 1972. The transformation of experience in narrative syntax. In: *Language In the Inner City*, 354–396. Philadelphia: University of Pennsylvania Press.

Ramig, L.A. 1986. Aging speech: physiological and sociological aspects. *Language and Communication*, 6, 25–34.

Sankar, Andrea. 1984. "It's just old age": old age as a diagnosis in American and Chinese medicine. In: D. Kertzer and J. Keith, eds. *Age and Anthropological Theory*. Ithaca: Cornell University Press.

Shadden, Barbara, ed. 1988. *Communication Behavior and Aging*. Baltimore: Williams and Wilkins.

Tannen, Deborah. 1984. *Conversational style: Analyzing Talk Among Friends*. Norwood, NJ: Ablex.

Tannen, Deborah. 1989. *Talking Voices: Repetition, Dialogue, and Imagery in Conversational Discourse. Studies in Interactional Sociolinguistics 6*, ed. John J. Gumperz. Cambridge University Press: Cambridge.

Tannen, Deborah, and Cynthia Wallat. 1983. Doctor/mother/child communication: linguistic analysis of a pediatric interaction. In: Sue Fisher and Alexandra Dundas Todd, eds. *The Social Organization of Doctor-Patient Communication*. Washington, DC: Center for Applied Linguistics, 203–219.

Ward, Russell. 1984. The marginality and salience of being old: when is age relevant? *The Gerontologist*, 24: 227–232.

WNET-13 movie. 1977. *Georgia O'Keeffe*. Produced by Perry Miller Adato.

CHAPTER 10

"I Can't Drive"

Painful Self-Disclosure in Intergenerational Talk

Shoko Yohena Okazaki[1]

The meaning of age and the elderly as a social category differs from one culture to another. How a certain communicative behavior of the elderly is perceived by the younger generation may be influenced significantly by the status of the elderly in the society. In intergenerational communication, even when the interlocutors try to establish a common ground in the conversation, lack of shared knowledge and different points of view may result in miscommunication, which further contributes to the development of stereotypes against the elderly speech and against intergenerational interactions.

This paper examines a case of "painful" self-disclosure, which was suggested by J. Coupland, N. Coupland, Giles, and Wiemann (1988) as one of the characteristic phenomena of elderly speech. The disclosure of information about one's misfortune and painful experience is found to be an essential mode of talk employed by the elderly even when they are talking with strangers. In the present study, I analyze an informal interview with an elderly woman, Mary. Her painful self-disclosure centers around the theme of her not being able to drive because of the stroke which affected her eyes four years prior to the interview. By applying Coupland and Coupland's notion of painful self-disclosure not only to the elderly talk but also to cross-cultural communication, I argue that certain variables in communication facilitate and even encourage the occurrence of the painful self-disclosure in intergenerational talk. Further, I claim that lack of age-relevant shared experience may cause miscommunication and develop stereotypes.

While painful self-disclosure can be one of the important strategies for creating rapport between participants, social meanings accomplished by the painful self-disclosure are different for the elderly and for the young. For this reason, a "cross-talk" (Gumperz 1982) or misinterpretation of communicative intent may occur in inter-generational conversation as is often found in cross-cultural interactions.

I also discuss the significance of certain social events such as giving up driving in one's later life. Such events may change the communication network for the elderly and influence the elderly identity and the way the elderly talk. Since age is a social category as well as a chronological category, it is important to take such socially significant events into consideration in research on the elderly.

In the sections to follow, I first review some of the previous work on language use and the elderly with an emphasis on intergenerational talk and painful self-disclosure, followed by method of data collection. Then I present the analysis of painful self-disclosure of being unable to drive as revealed in one intergenerational conversation. I apply and extend the notions of Coupland and Coupland's framework to cross-cultural communication, since intergenerational talk can be seen as a type of cross-cultural communication in a broad sense as argued in Giles, N. Coupland, J. Coupland, Williams, and Nussbaum (1992). After discussing the significance of giving up driving for the elderly in the U.S., I will show how phatic questions can facilitate painful self-disclosure. My question of "Do you like it here?", which was meant to be more or less a phatic question, lets Mary reveal various painful information about her life, including her inability to drive. The topic of Mary's family is also connected with the theme of "I can't drive," as she repeats that if she could drive, she would go and see her children and grandchildren more often. Then I discuss the ways Mary presents a more positive and independent identity by counter-balancing her loss of face. The final section of analyses deals with miscommunication found in mutual disclosure of painful information, followed by the conclusion of this study and suggestions for future research.

THE ELDERLY IN INTERGENERATIONAL TALK

In sociolinguistics, age has been one of the salient variables in research on communicative behavior of human beings, but it is often classified simply by informants' chronological age. Age is, however, a more complex, socially developed feature and a careful consideration of its social aspect is necessary for understanding the relationship between language and aging. Rosenfeld's study (this volume) as well as J. Coupland, N. Coupland, and Grainger (1991), for example, show a variation of talk by the same elderly speakers in relation to their elderly identity.

Ward (1984: 227) claims that the meaning of age changes across cultures and over time because "the life cycle is embedded within different and changing social contexts." In addition, Ward points out that informal social networks play an important role in shaping the personal implications of aging. As we will see in this study, giving up driving in later life could imply separation from one's former community and friends since my informant, Mary, moved to an urban city where she can depend on public transportation. Such a change in social networks influences the shape of her social identity and the meaning of aging. It is also reflected in the way she talks as she repeats her frustration about being unable to drive.

This aspect of old age as a social category which is culturally and socially shaped by various assumptions is crucial for understanding intergenerational communication. The status of old age in a society influences the development of stereotypes toward the elderly, and these stereotypes may be reflected in the way the young communicate with the elderly. Overaccommodation and underaccommodation of speech may be typical examples.

Speech accommodation theory, the framework developed by Giles and his co-workers, seeks to explain the speaker's motives and behaviors to accommodate their speech in relation to the addressee's speech characteristics. Ryan, Giles, Bartolucci, and Henwood (1986) applied the notion of speech accommodation to intergenerational communication. They found that the young accommodated their speech toward the old for such reasons as (1) physical/sensory handicaps of the elderly, (2) over-protective and directive attitudes toward the elderly because they are "dependent" or "needy," and (3) the stereotypical view by the young toward the elderly. The potential consequences of such overaccommodation are, as Ryan et al. (1986:16) argue, the predicament of aging characterized by a vicious cycle in which "the changes of aging (e.g. physical appearance, voice quality, hearing difficulties, slowness of movement, loss of role) elicit interpretations from others of diminished competence; and these inferences then lead to constraining conditions in which the older person has less opportunity to communicate effectively."

Further, N. Coupland, J. Coupland, Giles, and Henwood (1988) examine accommodative behaviors from bilateral perspectives, that is, from the old to the young and from the young to the old. This is an important addition to intergenerational communication because communication problems may well have their origin in both sides.

N. Coupland et al. (1988) find that there is a sociological basis of miscommunication between the younger person and the older person. For example, the elderly may find it difficult to respond appropriately to phatic expressions such as "How have you been? What's happening?" if that person does not go out or do new things because of his/her physical weakness. Similarly "How are you?" may invoke a lengthy and specific explanation of sickness and pain that the elderly person is suffering from. This may in turn make the younger interlocutors feel it is extremely difficult to relate to the elderly.

When "How are you?" was asked by doctors in medical contexts, it was found that elderly patients and their doctors negotiate as to when they are moving into medical inquiry from the socio-relational frame of conversational openings (Coupland and Coupland 1992). Since social aspects are as important as medical/physical concerns for the elderly, "how are you" questions serve as important conversational openings. Therefore, J. Coupland, Robinson, and N. Coupland (1994:120) claim that "doctors will need to negotiate medical outcomes in the context of social considerations." Coupland and Coupland's more recent analysis (this volume) also emphasizes that it is through the negotiation between doctors and their elderly patients that the elderly persons' identities regarding age and health are constructed and reconstructed.

Moreover, N. Coupland et al. (1988) claim that occasional strongly asserted contributions by the elderly to the conversation should be examined against the background of power relationship between the elderly and the young. The younger interlocutor, in their study, had a leading conversational role, and a large majority of new transactions are opened by her. The younger interlocutor's frequent follow-up moves are also regarded as an indicator of the extent of her conversational responsibility.

In a revised version of accommodation theory, J. Coupland, N. Coupland, Giles, and Wiemann (1988) videotaped intergenerational and intragenerational interactions in which the participants (N= 40; 20 elderly and 20 young females) met for the first time and were instructed to "get to know each other." It was found that the female elderly tended to disclose personal and "painful" information (such as being widowed for many years, losing eyesight, having pain, etc.) far more frequently than their younger counterparts did.

N. Coupland, Henwood, J. Coupland, and Giles (1990) further found that painful self-disclosure was often perceived negatively by the younger persons as a "conscious intent on the part of some elderly people." For example, one of the young stated to the researchers after the videotaping that "they are trying to make you feel sorry for them in some way." The labels for the painful self-disclosures given by the younger subjects are *depressing, moaning, boring, selfish, rambling, rattling on,* etc. These potentially negative evaluations are sometimes transformed into sympathetic evaluations through considerations of elderly stereotypes ("old age is often a fairly sad situation"). Subsequently these evaluations form learned or reproduced knowledge about the elderly and about intergenerational talk, and they further develop stereotypes.

These stereotypes are often reflected in the research on linguistic competence of the elderly. The notion of *decrement* assumes that linguistic competence declines as people get older. N. Coupland and J. Coupland (1990: 452) argue that "a whole tradition of existing work, the deficit tradition, is in danger of adopting a stereotypically based set of assumptions about how diachrony and decrement 'naturally' relate to aging as a process, and so to what is researchable and knowable about elderly populations."

The notion of "normalcy" or "what constitutes 'normal' behavior" has long been used in a confusing manner in research. Many of the psycholinguistic and gerontological studies on linguistic competence of the elderly have been conducted on experimental situations. The "normalcy" of the older subjects is determined according to criteria of general health. There was little consideration for other socially sensitive variables such as educational background, social status, and gender. Since many studies were conducted in experimental settings, there is a question about real-life implications of the results. Moreover, the motivational and attitudinal factors are not taken into account, and, as a result, it is hard to know how much of the test result is due to the circumstances of the experiments that the elderly people are placed under, and how much is the true reflection of the subjects' linguistic competence. The data collected from these experiments generally conform to the expectation of decrement.

In order to overcome the problems stated above and to explore real-life implications of intergenerational talk, interactional sociolinguistics and discourse analysis of data obtained in naturalistic settings provide useful tools for analyses. It is this approach that this study will take. Interactional sociolinguistics is the framework developed by Gumperz (1982) and further expanded by Tannen (1984), and its major concern is examinations of the interactive nature of conversation. As Tannen (1992) explains it, conversation is seen as a joint production of the interlocutors rather than the unilateral product of the speaker. It is through the interactive nature of naturally occurring discourse that people create and interpret meaning in actual conversations. Discourse analyses from this perspective typically use audio- or video-taped conversations with detailed transcriptions including intonational and prosodic contours, pauses, and laughter, since all of these could affect the establishment and interpretation of meanings.

Gumperz (1982) introduces the notion of "discourse strategies" which are used by both the speaker and the hearer in order to create and maintain conversational meaning. Gumperz suggests that participants of conversation attend to the information beyond grammatical and lexical knowledge: what conversational activities they are involved in (serious discussion or just chatting?), what communicative intentions are implied by the speaker's utterances, how to participate in conversational routine (how to take turns, how to use backchannels, and so on), and how to interpret linguistic and non-linguistic cues (intonational and prosodic contours, eye contact, etc.). In cross-cultural settings, Gumperz argues that even if both the speaker and the hearer speak the same language, these discourse strategies may be used differently. As a result, "cross-talk" may occur: Communicative intentions are interpreted differently, and repeated misunderstanding could cause creation of stereotypes against certain ethnic groups.[2]

Tannen (1984) further shows that each speaker has different conversational styles which are partly rooted in the interlocutors' subcultural backgrounds within the same culture. When participants do not share communicative presuppositions about how conversation is created and maintained, they often misunderstand each other's communicative intentions. Moreover, because of the multiple levels and dimensions involved in communication, N. Coupland, Wiemann, and Giles (1991) see communication as pervasively miscommunicative and problematic.

Based on these findings from interactional sociolinguistics, then, careful examinations of the backgrounds of informants, communicative behaviors, and the conversational settings in which data are obtained are crucial for understanding intergenerational talk. It is also important to look for recurring patterns and strategies in interactions, as they provide essential clues to understanding what is actually going on in conversations.

Hamilton (1989, 1994) conducted sociolinguistic analyses of naturally occurring discourse with an Alzheimer's patient. By examining the data recorded at a nursing home for the elderly over the period of five years, she found significant changes in the discourse strategies of the interlocutors and the way questions and answers were handled in conversations. As the patient's ability to comprehend and maintain conversations decreased, the healthy partner's conversational strategies were also changed so that conversational routines could be maintained on the surface. Her study suggests the importance of minute analyses of elderly discourse from an interactional perspective as well as a longitudinal perspective.

Further in discourse analysis, Boden and Bielby (1986: 85) emphasize the importance of a research agenda located in natural settings, stating that "communication is not merely episodic exchange between patient and health care provider, nor between general service providers and the senior community, but rather an ongoing daily activity which needs to be studied as such." They analyzed conversations between elderly persons who were instructed to get to know each other, and they found that topic selection and formulation in the conversations between the elderly were closely related to their present identity.

> Elderly interactants employ shared historical life-events, time periods and social experiences as topic-organizing units. These long-past slices-of-life are frequently used interactively to contrast "the way it was" with "the way it is." (Boden and Bielby 1986: 75)

Thus, personal history and experience in the past are used to negotiate the present identity of the elderly person, and therefore "talking about the past" is a functional and effective form of communication for the elderly. Many researchers, for example Shadden (1988), identify the later life stage as the time to review one's life and evaluate past experiences. Many elderly individuals, therefore, often talk about their past as they go through this process of life review. Talking about shared historical life events not only contributes to the establishment of the identity and the creation of intimacy between the elderly interlocutors, but it also has an important function in evaluating one's life in the later stage. In intergenerational conversation, however, the young interlocutors may lack the shared historical life events to establish a common ground for communication. Talking about the past may rather function to emphasize the differences between the interlocutors.

DATA COLLECTION AND THE DESCRIPTION OF THE PARTICIPANTS

The data for this study were obtained from an informal interview of an elderly person (Mary) by a non-native English speaker who is a graduate student in linguistics (Shoko). Mary was asked by a friend of hers to meet with me for my project on linguistics. Prior to the interview, she was not told the specific purpose of the interview. Mary and I met in her apartment, and the conversation was audio-recorded with her permission by a small tape recorder placed on the coffee table in front of her. The interview consisted of two general parts, an introductory stage of "getting to know each other," and Mary's narrative discourse about nursery stories and children's books which she tells or reads to her grandchildren.

After the conversation was recorded, I transcribed it. I tried to write down not only the verbal forms of utterances but also some paralinguistic features such as rising intonation, pausing, laughter, overlapping speech, and so on. I used the following conventions in order to show certain paralinguistic features in the transcripts. These are based on Tannen (1984).

CAPS	emphatic stress
?	yes/no question rising intonation
!	exclamation
:	lengthened vowel sound
.	sentence final falling intonation
. . .	noticeable pause or break
(2.0)	2 seconds pause
[laugh]	laughter
|_	overlapping speech (two speakers are talking at the same time)
/?/	unintelligible utterance

The transcribed data including such paralinguistic features provided important information for understanding the dynamics of the intergenerational talk.

At the time of data collection, Mary was a sixty-eight-year-old white American. She had three children and seven grandchildren. Her husband had died four years earlier, and, at about the same time, she had had a mild stroke which affected her eyesight. She used to live in southern Virginia, but when the interview was conducted, she was living in Washington, DC, by herself in an apartment complex for the elderly. Because she could not drive anymore and because there was no public transportation in the area where she used to live, she moved to Washington, DC, so that she could travel by public transportation. Other than poor eyesight, she did not have major sensory or cognitive problems.

At the time of recording, I was thirty years old, a Japanese graduate student at Georgetown University. I had studied in Los Angeles, California, from 1984 to 1987 and came to Washington, DC, in 1990, where I lived for two years.

THE THEME OF "I CAN'T DRIVE"

One of the recurring topics during our conversation was that of Mary being unable to drive because of her weak eyesight. It resulted in her feelings of loneliness due to lack of transportation. Eckert (1984) suggests that the time of retirement has a significant social meaning in one's life. Since it changes the kind of communication network people participate in, sociolinguists should pay more attention to the language change around this stage of life. I want to propose that immobility also contributes to the identity of elderly persons. In the United States, in addition to retirement, giving up driving creates a significant change in the life of the elderly. Bruce (1994: 49) states that, in 1990, 22 million of the 167 million licensed drivers (13%) were over sixty-five. This number is expected to grow in the future; the number of drivers eighty-five years of age will more than double, increasing from 3.1 million in 1990 to 8.1 million in 2030. According to Campbell, Bush, and Hale (1993), who studied older adults aged seventy to ninety-six in Florida, 17% had quit driving. Among these, 50% of the decisions could be related to health conditions of the elderly. Kington, Reuben, Rogowski, and Lee (1994) further report that those who have better self-perceived health are more likely to drive, but persons who live with other adults tend to rely on the others for transportation, and therefore they are less likely to drive. Self-restriction of driving after dark seems to be an intermediate stage before quitting driving completely. It is also found that women tend to quit driving more often than men. NHTSA (National Highway Traffic Safety Administration) statistics (cited by Bruce 1994) show that almost one fifth of women between seventy-five and eighty-four quit driving. Only about half of the women over eighty-five, compared to two-thirds of the men over eighty-five, are still licensed to drive.

Those who cannot drive must choose among being dependent on younger people for transportation, having to move to urban areas where they can use public transportation in order to maintain their independence, staying at home, or moving into senior citizens' housing/nursing homes. Bruce (1994) comments that removing a driver's license from an elderly individual is a serious step, because it often means loss of mobility and freedom, particularly for those living in suburban and rural areas.[3]

Loss of mobility may change the communication network and social roles of elderly persons as well as the self-image and social identity of the elderly. Those who cannot drive are what J. Coupland, N. Coupland, and Grainger (1991) call "members of a disadvantaged group of society," because of their limited mobility and dependence on other members of the society. It is "the end of independence" (Bruce 1994:49). Further, one National Transportation Safety Board researcher (cited by Bruce 1994:49) points out that denying a driver's license to an older person can be an extremely traumatic event psychologically, especially for some retired men. When men stop driving, some of them may even die soon thereafter.

In the present study, Mary chose to move to Washington, DC, because of its better public transportation system. Moving to a new area in later life can be a very "painful" event for the elderly. Even if public transportation is available, being unable to drive makes it more difficult for the elderly persons to go back to their former community than for the young. She states her wish to drive and visit her family members and friends in Southwestern Virginia in the following conversation.

Example 1

Mary:	I MISS driving
	NOT because I would want to drive HERE,
	but I miss it when it comes to see my grandchildren
Shoko:	mmm
Mary:	or going back to where I lived before I came here
	or visiting friends.
Shoko:	Yes.
Mary:	Not being able to drive makes
Shoko:	uhuh
Mary:	makes it uh difficult.

Even if airplanes, taxis, and buses are available, not being able to drive sometimes limits the time of the year that the elderly persons can travel long distances. Mary states in another part of the conversation that she has to travel during the summertime so that she does not need to carry heavy winter clothes. She thinks that if she could drive, she could put her belongings in the car and could visit her children even for Christmas:

Example 2

Mary:	and when I'm traveling
	I'm alone,
	and I can't carry all that much.
Shoko:	No.
Mary:	If I could drive,
	I might even go up for Christmas sometime because
	I could put my clothes in the car.

All of these difficulties in traveling or visiting families and friends contribute to feelings of loneliness and separation. When Mary talks about the frustration of not being able to drive, her statements are closely related to her desire to spend more time with her children and grandchildren. She repeatedly states that she does not see them often and she misses them:

Example 3

Mary: I don't see them very often because . . .
        and I miss them.
Shoko: Oh, I'm sure.
Mary: I would, I wish I were close enough to see them
Shoko: Uhuh uhuh.
Mary: and if I had a CAR,
        I could drive, I would get in my car,
        go up, and VISIT.

Later—

Mary: I don't, as I said I don't see them
        very often,
Shoko: Uhuh uhuh.
Mary: since I can't drive.

As can be seen in examples 1–3, the theme of "I can't drive" is prevalent in this interaction, and it indicates the significance of driving cars in U.S. society. Not driving seems to be closely integrated into the identity of this older American woman, especially since she lived in a rural area.

In the sections to follow, I examine how this theme of "I can't drive" is raised and maintained and what social and communicative meanings it conveys. First, I examine phatic questions. The different points of view between Mary and me concerning driving create a slight miscommunication or "cross-talk" in the intergenerational conversation, and they further facilitate the recurrence of the theme. The negative image about her not being able to drive is emphasized as a result.

PHATIC QUESTIONS AND PAINFUL SELF-DISCLOSURE

J. Coupland, N. Coupland, Giles, and Wiemann (1988) found that the disclosure of personal and "painful" information is a potentially significant mode of elderly talk. The types of painful information were categorized into *ill health, bereavement, immobility, disengagement and loneliness,* and others (such as failing marriage). In my data, Mary discloses most of the information indicated above in spite of the fact that she and I had met for the first time. Moreover, she connects all of these painful experiences to the fact that she cannot drive. For example, she talks about her stroke and weakening of her eyesight (ill health), her husband's death (bereavement), immobility caused by giving up driving, and disengagement and loneliness as a result of being unable to see her children and grandchildren frequently.

J. Coupland et al. (1988: 211) consider utterances such as *how are you?* and *are you keeping well?* as "likely elicitation of disclosure rather than as mere phatic openings . . . by virtue of some elderly's apparent propensity to define potentially phatic questions as contentful elicitations." They categorize these questions as direct elicitations of painful self-disclosure. In medical situations, J. Coupland and N. Coupland (1992) and J. Coupland, Robinson, and N. Coupland (1994) find that both elderly patients and their doctors negotiate when "how are you?" is intended to elicit the information about medical symptoms and when the interlocutors are still in a socio-relational frame of talk. J. Coupland and N. Coupland (1992: 226) claim that although disclosure of personal medical troubles is face-threatening, "there are some elderly people for whom other priorities (e.g., felt indignation or bitterness or a desire to disclose cathartically) supersede the need to respect face[4] needs." In addition, a question about the elderly person's family or life circumstances may also allow painful self-disclosure even though it does not specifically invite it. J. Coupland et al. (1988) call this an indirect elicitation. Thus, questions such as *do you have any children?* and *where are your family living now?* may indirectly invite speech about separation from family members or misfortune.

In Example 4, in response to my question of whether Mary was originally from Washington, DC, or not, she explained that she used to live in Washington, DC, when she was a child, but she moved to different places, and then she came back to Washington, DC, four years ago. My question "do you like it here?" (line 7) invokes Mary's whole narrative of the reason why she came back to Washington, DC, and why she did not like living in this area. The narrative includes her disclosure of her husband's death, her ill health and giving up driving (indicated by arrows in the transcript).

Example 4

1	Mary:	I, I never lived in Washington again after
2		that.
3	Shoko:	mmm
4	Mary:	until four years ago [laugh]

5	Shoko:	Oh, I see.
6	Mary:	Yes.
7	Shoko:	And do you like it here?
8	Mary:	Not really.
9		I, I don't like cities. [laugh]
10	Shoko:	Oh, I see.
11	Mary:	I like living in the country.
12	Shoko:	mhm
13	Mary:	But uh but it's I mean, cities are all right
14		and I have to be where I can get public
15		transportation.
16	Shoko:	mhm
17	Mary:	And in the small
18		town that I lived in uh

-> 19   at that time my husband died,

-> 20   I had a mild stroke that affected my eyes.

| 21 | Shoko: | Oh |

-> 22   Mary: so that I can't get a driver's license.

23	Shoko:	uhuh
24	Mary:	And so uh
25		if you live in a small town in southwestern
26		Virginia, you don't,

-> 27   you can't live there if you can't drive

28	Shoko:	Right.
29	Mary:	There's no, no public transportation.
30	Shoko:	That's right.
31	Mary:	So, that's why I'm in Washington.

My question in line 7 ("do you like it here?") was meant to be more or less a general phatic question, and I did not expect a specific and elaborated explanation about the reason why Mary liked or disliked living in Washington. Mary answers "not really" and states that she likes living in the country rather than in cities. Then she further elaborates her answer by telling me why she lives in the city of Washington, DC, despite the fact that she does not like living there. Her reason is that she has to be where she can depend on public transportation since she can not drive any more as a result of the mild stroke. In line 19, she reveals the fact that her husband died and, in line 20, that she had a mild stroke, both of which disclose personal and painful experience.

J. Coupland et al. (1988) argue that the disclosure of such information to a stranger may be one of the characteristics of women's speech in general when both the speaker and the hearer are women. Moreover, the tendency to do so is found among elderly women more frequently than among young females. Mary may have disclosed her personal information because both she and I are female. In addition, Mary may have felt obliged to provide the specific reason for her negative answer because "not really" was not a preferred answer to such a phatic question, and it could create what Brown and Levinson (1987) call "positive face threat." Positive face is one of the basic needs in maintaining human relationships. It is the desire to be accepted and liked by others as well as claiming commonalties with others. Giving an unpreferred answer to a question in a socio-relational frame of talk potentially threatens this positive face. Therefore Mary provides the reasons why she does not like Washington, DC ("I like living in the country"). She also provides the reason why she moved to Washington, DC. That is, she had a mild stroke which caused her to give up driving.

My response to Mary's self-disclosure in line 21 was a sympathetic exclamation of "Oh," which falls into the category of "minimal moves" in J. Coupland et al. (1988). The minimal moves are the minimal response (such as *oh dear, good heavens* and *mm*) to the elderly person's "painful" self-disclosure. The affective force of such minimal moves seems to be "heavily dependent upon non-verbal and prosodic/paralinguistic realizations," and some responses such as *oh dear* "may be taken to encode sympathy, at least in their unmarked realization" (J. Coupland et al. 1988: 226). My tone of voice (and perhaps my facial expression, too, although the data are not available as the conversation was not videotaped) seems to encode my sympathetic attitude toward her losing her husband and having a stroke at about the same time. This move may have encouraged Mary's further self-disclosure of the negative information in her next turn: "so that I can't get a driver's license" (line 22).

TALKING ABOUT FAMILIES

Topics which were related to Mary's children or grandchildren also initiated her painful self-disclosure about not being able to drive and not having many opportunities to see them. In talking about where her children live, Mary reintroduced the theme of "I can't drive" in relation to her feelings of loneliness.

Example 5

1	Mary:	That, my older boy has four children,
2	Shoko:	uhuh
3	Mary:	and my younger boy has three.
4	Shoko:	Wow.
5	Mary:	But they all live
6		pretty far away.
7	Shoko:	uhuh
8	Mary:	um the older boy lives in New Hampshire
9	Shoko:	uhuh
10	Mary:	and the younger boy lives in Connecticut
11		and our daughter lives in uh Pennsylvania
12	Shoko:	I see.
13	Mary:	So, it's, it's not easy.
->14		I don't see them very often because . . .
->15		and I miss them.
16	Shoko:	Oh, I'm sure.
17	Mary:	I would, I wish I were close enough to see
18		them
19	Shoko:	uhuh uhuh
->20	Mary:	And if I had a CAR,
->21		I could drive, I would get in my car,
->22		go up, and VISIT.
23	Shoko:	Oh yes.

After mentioning how many children each of Mary's sons has, Mary comments "but they all live pretty far away" (lines 5 and 6). This comment is followed by a list of places where her children live and the disclosure of the fact that she does not see them often. This in turn invited the statement of her wish to be able to drive a car so that she could visit her children (lines 17, 18, 20, 21, and 22).

What is interesting here is that in line 14, when she says "I don't see them very often because . . .," she does not complete her utterance, and *because* is said in a very low and soft voice. She could have said something like "I don't see them very often because *I can't drive*," but, instead of talking about driving, she continues her turn, saying "and I miss them." It could be the case that she might have been afraid of damaging her positive face since she had already talked about giving up driving twice prior to this interaction.

My response in line 16 ("oh I'm sure") again conveyed a tone of voice which signals my sympathy to her, and it encouraged Mary to continue. The sympathetic attitude created a supportive atmosphere in which Mary could talk about her difficulty and loneliness of not being able to see her family frequently. The disclosure of personal information and sharing the feelings of pain contribute to the creation of involvement (Tannen 1990). As N. Coupland et al. (1990) argue, the listener's response seems to facilitate the context for the elderly to continue disclosing painful and personal information. My sympathetic tone of voice (and probably facial expressions as well) resulted in encouraging more of her self-disclosure. My conversational style may also have put some pressure on her to disclose further information; being a non-native speaker of English and being a Japanese woman, my utterances are generally very short and full of backchannels, which encourage the current speaker to continue to talk[5]. It may have signaled "Keep talking. I am listening to you, and I am interested in your talk." It resulted in reassuring her that she could continue to disclose her "painful" information. So, she talks about it in lines 20 to 22.

Duranti (1986) suggests that listeners can be seen as co-authors of a conversation since the speakers direct and the listeners ratify the speech, and thus the conversation is maintained jointly. In interactional sociolinguistics, a conversation is seen not as a unilateral product of the speaker but as a complex interaction of the relationships of interlocutors, culture, pragmatic concerns, and society. Thus, it is not just the elderly person's communicative style or tendency to disclose personal information, but the combination of the listener's response pattern and interactional expectations which allows an extended occurrence of painful self-disclosure.

COUNTER-BALANCE AND RATIFICATION

After the elderly disclose their personal and negative information to the listener at the risk of damaging their positive face and threatening the listener's negative face (the needs for not being imposed upon), they sometimes try to compensate for the loss of face as discussed in J. Coupland et al. (1988). During the conversation, Mary counter-balances her loss of face by stating something more positive such as visiting her children once a year. She also avoids taking full responsibility for not being able to visit her children for Christmas by implying that it is the cold weather, rather than her physical problem, which prevents her from traveling in winter.

Example 6

1	Mary:	and if I had a CAR,
2		I could drive, I would get in my car,
3		I go up, and VISIT.
4	Shoko:	Oh yes.
5	Mary:	but uh,
6	Shoko:	That's too bad.
-> 7	Mary:	um, I, I do go up once a year, I go up.
8	Shoko:	mhm
9	Mary:	and and
10	Shoko:	for Christmas?
11	Mary:	No, no, in the summer.
12	Shoko:	uhuh
-> 13	Mary:	It's too cold to go up THERE for Christmas
14		[laugh]
15	Shoko:	Oh I see, oh yeah, that's right.

After hearing Mary's wish to drive for the third time in the interaction, I said "that's too bad" (line 6) which is an explicit acknowledgment of her misfortune and difficult life. This utterance can be a potential threat to Mary's positive face since it may imply "I admit that your situation is very bad. I feel sorry for you because you cannot visit your children even though you want to." While my utterance is meant to be sympathetic, it also places her in the position of a passive and unfortunate person who cannot do what she wants to do.

In line 7, however, she mentions that she goes up and visits her children once a year, counter-balancing her loss of face with the positive statement. Then I ask her a follow-up question, "for Christmas?" Christmas is a common time for family gatherings in the U.S. But this question invited another negative answer from Mary ("no, no, in the summer"), which is followed by her reasoning ("it's too cold to go up THERE for Christmas.") This utterance seems to be functioning as the counter-balance against her face threat. By referring to the cold weather, she seems to indicate that she is not fully responsible for avoiding a trip in winter but that it is the weather which prevents her from spending Christmas with her family.

In another instance, the counter-balance occurs in relation to her not wanting to drive in Washington, DC. In the following example, I tell Mary that I had a hard time getting around in Los Angeles since I did not have a car, and therefore I like Washington, DC, in terms of the public transportation system.

Example 7

1	Shoko:	So, it was really hard for me.
2		and so, with that part, I really like
3		Washington, DC.
4	Mary:	Oh, Washington is much,
5		it's really easy to get around.
6	Shoko:	mhm mhm
7	Mary:	I find it, not me,
8		not,
9		I MISS driving
->10		NOT because I would want to drive HERE
11		but I miss it when it comes to see my
12		grandchildren
13	Shoko:	mmm
14	Mary:	or going back to where where I lived before
15		I came here or visiting friends.
16	Shoko:	Yes.
17	Mary:	Not being able to drive makes
18	Shoko:	uhuh
19	Mary:	makes it uh difficult.
20	Shoko:	Yeah, oh yes. I understand.
21	Mary:	But while I'm here in the city,
22	Shoko:	mhm right.
->23	Mary:	I wouldn't want to drive.
24	Shoko:	[laugh] That's right.

Even though Mary agrees with me in lines 4 and 5 that it is very easy to get around by public transportation in Washington, DC, she still states that she misses driving and elaborates the reason for that in her next turn. That is, she misses driving *not* because she wants to drive in the city but because she wants to visit her family members and friends who live far away. Mary further states in line 23 that she would not want to drive in the city even if she could drive. Her utterance seems to imply that it is her choice (rather than the unfortunate circumstance) that leads her not to drive in Washington, DC. This factor of intentionality and independence on making a choice to drive or not presents a very different image of her from someone who is forced to give up driving in spite of the desire to drive. In her study of conversations with an Alzheimer's disease patient, Hamilton (1996) also points out that creation and reflection of identity as "patient" is closely related to the way a patient is positioned as either dependent or being unable to carry out certain tasks.

MUTUAL DISCLOSURE AND MISCOMMUNICATION

As has been seen, Mary reveals her personal and negative information to me frequently and most of her disclosures are related to the fact that she cannot drive. In response, I show sympathy for her and try to relate to her feelings of difficulty by disclosing my own personal experience. Tannen (1990) points out that one of the characteristics of women's trouble talk is that women show sympathy by matching experiences, reinforcing similarity of their experiences, and then encouraging the speaker to tell more. However, in the present study, I was born and raised in Japan, where the public transportation is well developed and many people may never own cars during their lives. In addition, I am much younger than Mary. Therefore it becomes difficult for me to relate to her frustration of giving up driving *in the United States* in one's *later life.*

The following conversation is an example of this mismatch in perspectives. When Mary says that she has to visit her children in the summer because she cannot carry heavy winter clothes by herself, I try to relate to her by revealing the fact that I cannot carry heavy things either because of surgeries on my arm. Prior to this conversation, Mary mentioned that if she could drive, she could put heavy clothes in her car, so it would not be a problem to travel in winter. She ratifies my statement of having a problem with my arm, but she also distinguishes the difference between traveling light because of one's arm and because of giving up driving:

Example 8

   1   Mary: You, you just can't carry all of the stuff.
   2   Shoko: Yes, yeah.
   3   Mary: So, I, I travel very light in summertime

4		[laugh]
5	Shoko:	mhm that's a good idea.
6		Yeah, I understand.
7	Mary:	—It makes the difference.
8	Shoko:	Yes. See, I have a problem with my arm, too.
9	Mary:	—mm—
10	Shoko:	I had surgery twice,
11	Mary:	mhm
12	Shoko:	on my arm,
13		um, it was, I had um some kind of tumor.
14	Mary:	mhm
15	Shoko:	And so, um, it's now okay,
16		but I cannot carry heavy things,
17	Mary:	carry heavy things, no.
18	Shoko:	So, I, I usually try to, you know, travel
19		light.
20	Mary:	Yes, well you have to.
21	Shoko:	I understand.
22	Mary:	because there's no no way you can carry /?/
23	Shoko:	No, mhm
24	Mary:	just by yourself.
25	Shoko:	Right.
–>26	Mary:	Even if, even if your, your arm's strong
–>27		there's a limit to what you can carry.
28	Shoko:	That's right.
29	Mary:	So um, summer time works out well. [laugh]

Mary states that she travels very light in summertime because she cannot carry heavy winter clothes. I agree with her and show understanding ("that's a good idea. Yeah, I understand"). Mary further approves herself by stating "it makes the difference" which overlaps with my utterance.

Then I disclose my problem with my arm and mention that I cannot carry heavy things either (lines 8, 13, and 16). Here I try to establish common ground with Mary in terms of having to travel light. I also try to match up with Mary in disclosing painful information (having a tumor and two surgeries, being unable to carry heavy things). J. Coupland et al. (1988) observe a competitive painful self-disclosure in their analysis. After the elderly persons did painful self-disclosure, the conversational partner sometimes disclosed her personal information also. In their study, they found that the elderly conversational partners provided painful information more frequently than the younger partners in response to the other person's self-disclosure. In fact, the elderly persons may disclose it as if they were in competition. The mutual disclosure of painful information in the present interaction, however, seems to create the feelings of involvement and rapport as suggested by Tannen (1990): "I disclose my personal information because you did too. We can trust each other and share personal experiences."

What is also interesting here is the frequent occurrence of overlap right before and after my self-disclosure about my arm. For example, in line 17, most of Mary's utterance ("carry heavy things, no") overlaps with my utterance in line 16 ("but I cannot carry heavy things"), indicating her rapport and understanding of what I said. Then in line 21 ("I understand"), I overlap with Mary's utterance "yes, well you have to," emphasizing my understanding of her problem. These overlaps seem to be examples of what Tannen (1984) calls "supportive overlap," which contributes to the creation of involvement rather than interruption and competition for the conversational floor. These overlaps also indicate a supportive attitude for self-disclosure.

On the surface, it seems that Mary and I are building solidarity because both of us revealed some negative information about ourselves which related to the same topic of traveling light. The difference in our points of view, however, soon becomes apparent when Mary says "even if your, your arm's strong, there's a limit to what you can carry" (lines 26, 27). My point is that "since my arm is weak, I cannot carry heavy things. If my arm were stronger, I could carry more stuff." On the other hand, Mary's point of view is that "it does not matter whether your arm is strong or not. What is crucial is that there is always a limit to the amount that you can carry by yourself, if you are not traveling by car." Her utterance, then, seems to imply "so, it's okay that your arm is weak. Do not worry."

While Mary's reasoning is consistent with her frustration about giving up driving and being unable to visit her children and friends freely, my point of view has nothing to do with giving up driving or the feeling of separation or loneliness; it is just a matter of convenience. This kind of cross-talk may sometimes leave the interlocutors with a feeling of dissatisfaction. As Gumperz (1982) found in cross-cultural settings, cross-talk often occurs without being clearly identified as such by the interlocutors. Even so, misinterpreted communicative intentions could cause severe damage to the feeling of rapport and satisfaction in conversations. In the interaction between Mary and me, the cross-talk seems to encourage Mary to talk repeatedly about not being able to drive in order to clarify and reinforce her point.

Similar cross-talk is also found in the following interaction. Prior to this conversation, I told Mary that I did not drive because public transportation was well developed in Japan. I also told Mary that the bus system in Los Angeles was very bad, and therefore I had a difficult time getting around in Los Angeles.

Example 9

	1	Shoko:	so I never learned to uh drive, and so when
	2		I was in California, [laugh]
->	3	Mary:	and in Los Angeles, the roads aren't narrow
	4		but they're they're packed so close with cars,
	5		I think I'd be scared to death to drive out
	6		there. [laugh]
	7	Shoko:	Yes, yes.
	8		It was really hard for me, and so,
	9		with THAT part, I really like Washington, DC
	10	Mary:	Oh, Washington is much,
	11		it's really easy to get around.
	12	Shoko:	mhm mhm
	13	Mary:	I find it, not me,
	14		not,
	15		I MISS driving
->	16		NOT because I would want to drive HERE
	17		but I miss it when it comes to see my
	18		grandchildren
	19	Shoko:	mmm
	20	Mary:	or going back to where where I lived before I
	21		came here or visiting friends.
	22	Shoko:	Yes.
	23	Mary:	Not being able to drive makes
	24	Shoko:	uhuh
	25	Mary:	makes it difficult.
	26	Shoko:	Yeah, oh yes. I understand.

In line 1, I state that I never learned how to drive, a message which is meant to claim the common ground of living in the United States without a car. In lines 3 to 6, however, Mary claims her reluctance to drive in a big city such as Los Angeles, where the roads are packed with cars. Here, her utterance implies that even though she *knows* how to drive, she does not have any intention of driving in Los Angeles, and therefore, it is okay for me also that I did not drive there. By saying that she would be scared to death to drive in Los Angeles, she tries to sympathize with me. It also helps to maintain my positive face. Disclosure of not knowing how to drive in Los Angeles is possibly face threatening since it may signal that "I am not a capable person." But Mary's utterances communicate that "it is okay not to drive anyway. Even those who know how to drive would not want to drive there." Her view, however, contrasts with my line of argument. The reason why I did not drive is because I did not know how, regardless of my intention.

In line 7, I try to build rapport with her by agreeing with her ("yes, yes") and I further admit the difficulty of not being able to drive in Los Angeles ("it was very hard for me") in order to establish a common ground for the communication once again. Then I continue my utterance mentioning that I like Washington in terms of the public transportation system.

Mary agrees with me about the easiness of getting around using public transportation in Washington ("oh, Washington is much, it's really easy to get around"), but she comes back again to the theme of "I can't drive." Thus, she states that she misses driving in line 15, even though she does not like driving in cities. She misses it because "not being able to drive makes, makes it uh difficult" (lines 23 and 25) to visit her family and friends who live far from Washington.

Mary's point is not simply the question of being able to drive or not, but it is closely related to the feeling of loneliness and separation. Moreover, as mentioned before, not driving is connected with many other painful experiences such as her husband's death, ill-health, immobility, and so on. This may have contributed to the vocalization of the "I can't drive" theme in this discourse. Being unable to drive seems to have some symbolic value of a drastic change in Mary's later life.

Obviously I not only come from a culturally different background but also have never experienced what it is like to be elderly in the U.S. (with or without a car). Even though I try to establish a shared ground for communication and to be supportive, I cannot relate to her problem as one of the "elderly"; all I can do is to share my problems which seem to have some commonalties with Mary's. But they are not exactly the same, and therefore the difference in our points of view created the cross-talk.

CONCLUSION

Even though this is a study of just one intergenerational interaction, sociolinguistic analysis of naturally occurring discourse revealed the subtlety as well as complexity of various factors which may contribute to miscommunication in intergenerational conversations.

This study showed that intergenerational communication has a certain resemblance to cross-cultural communication. The interlocutors may speak the same language and may have every intention to understand each other to communicate successfully. But because of different communicative styles, discourse strategies, and lack of shared background knowledge, communication breakdown may occur. Therefore, participants need to negotiate different agendas in communication: What does the speaker really mean? How do I want to present myself in this conversation? As Coupland and Coupland (this volume) demonstrated in medical settings for the cases of doctors and elderly patients, it is both the young and the elderly interlocutors who work on the process of negotiating an elderly identity. In other words, the elderly identity is "relative to projected identities of others" (J. Coupland, N. Coupland, Giles, and Henwood, 1991).

Recurring patterns of language use may contribute to the construction of stereotypes against a particular group of people who are "different." Researchers such as Gumperz (1982), Tannen (1984), Young (1982), and Okazaki (1993), for example, demonstrated how different communicative conventions such as stress, lexical, and syntactic choices, and sequencing strategies can influence contextual interpretation in cross-cultural encounters (including subculturally different participants). Different ways of using these conventions often result in misinterpretation of communicative intent.

Elderly people may talk frequently about their past or about their personal problems and pains even to a stranger. In my study, the theme of "I can't drive" was noticed frequently, and it was often followed by expressions of a feeling of loneliness. This communicative behavior may seem deviant from the "norms" of communication found among the younger generation, and therefore the elderly may be negatively regarded as difficult people to relate to. When we judge another person's communicative style using our own style as a criterion or standard of communication, the value judgment often creates negative stereotypes as often found in the cases of cross-cultural communication.

J. Coupland, N. Coupland, Giles, and Henwood (1991:88) suggest that the elderly constitute a "distinct *cultural* group, with particular experiences and characteristics of talk, and also particular identifiable needs, predispositions, and values for talk." Giles et al. (1992) also point out that the older and younger people inhabit different historical cohorts which are often associated with different values, predispositions, and problems to adjust (p. 292). In the present study, one of the sociological contexts of miscommunication for intergenerational interactions seems to lie in the fact that not only are Mary and I from different ethnic and social backgrounds, but also I was unable to share Mary's age-relevant perspective. In this sense, my conversation with Mary was cross-cultural on multiple levels.

During the interaction, both Mary and I tried to be supportive of each other and signaled understanding frequently. On the surface, in spite of cultural and generational differences, it seemed that Mary and I shared certain social and physical factors in common, such as not driving cars and not being able to carry heavy things. But the reasons for not driving or not being able to carry heavy things were different for Mary and for me. For Mary, it was because she had a mild stroke and weak eyesight, and she was forced to give up driving. She also has to travel light because there is a limit to the amount which one can carry unless the person travels by car. On the other hand, I cannot drive because I did not need to learn how to drive in Japan. Driving has a different meaning and social significance for Japanese and Americans. Moreover, I cannot carry heavy things because of the surgery on my arm, which has nothing to do with driving or my age. Because of these differences, the same theme was reintroduced to clarify the slightly different points of view between Mary and me. Thus, the "I can't drive" theme appeared again and again, resulting in shaping and emphasizing Mary's elderly identity.

My frequent backchannelling to Mary and the characteristics of women's speech[6] in general may have also affected Mary's repeated reference to driving. Women tend to disclose personal information more often than men do, and my communicative style (frequent backchannels and short utterances) encouraged further disclosure. Moreover, my disclosure of the surgery was meant to create a supportive atmosphere for Mary's painful self-disclosure.

As N. Coupland, Henwood, J. Coupland, and Giles (1990) point out, evaluations of communication with the elderly may reconstruct knowledge about the elderly identity and about intergenerational talk, and they may further reinforce stereotypes. Although the elderly disclose their painful information to peers more frequently than to the young interlocutors (J. Coupland et al., 1988), the young listener's communicative behavior and a lack of shared background experience may also facilitate the context for the occurrence of painful self-disclosure. The elderly may reinforce the information which is not shared by the young conversational partners in order to make their point. In Mary's case, she clarified the difference between giving up driving due to age-related ill-health and not driving because of a lack of desire to drive.

In order to understand intergenerational communication and possible sources of breakdowns and stereotypes, more studies of naturally occurring conversations are necessary. Research on gender difference in painful self-disclosure and the relationship between language change and socially significant events of life (such as giving up cars and retiring from jobs) would also be important. Since age is a social category as well as a chronological category, the integration of socially sensitive features into sociolinguistic research is essential.

NOTES

1. I am greatly indebted to Dr. Heidi Hamilton for her constructive criticism and insightful comments on the earlier draft of this chapter. It was through her teaching that my view was widened toward language and aging.

2. The term, "cross-talk," became well known through an educational video on cross-cultural communication made by Gumperz, Jupp, and Roberts (1979). The video clearly showed how conversational cues (such as tone of voice, intonation, selection of lexical items, and so on) could lead to misunderstanding of intentions in real life situations.

3. Lynn Thiesmeyer (p.c.) points out that characteristics of the area where a person lives change the meaning of giving up driving. In New York City, for example, where public transportation is well developed, not driving does not affect the mobility of the elderly too much. Not having a car is considered to be preferable for the elderly, and many people live without cars because driving in the city can be dangerous and frustrating even for the young.

4. "Face" is a term derived from Goffman (1967, 1971) and further developed by Brown and Levinson (1987). Relating to the expression "lose

face," it means individuals' self-esteem in human relations (Brown and Levinson, 1987:2). Brown and Levinson distinguish two types of face, namely, positive face and negative face. Positive face needs are basic desires to be liked and accepted by others, while negative face needs are fundamental needs to protect one's territory or not to be imposed upon.

5. LoCastro (1987), Mizutani (1982), White (1989) and Maynard (1989, 1990) all indicate a high frequency of backchannels (short responses such as "uhuh" and "yeah") in Japanese discourse. These backchannels, called *aizuchi* in Japanese, are used to show the listener's willingness to co-operate in the conversation and show support of the speaker.

6. Tannen (1990), for example, points out that women tend to approach conversations as a means to negotiate closeness, whereas interlocutors try to exchange confirmation and create rapport.

REFERENCES

Boden, Deirdre and Bielby, Denise. 1986. The way it was: topical organization in elderly conversation. *Language and communication* 6. 73–89.

Brown, Penelope and Levinson, Stephen. 1987. Politeness: Some universals in language and usage. Cambridge: Cambridge University Press.

Bruce, Juliet. 1994. To drive or not to drive. *Aging* 366. 49–51.

Campbell, Miriam, Bush, Trudy, and Hale, William. 1993. Medical conditions associated with driving cessation in community-dwelling, ambulatory elders. *Journal of Gerontology* 48. 25–32.

Coupland, Justine, Coupland, Nikolas, Giles, Howard, and Wiemann, John. 1988. My life in your hands: processes of self-disclosure in intergenerational talk. In Nikolas Coupland, ed., *Styles of Discourse*. New York: Croom Helm.

Coupland, Justine, Coupland, Nikolas, Giles, Howard, and Henwood, Karen. 1991. Formulating age: dimensions of age identity in elderly talk. *Discourse Processes* 14. 87–106.

Coupland, Justine, Coupland, Nikolas, and Grainger, Karen. 1991. Intergenerational discourse: contextual versions of ageing and elderliness. *Ageing and Society* II. 189–208.

Coupland, Justine, Nussbaum, Jon F., and Coupland, Nikolas. 1991. The reproduction of aging and agism in intergenerational talk. *"Miscommunication" and Problematic Talk*. Newbury Park: Sage.

Coupland, Justine, and Coupland, Nikolas. 1992. "How are you?": Negotiating phatic communion. *Language in Society* 21. 207–230.

Coupland, Justine, Robinson, Jeffrey D., and Coupland, Nikolas. 1994. Frame negotiation in doctor-elderly patient consultations. *Discourse and Society* 5,3. 89–124.

Coupland, Nikolas, Coupland, Justine, Giles, Howard, and Henwood, Karen. 1988. Accommodating the elderly: invoking and extending a theory. *Language in Society* 17. 1–14.

Coupland, Nikolas, and Coupland, Justine. 1990. Language and later life. In H. Giles and P. Robinson, eds., *Handbook of Language and Social Psychology.* New York: John Wiley & Sons Ltd.

Coupland, Nikolas, Henwood, Karen, Coupland, Justine, and Giles, Howard. 1990. Accommodating troubles-talk: the management of elderly self-disclosure. In G. McGregor and R.S. White, eds., *Reception and Response.* London: Routledge.

Coupland, Nikolas, Wiemann, John M., and Giles, Howard. 1991. Talk as "problem" and communication as "miscommunication": an integrative analysis. Nikolas Coupland, Howard Giles and John M. Wiemann, eds., *"Miscommunication" and Problematic Talk.* Newbury Park: Sage.

Coupland, Nikolas, and Coupland, Justine. 1998. Ageing, ageism and anti-ageism: Moral stance in geriatric medical discourse. In Heidi Hamilton, ed., *Language and Communication in Old Age: Multidisciplinary Perspectives.* New York: Garland.

Duranti, Alessandro. 1986. The audience as co-author: an introduction. *Text* 6, 3. 239–247.

Eckert, Penelope. 1984. Age and linguistic change. In D. Kertzer and J. Keith, eds., *Age and Anthropological Theory.* Ithaca: Cornell University Press.

Giles, Howard, and Ryan, Ellen. eds. 1986. Language, communication and the elderly. Special issue of *Language and Communication.*

Giles, Howard, Coupland, Nikolas, Coupland, Justine, Williams, Angie, and Nussbaum, Jon. 1992. Intergenerational talk and communication with older people. *International Journal of Aging and Human Development* 34, 4. 271–297.

Goffman, Erving. 1967. *Interaction Ritual.* New York: Anchor Books.

Goffman, Erving. 1971. *Relations in Public.* New York: Harper and Row.

Gumperz, John. 1982. *Discourse Strategies.* Cambridge: Cambridge University Press.

Gumperz, John, Jupp, T.C., and Roberts, Celia. 1979. *Cross-Talk: A Study of Cross-cultural Communication.* Southall: National Centre for Industrial Language Training.

Hamilton, Heidi. 1989. Conversations with an Alzheimer's patient: an interactional examination of questions and response. Ph.D. dissertation. Washington, DC: Georgetown University.

————. 1994. *Conversations with an Alzheimer's Patient: An Interactional Sociolinguistic Study.* Cambridge: Cambridge University Press.

————. 1996. Intratextuality, intertextuality, and the construction of identity as patient in Alzheimer's disease. *Text* 16, 1. 61–90.

Kington, Raynard, Reuben, David, Rogowski, Jeametter, and Lee, Lillard. 1994. Sociodemographic and health factors in driving patterns after 50 years of age. *American Journal of Public Health.* 84. 1327–1330.

LoCastro, Virginia. 1987. Aizuchi: A Japanese conversational routine. *Discourse Across Cultures,* Larry E. Smith, ed. London: Prentice Hall. 101–113.

Maynard, Senko. 1989. *Japanese Conversation: Its Structure and Interactional Management.* Norwood, New Jersey: Ablex.

————. 1990. Conversation management in contrast: Listener response in Japanese and American English. *Journal of Pragmatics* 14. 397–412.

Mizutani, Nobuko. 1982. The listener's response in Japanese conversation. *Sociolinguistic Newsletter* 13.1: 33–38.

Okazaki, Shoko. 1993. Stating opinions in Japanese: Listener dependent strategies. Georgetown University Round Table on Languages and Linguistics, 1993. Washington, DC: Georgetown University.

Rosenfeld, Elif T. 1998. When and how old age is relevant in discourse of the elderly: A case study of Georgia O'Keeffe. In Heidi Hamilton, ed., *Language and Communication in Old Age: Multidisciplinary Perspectives.* New York: Garland.

Ryan, Ellen, Giles, Howard, Bartolucci, Giampiero, and Henwood, Karen. 1986. Psycholinguistic and social psychological components of communication by and with the elderly. *Language and Communication* 6, 1/2. 1–24.

Shadden, Barbara. 1988. Interpersonal communication patterns and strategies in the elderly. In B. Shadden, ed., *Communication Behavior and Aging.* Baltimore: Williams & Wilkins. 182–196.

Tannen, Deborah. 1984. *Conversational Style: Analyzing Talk Among Friends.* Norwood, New Jersey: Ablex.

Tannen, Deborah. 1990. *You Just Don't Understand: Women and Men in Conversation.* New York: William Morrow.

Tannen, Deborah. 1992. Interactional sociolinguistics. In William Bright, ed., *The International Encyclopedia of Linguistics.* New York: Oxford University Press. 9-12.

Ward, Russell. 1984. The marginality and salience of being old: When is age relevant? *The Gerontologist* 24. 227–232.

White, Sheida. 1989. Backchannels across cultures: a study of Americans and Japanese. *Language in Society* 18. 59–76.

Young, Linda Wai Ling. 1982. Inscrutability revisited. In John Gumperz, ed., *Language and Social Identity*. Cambridge: Cambridge University Press.

Social Norms, Values, and Practices in Old Age

CHAPTER 11

Gossip in an Older Women's Support Group

A Linguistic Analysis[1]

Pamela A. Saunders[2]

INTRODUCTION

During 1992–1993 I conducted fieldwork at a geriatric center in urban Philadelphia. I spent 18 months attending weekly meetings with a support group of older women who called themselves the "SOWN group" (Supportive Older Women's Network).[3] I was interested in the gender identity of older women and the social construction of gender identity through forms of talk. In participating in this group I was able to observe how older women talked to each other and what they talked about.

As my fieldwork developed I began to notice that gossip was a recurrent form of talk in the support group. The women gossiped about fashion, dating, sex, and problems of living in an institution. Targets of their gossip included their own group members, service employees, other people in the local speech community, and celebrities. From my observations, they appeared to enjoy gossiping, but they were aware that it wasn't always appropriate. Group members might introduce a gossip narrative by saying, "I won't mention any names, but. . . ." If asked, they would deny participating in gossip. This awareness of gossip's negative connotations was supported by a group policy against gossip. The policy as stated by the group facilitator discouraged gossip about the content of group meetings with non-SOWN group members. In spite of this policy and despite their awareness of gossip as a sometimes inappropriate activity, it happened anyway. To fully understand their negative attitude towards gossip, it is important to know the historical derivation of the word as it refers to women and their talk.

Starting in the nineteenth century, gossip acquired the meaning "lazy small talk" or "the idle chit-chat of women." Where did gossip get its negative connotation? Historically, gossip had nothing to do with women or talking. According to Rysman (1977) gossip developed out of an Old English phrase "God sib" which originally referred to a god-parent or family friend. By the Elizabethan period (late 1500s), the meaning of "gossip" moved from a family relationship to an individual relationship. By the eighteenth century, Samuel Johnson identifies two newer meanings in addition to the older one. Gossip could now be used to refer to a "tippling" or "drinking companion." Johnson also identifies another meaning for "gossip" (i.e., "one who runs about tattling like women at a lying [birth].") Since hospital deliveries were virtually unknown at the time, births were generally at home among friends, family, and "gossips." A home delivery was a general coming-together of women in the community. This is how gossip started to refer to women in particular. By 1730, Bailey's dictionary reports gossip as referring negatively to women. The word "gossip" acquires its negative connotation only after it starts to be applied to women. It is not until the nineteenth century that the noun starts to be a description for idle talk. When used to describe a man, the connotation carries feelings of warmth and the good companionship of a drinking partner; when applied to the female the connotation is more hostile. According to Rysman (1977), by the twentieth century the use of gossip to mean "drinking companion" has become rare. The meaning of "idle talk" emerged in the nineteenth century and remains current; however, when used as a derogatory term, it is usually applied to women.

Given the nineteenth and twentieth century's definition of "gossip," it is easy to see how this group of women would view gossip as an inappropriate behavior for women. They have internalized this negative definition and proclaim to avoid this speech activity. Yet frequently during support group meetings, these women shared gossip about each other and about strangers. This chapter shows what older women in a self-help group setting gossip about and how they go about it. I illustrate that gossip is not idle or lazy small talk but is a process through which older women create group cohesiveness and establish feelings of solidarity.

GOSSIP

While past and present definitions of gossip point to women as likely candidates for idle and lazy talk or gossip, current research across a variety of disciplines demonstrates the positive social and interpersonal functions of gossip. Gossip is researched from a variety of disciplines including social anthropology, linguistic anthropology, and communication studies. Each discipline focuses on a different aspect of the form or the function of this speech activity and contributes something unique to the findings in this area of social interaction.

Social Anthropology

Three prominent views of gossip stem from British social anthropology. One group of researchers called functionalists are interested in explaining the social function of gossip (Almirol, 1981; Colson, 1953; Epstein, 1969; Frankenberg, 1957; Gilmore, 1978; Harris, 1974). In this functionalist view, gossip is one way for a group to establish unity and cohesion. Gluckman (1963:313) states that "the right to gossip about certain people is a privilege which is only extended to a person when he or she is accepted as a member of a group or set. It is a hallmark of membership. Hence rights to gossip serve to mark off a particular group from other groups."

Group membership is established through the assertion of collective values. Gluckman characterizes gossip as maintaining "the unity, morals, and values of social groups" (1963: 308). Gossip reinforces the values of a particular group thereby establishing social norms for the group. Those people who have knowledge of group values are identified as group members. Those who do not know the values of the group are outsiders or non-group members. Later in this chapter, I examine gossip in which SOWN group members assert their beliefs about fashion and femininity. Through their gossip, they mark themselves off from other groups of women, for example, in their praise of Barbara Bush.

Another group of social anthropologists calling themselves transactionalists proposed that gossip serves individual rather than group motivations (Campbell, 1964; Cox, 1970; Gilmore, 1978; Hannerz, 1967; Hotchkiss, 1967; Szwed, 1969; Paine, 1967). Paine (1967:279) states that "gossip is a genre of informal communication [and] is a device intended to forward and protect individual interests." Gossip is a self-serving tool through which particular individuals seek to further their self-interests at the expense of others. People gossip in order to promote themselves in the eyes of others by bolstering themselves while putting others down.

Similar yet slightly different from the transactionalists is what Fine (1985) calls the conflict perspective. While the transactional perspective focuses on the relationship between individuals, the conflict perspective emphasizes that gossip and rumor may be used as a political strategy by groups. Paine describes the connection between gossip and communication as "information management" (Campbell, 1964; Cox, 1970; Hannerz, 1967; Paine, 1967). Cox (1970) proposes that gossip is a way to manage the impression of oneself and others. People gossip to manage or share information with which to compare themselves with others and their achievements. For example, when Republican Party members gossip about the Democratic First Lady, they are sharing as well as managing information. In the same vein, when an older woman compares herself to the former Republican First Lady, Barbara Bush, she may be trying to construct an impression of herself as a supportive wife and mother as well as ally herself with a political group.

Linguistic Anthropology

While social anthropologists concentrate on the function of gossip in social interaction, linguistic anthropologists analyze both the form and the function. Both Goodwin (1990) and Besnier (1989) recognize the debate over the function which gossip plays in the social organization of a group, noting that what is missing from this debate is how gossip is conducted at micro-levels of organization.

Besnier (1989) studies the organization and function of information-withholding sequences, a conversational strategy used by participants in gossip interactions on Nukulaelae, a Polynesian atoll of the Central Pacific. Besnier describes gossip activity taking place in open-walled houses in multiparty interactions. Nukulaelae gossip is also dyadically focused, in that a clear distinction is drawn between primary and secondary participants. Primary participants are usually two people of the same gender. Secondary participants contribute to the conversation sporadically. Among primary participants, a division of labor between the principal speaker and the audience is often clearly demarcated. A broad range of topics may be addressed in gossip sessions such as actions of absent persons, everyday events, and community scandal. Nukulaelae gossip is less evaluative or interpretive and speakers do not speculate on the reasons or motivations that underlie the behavior of others (Besnier 1989). Besnier shows that gossip in Nukulaelae is both self-serving and group-serving, unlike Gluckman or Paine who claim one or the other. Besnier calls for research which incorporates both macro-social and micro-linguistic levels of analysis.

Using a similar framework, Goodwin (1990) examines a speech activity called "he-said-she-said" which is a gossip dispute process practiced by African American adolescents in urban Philadelphia. Goodwin pays "special attention to how the structure and internal organization of a story are shaped by the way in which its telling is embedded within larger activities such as disputes" (1990:9). Goodwin includes a depiction of the time line for the dispute process including an initial gossip stage in which the current defendant is alleged to have talked about her accuser in her absence, an intermediate stage in which the girl who was talked about learns about the offense committed against her from a third party, and the confrontation itself (1990:190). While Goodwin examines the entire chronology preceding and following the gossip narrative, the present study examines gossip interaction at only one moment in time (i.e., during the self-help group meetings) and does not provide the historical background into the construction of the gossip interaction. The present study is informed by Goodwin's micro-analytic framework by looking at specific discourse devices.

Communication Studies

Communication studies offer definitions of gossip, rumor, and self-disclosure which help to operationalize the study of gossip (Rosnow, 1974; Rysman, 1977; Ting-Toomey, 1979). What distinguishes gossip from other speech activities such as rumor or self-disclosure? In her review of the literature, Ting-Toomey (1979:4) offers the following definition of gossip: "Gossip is the communication process whereby information about another person's affairs or activities is disclosed and circulated in an exclusive manner." This is a very general definition and does not help to distinguish gossip from other speech activities such as rumor, self-disclosure, or narrative.

How is gossip different from rumor? There are three basic distinctions between gossip and rumor. First, in gossip the information being disclosed is closely connected to the affairs or activities of a third person, while in rumor the information disclosed may be on any issue or subject from world politics and economics, to individuals with whom they may have no direct contact or involvement. Second, in gossip, the act of "disclosure" is the essence of the process. It is "disclosing" news about a third person whom gossipers know, and through the process of gossiping the news is made available. In rumor, the process of "diffusion" is the key. Information is circulated freely through different channels. Third, in gossip the information disclosed may or may not be factual. In rumor, that which is being diffused is unsubstantiated, without the basis of truth. Rumor is unauthenticated information (Rosnow, 1974; Klapp, 1968).

Ting-Toomey (1979: 3) points out that gossip also differs from self-disclosure. She defines self-disclosure as "the private disclosure of information about the self to another person." Gossip, on the other hand, is "the disclosure of information between person A and person B about person C. In self-disclosure, information about the 'self' is being disclosed, whereas in gossip, it is information about a third person that is disclosed" (1979: 3). While this definition is primarily geared toward dyadic communication, it can be applied to gossip in the self-help group setting where one or more gossipers talk about a third person.

Whom and what are gossiped about? Another study by Levin and Arluke (1987) of gossip in college settings found both positive and negative gossip concerning personal habits, manners, appearance, and role performance. On the negative side, students complained about public displays of "gross" personal habits: nail biting, eating with open mouth, belching in public, teachers who are clumsy and who fail to comment on papers, rudeness on a train, an ugly girl who walks awkwardly. Among the nice things said: praise for a student athlete, appearance of a classmate, kindness to friends, virtues of a popular girl (1987:19). Levin and Arluke found sex differences in what people talked about. They found that women were more likely to gossip about other people than men were. "Women were more likely than men to talk about close friends and family members, whereas men were likely to talk about celebrities, including sports figures, as well as about other acquaintances on campus" (1987:21).

Given that people gossip about certain topics, what is it that they say about these topics? Levin and Arluke (1987) observe that during the 1920s–1950s people used to gossip about the jobs of celebrities, but more recently gossip focuses on celebrities' private lives: relationships with children or spouse, their daily habits at home, or their love affairs. Levin and Arluke see a pattern where gossip was once descriptive and simple but now is judgmental and complex.

This paper follows in the tradition of the linguistic anthropologists by taking a multi-functional view of gossip. The gossip examples in this chapter will illustrate that gossip creates and establishes group boundaries while, at the same time, gossip is a way to further one's own self-interests. Gossip is both an individual and group process whereby group solidarity and individual relationships are established and maintained by gossip interactions. This paper illustrates that gossip among older women functions in two ways: (1) to share information and (2) to reinforce social norms.

DISCOURSE DEVICES: OVERLAPS AND QUESTIONS

This chapter follows the frameworks of Besnier and Goodwin by integrating social analysis with micro-analysis of discourse features. I decided to examine overlap and questions because these devices were prevalent in the talk of the support group and because prior research illustrates that overlaps and questions work in conversation to build interpersonal solidarity (Tannen, 1984). By looking at how overlap and questions establish solidarity, I provide a picture of how gossip creates group cohesiveness and feelings of solidarity.

Overlaps

An overlap occurs when two speakers talk at the same time. An overlap may be when speaker 2 overlaps with just the last word of speaker 1's utterance or it may be when speaker 2 overlaps with all of the words in speaker 1's utterance. An overlap is identifiable by its acoustic properties such that one could measure sound waves and fundamental frequencies to define two simultaneous voices. While the occurrence of an overlap may be easier to identify than a question, establishing the meaning of an overlap requires a functional analysis.

An interactional sociolinguistic perspective of language use proposes a variety of functions for overlap. On the one hand, an overlap may signal that another interlocutor wants to take over the conversational turn (Edelsky, 1981; Fishman, 1978; Greenwood, 1989; Kalcik, 1975; Murray, 1985; Tannen, 1984; West and Zimmerman, 1983; Maltz and Borker, 1982). This kind of overlap (i.e., interruption) may be a hostile conversational move. For example, Tannen describes

an interruption as "a hostile act, a kind of conversational bullying . . . .
An interruption is an intrusion, a trampling on someone else's right to
the floor, an attempt to dominate" (1990:189). On the other hand,
overlaps can be signs of cooperative construction of ongoing talk.
Overlaps might occur when high-involvement speakers chime in to
show support and participation (Tannen, 1984). Cooperative overlap
occurs when one interlocutor is showing her enthusiastic support and
agreement with another. Cooperative overlap occurs when the speakers
view silence between turns as impolite or as a sign of a lack of rapport.
While an overlap may be construed as cooperative in a conversation
between two friends, it may be construed as an interruption when
between boss and employee. Overlap and interrogative have different
meanings depending on the speakers' ethnicity, gender, and relative
status differences. For example, when a teacher, a person of higher
status, overlaps with her student, a person of lower status, typically the
overlap is interpreted as an interruption.

Questions

A question is typically a sentence by which a speaker asks a hearer to
give information (Leech and Svartvik, 1975). As outlined in the
literature (see Schiffrin, 1994), questions are difficult to identify. A
variety of criteria have been suggested as defining aspects of questions
including sequentiality, grammar, and function.

Conversation analysts contend that question-answer sequences are
readily identifiable from the relationship between the first and second
part of the question-answer or adjacency pair. The question is the first
part of the adjacency pair and is always followed by the answer which
is always the second part. One problem with this criteria is that not all
questions are followed by answers and not all answers are preceded by
questions (Schiffrin, 1994).

Another set of criteria for identifying questions includes
grammatical or syntactic cues. For example, subject-verb inversion of
an interrogative (e.g., Do you like cheese?) and wh- words (e.g., Which
cheese do you prefer?) are primary grammatical clues to identifying
questions. Once again, the problem is that questions can occur without
the presence of interrogative syntax and wh-words. For example, a
speaker can utter the words, "eating lunch" which in elliptical form is a
declarative statement, not an interrogative, yet it can be interpreted as a
question about the desire to eat lunch.

So utterances such as "eating lunch" that are not clearly questions by syntactic criteria could be expanded to fuller interrogative utterances: "Are you eating lunch today?" "Do you want to each lunch now?" The utterance, "Eating lunch?" does not have interrogative syntax, thus is not unequivocally a question, but when uttered with rising intonation may be a question. As illustrated by Schiffrin (1994) rising intonation may not always provide sufficient evidence for identifying a question. She provides the example "Do you want to have lunch." with final falling intonation (indicated by a period) typical of a declarative sentence. Schiffrin (1994:30) notes "the word order is typical of interrogatives, but the intonation seems more typical of declarative sentences."

A third set of criteria for identifying questions comes from a more functional perspective which analyzes the interpersonal goals and social meanings of language use (Jacobson, 1960; Hymes, 1961; Halliday, 1973). In examining the functional criteria of a question-answer pair, one might look at the interpersonal goals of the speakers. If speaker A says, "Eating lunch?" she might be asking for information about speaker B's schedule or she might be making an offer or invitation for lunch (Schiffrin, 1994). It is important to have information regarding the speaker's relative social status, the relationship between the participants, the setting, and their usual ways of interacting in order to identify the function of an utterance.

Questions can have a variety of functions. They can be requests for information (e.g., "Where is my book?"), or requests for confirmation (e.g., "You locked the door, didn't you?"). Leech and Svartvik (1975) describe tag questions as requests for confirmation and when "added to the end of a statement they ask for confirmation of the truth of the statement. . . . The answer expected is 'yes' if the statement is positive, and 'no' if the statement is negative" (1975:112). Questions can be requests for action in the form of indirect speech act (e.g., "Can you pass the salt?") (Searle, 1975; Ervin-Tripp, 1976). Echo questions (e.g., "Pass the what?") are requests for repetition "in which we ask the speaker to repeat some information usually because we failed to hear it, but sometimes also because we can't believe our ears" (1975:115). Besides functioning as requests, questions can also express surprise or an opinion (Hamilton, 1994; Greenwood and Freed, 1992). For example, Quirk and Greenbaum (1972) suggests that questions can be a way of exclaiming over something.

Given the difficult nature of identifying questions, I use a variety of formal (e.g., interrogative syntax, wh- words, intonation) and functional criteria (e.g., interpersonal goals). In addition I use sequential cues such that I identify questions in part by locating them in relation to their answers. In this chapter, I identify six questions that function in gossip interactions including: requests for information, requests for clarification, introduction of a new topic, expression of an opinion, expression of encouragement, and expression of exclamation. SOWN group members used these questions to engage their interlocutors and to display solidarity within the support group.

This section described the form and function of overlaps and questions. I illustrated that both of these discourse devices are contextually identified and defined. Overlaps can be cooperative and competitive depending on the context. Questions can function as requests, exclamations, and statements. In the analysis section of this chapter I illustrate examples of overlaps and questions which achieve interpersonal and intragroup goals.

SUPPORT GROUP/SOWN

The data for this study were collected in a support group setting. I chose to examine this women's support group because it provided an opportunity to observe the talk of older women. Talk in the support group setting revolves around the problems and concerns of the participants.

Definition of support groups

The basic definition of a support or self-help group is a group that forms around people who have some specific concern or disorder or who face some definitive life crisis—for example, panic disorder, bereavement, AIDS and HIV, dementia, dementia caregiving. In addition to offering mutual support, these groups generally utilize an approach which offers explicit instruction about the nature of the person's illness or life situation and examines patients' misconceptions and self-defeating responses to an illness or situation (Yalom, 1995: 9). Now groups are forming around people of a specific age cohort who face similar issues surrounding a life stage such as retirement, institutionalization, and aging in general. This SOWN group formed as a specialized group for older women living in the same institution.

The extensive literature on support and encounter groups describes both the advantages and disadvantages. The advantages for participants are, for example, reducing isolation, learning from and modeling on one another, and creating a permissive atmosphere for expression of emotions (Yalom, 1995). Currently, most published reports on self-help groups have emphasized sharing information and emotional release as the primary foci (Clark and Rakowski, 1983). There are also drawbacks to support groups. For example, the leader may lack the skills to establish and maintain appropriate therapeutic norms or there may be difficulty integrating severely distressed participants into the group (Lieberman, Yalom, and Miles, 1973; Zarit, Anthony, and Boutselis, 1987).

The SOWN group members at the Philadelphia Geriatric Center describe themselves as a support group which gives people the opportunity to really share with other people about personal things. It is a place to discuss current events as well as matters of personal concern to the members.

According to Yalom (1995: 284) groups need to establish certain ground rules, the most important having to do with confidentiality. "For members to speak freely, they must have confidence that their statements will remain in the group." A self-help group is a place to talk about feelings and ideas without the threat of being exposed. The threat of gossip may deter members from revealing their true feelings. Thus gossip is detrimental to the success of a self-help group.

While confidentiality is important in regard to what is said during meetings, there is no rule against gossip during meetings. While gossiping outside the group was prohibited, it still occurrs during group meetings about non-group members. I propose that gossip during meetings is not detrimental to this self-help group and serves as a form of support.

Organization of SOWN organization

This self-help group is one branch of the Supportive Older Women's Network (SOWN), which is an organization throughout southeastern Pennsylvania's greater Delaware valley. The primary services provided by SOWN are ongoing support groups for older women, leadership seminars which train older women to be group facilitators, consultative and outreach service, a newsletter, and networking. Kaye (1995) reports that over 750 older women are now served annually in over 50 groups in different locations. The average group was comprised of 13.5 members, met on a weekly basis, and had been operational for 4.4 years. SOWN services were developed based on a self-help delivery model. According to Kaye (1995) SOWN members are a mean age of 76.1 and most are widowed. Most members were either white (72.9%) or African American (25.6%). The mean number of years of education attained by group members was 10.9 with 50% having graduated from high school. The majority of group members were retired. Approximately 85% of SOWN members had one or more children.

According to Kaye's survey research, SOWN organization members report a variety of gains and benefits from group membership. "The most frequent increases in support are realized in women's relations with relatives and friends and in terms of the degree of telephone contact maintained with other SOWN group members" (Kaye, 1995:24). The most common gains from group participation are the ability to listen to others better, building new friendships, and receiving support as an older woman. Most groups maintain an agenda but focus on feelings and problems of members. Kaye describes the topics most commonly dealt with to include life review, relationships with children, health issues, friendships, communicating better, and grandparenting. In my experience in attending one SOWN group, speakers focused on current events with occasional discussions of feelings and problems of members. When a serious life event occurred, such as the death of a child, the group shared their own experiences to offer sympathy and comfort.

THE STUDY

Setting

The data were collected during meetings of a self-help group which met weekly at the Philadelphia Geriatric Center. The Philadelphia Geriatric Center is home for 1100 older people who live in assisted living apartments and in a nursing home. Residents eat meals together and participate in social and religious activities organized by the Center. The Center functions as a speech community where most residents know each other.

Participants

The Philadelphia Geriatric Center branch of the SOWN organization consists of ten residents and the group facilitator. The members' ages range from seventy-five to one-hundred-and-two, except for the facilitator who is in her mid-forties. Since the Center catered to Jewish elderly, all of the SOWN group members are Jewish. All but one are widowed and all are retired. This specific group of women had been meeting consistently for a year when I joined them.

The group facilitator is another important member of the SOWN group. In this case the group facilitator is the Activities Director from the Center. Other SOWN groups are led by one of the group members. This facilitator's duties include suggesting a topic for each weekly meeting (e.g., current events from the news, Geriatric Center activities, living wills). She launches the topic and allows the members to shape the discussion. The facilitator moderates turn-taking between members, allowing less talkative members to have their turn.

Types of Speakers

A gossip participant is an individual who pursues the activity of gossiping.[4] According to my observations, there are three kinds of gossip participants in this self-help group: active gossipers, passive gossipers, and non-gossipers. The active gossipers initiate topics about SOWN group members as well as other people. Passive gossipers listen and sometimes respond and participate in the gossip initiated by the active gossipers but do not initiate any topics on their own. The non-gossipers neither start gossip nor respond to gossip initiated by other people. Often non-gossipers actively discourage any mention of gossip by calling the group's attention to the inappropriateness of the gossiping activity.

The Status of Gossip

The issue of gossip is a topic of discussion for the SOWN group. In one of the first meetings I attended, the group talked about gossip. They emphasized that one important rule of the SOWN group is to keep all information about the happenings of the group confidential. They provided their own position on gossip. In this first example the facilitator, Andra, discusses the idea of a self-help group for the benefit of a new member.

The following example illustrates two points that are relevant for the group: (1) the group's definition of self-help group, and (2) the rule governing gossip.

Example 1—Definition of Gossip[5]

Andra:	This is a support group.	1
	Meaning that,	2
	this is an opportunity for when people really have something	3
	that they want to share with other people.	4
	This is a place to share personal things.	5
	In addition to having discussions about current events,	6
	and things that are more general.	7
	This is a place where you can maybe bring up a subject that is more personal.	8
	And we have a rule in the group,	9
	that no one is really allowed to repeat what anyone in the group says,	10
	outside the group.	11
	So whatever happens here is not to be discussed or gossiped about or anything.	12

First, on lines 1–8, Andra describes the advantages a self-help group provides, such as the opportunity to share personal thoughts and feelings. On lines 9–12, Andra states that gossip is prohibited by SOWN group members about each other when outside the group. Here, Andra is describing just one permutation of how gossip could happen, but implicit in Andra's statement are three other ways that gossip can occur.

Gossip Situations

There are at least four kinds of situations in which gossip may happen. These gossip interactions are cross cut by two dimensions, (1) where gossip happens: either inside or outside SOWN group meetings and, (2) the gossip target (i.e., SOWN group members or non-group members) (see Figure 1).

Figure 1. Gossip Situations

	Group Members	Non-Group Members
Outside meetings	A) +	B) +
During meetings	C) +	D) +

The first type of gossip is gossip about SOWN group members outside group meeting time (see box A). As seen in the text example above, Andra explicitly states that SOWN group members should not gossip about group members or meeting topics with anyone when outside the group. This is the only situation that Andra as group leader comments on as unacceptable. There is little control over what group members gossip about during their free time, and, presumably, group members gossip about non-group members and their activities. Given the group's propensity for gossip during group meetings, it is probable that they gossip at other times as well.

Gossip may also occur outside meetings by SOWN group members about non-group members (see box B). My research focused on the workings of the support group rather than on the general social activity of the Center. While I noticed conversations among residents in the front hall and in the dining room which may have included gossip narratives, I did not record any.

Another permutation (see box C) is gossip by group members during meetings about other group members. Gossip about group members by other group members occurs in two ways. First is gossip about group members by other group members when those members are absent from the meetings. Second is gossip about group members by other group members when those members are present during the meeting. I have only one example of this latter scenario. When this type of gossip happens, it takes place in the form of moralistic messages that portray the concern and support of the teller (see below in Example 4). This type of gossip is different from stereotypically negative or sensational gossip. I submit that gossip is not always divisive but can also be supportive.

Gossip can also occur during meetings about people who are residents of the Center but not members of the self-help group (see box D). While SOWN group members frown on this kind of gossip, there is no stated policy against it. Example 3 about the sexual practices of other residents illustrates this later in this chapter.

ANALYSIS

Self-help group members gossip about personal relationships as well as strangers. The people who are targets of the gossip fall into three categories. First, gossip subjects are other SOWN group members. Second, gossip subjects are non-SOWN group members such as Center employees or other Center residents. Third, gossip subjects include famous personalities and political figures. This category differs slightly from the first two, because SOWN group members do not personally know these famous personalities and political figures. Yet due to media exposure, these personalities become members of a larger common speech community. Everyone knows something about these personalities and can refer to them as topics of common knowledge.

While specific individuals are often the topic of gossip, gossip also included more general topics. The content of their gossip varies widely from "looking good" over sixty-five years old, to dating, to life and its many problems. In this self-help group, gossip activity focuses on three general topic areas: fashion, dating, and problems at the Center. The following discussion describes these topic areas and gives examples of gossip interactions. This section examines the function of the gossip interaction and how the discourse devices of overlap and questions facilitate gossip activity.

Celebrity Gossip

Group members enjoy gossiping about political and entertainment figures. In one gossiping incident, Eva introduces the subject of Mrs. Bush's wardrobe that, in turn, initiates a discussion of previous First Ladies. Eva, Anne, and Andra join the discussion of hairstyles and self-presentation. They praise Barbara Bush for being lady-like. Andra in her role as Activities Director asks several questions in this gossip interaction that facilitate the flow of talk.

Example 2—Celebrity Gossip

Anne:	I think she's a beautiful woman, Mrs. Bush.	1
	She's very different from Nancy Reagan.	2
Eva:	It's a beautiful article in Sunday's *Inquirer.*	3
Anne:	She has that lady look.	4
	You know what I mean?	5
Andra:	What's a lady look, Anne?	6

Anne:	Well the way she dresses,	7
	the way she wears her hair,	8
	[the way she]	9
Eva:	[the way she] carries herself.	10
Anne:	The way she carries herself.	11
Andra:	And you don't think Nancy Reagan had that look?	12
Anne:	No she looked to me like just a society,	13
	she wanted to know that she dresses better than anybody,	14
	she looked better than anybody,	15
	and she was bossy and domineering.	16

This example illustrates the habits and lives of famous people outside the immediate speech community of the Center. Gossip about famous people is somewhat different from gossip about people in the local speech community. In this example about famous individuals, a discussion ensues about appropriateness and social norms, thus allowing the group to moralize without referring to people in their own social circles which might provoke a confrontation. Gossip about famous people and their life styles occurs in this self-help group.

In Example 2, the use of overlap illustrates the collaborative nature of gossip. On line 10, Eva overlaps with Anne to give her own evidence of Mrs. Bush's lady-like manner. While Anne comments on Mrs. Bush's hair style, Eva offers a comment about her deportment. Both women are talking about Mrs. Bush's appearance. This overlap shows Eva's support of Anne's gossiping activity and of Anne's assessment of Mrs. Bush. Overlap is a way for one speaker to show mutual support and interpersonal solidarity with an interlocutor. The use of overlap is significant since the use of overlap constructs gossip as a multiparty interaction.

Example 2 also describes questions asked by Anne and Andra which illustrate the collaborative nature of the gossip interaction. On line 5, Anne asks whether the group understood her statement about Barbara Bush. Her question functions as a request for confirmation from the group. Andra asks two questions, one on line 6 and another on line 12, each fulfilling a different function. On line 6, Andra responds to Anne's question on line 5 with another question. Andra's question/response to Anne essentially says, "No we don't know what you mean, tell us." Andra's question serves as a request for information as to the exact meaning of the phrase "lady-look." On line 12, Andra's question is a request for clarification. Andra is elaborating on Anne's statement on line 2 by asking Anne about Nancy Reagan's look.

How does the role of the speaker influence the meaning of the discursive device? Andra is in a high-status position as the group facilitator. Andra's use of questions exhibits a high-involvement style through which she shows support and enthusiasm of the gossip interaction and in turn facilitates the flow of talk (Tannen, 1984). Andra may be using her role as facilitator to understand the values of older people. In addition, Andra may be employing questions as a discursive device to create group cohesiveness. As seen in example 2, Andra asks a number of questions which identify her as a facilitator of talk in the group. This gossip example identifies Andra as a group leader and reinforces her role within the group. Gossip is encouraged by the group facilitator and appears to be productive rather than lazy or idle talk.

Example 2 has illustrated that questions serve as requests for confirmation and requests for information. A request for confirmation constructs the gossip narrative as a multiparty interaction. A request is often followed by a response from the group and in asking for confirmation, a speaker facilitates the flow of gossip. This is also true of questions that serve as requests for information. As a request for information is followed by a response or answer, a speaker perpetuates the gossip interaction by asking for more information. This exchange of information between members of the group allows for an exchange of ideas on shared social values about fashion and femininity. This communication of shared values is a basic component of gossip. As expressed by Gluckman (1963) gossip reinforces the values of a particular group thereby establishing social norms for that group. Gossip functions to express shared values and thus to create solidarity and cohesion within the group.

Sex at the Center

Sex and dating are popular topics of gossip within the SOWN Group. There are several examples in which the self-help group members talk about residents of the Center who date members of the opposite sex. SOWN group members discuss the dating habits and marital situations of other male and female residents. In the next example, Anne describes an incident when a male resident propositioned her for sex. Ceil, Eva, and Fran question Anne's interpretation of the man's comment.

Example 3—How 'bout some sex, honey?

Anne:	I know about two men who actually came out with it	1
Andra:	What did they come out with? (laughter)	2
Anne:	"How 'bout some sex,	3
	how 'bout some sex, honey"	4
Ceil:	They came out of the bathroom (laughs)	5
Andra:	They came out=	6
Anne:	=I won't tell you their names.	7
Andra:	They said it to you?	8
Anne:	Yeah and to somebody else.	9
Andra:	They did?	10
Anne:	One man said [to this lady]	11
Eva:	[Do you think] it's all in his mind?=	12
Anne:	=One man said to the lady,	13
	"I only want sex from you.	14
	That's all I want is sex."	15
Eva:	Anne, don't you think it's all in his mind?	16
Fran:	I think so. (laughter)	17
Anne:	Of course it's in their mind.	18
Eva:	It's all in his mind.	19
Andra:	WELL	20
	It can't be all in his mind.	21
Eva:	All in his mind.	22
(laughter)		

This is an example of gossip because the group members are talking about an individual who is not present and the tone of the exchange is moralistic and sensational. Anne acknowledges on line 7 that this exchange is a non-sanctioned activity by stating she would omit specific individual's names. While gossiping in general is looked down upon, gossip about non-self-help group members does occur in the context of the self-help group. In this instance Anne omits the gossip subject's name yet continues with the gossip activity.

The use of overlap illustrates that gossiping is collaborative. On line 12 Eva overlaps with Anne who is just about to tell the exciting part of her story. Eva overlaps with Anne to give her own analysis of the situation. She is showing her enthusiasm and personal understanding of Anne's story by overlapping with her and by questioning her.

On lines 12 and 16, Eva queries Anne about the viability of this man's proposition. Eva's questions extend the gossiping activity by asking for and expressing opinions (Greenwood and Freed, 1992). Eva's questions are cooperative moves that sanction the gossiping activity.

Again Andra fulfills her role as group facilitator by asking questions. On line 2, Andra requests further information about the men's activities. Andra's question encourages Anne to continue an obviously sensational narrative. On lines 8 and 10, Andra's questions are expressions of surprise, "They said it to you?" and "They did?" These questions serve to move the interaction forward by an emotional involvement in the gossip narrative.

In this example, questions function to request clarification and to express encouragement. This gossip narrative moralizes about other members of the speech community. By gossiping about the sexual proclivities of other residents, the group expresses its disapproval of this activity and in so doing they establish a basis of opinion for group unity. Asking questions in this way, Andra encourages this gossip interaction. While she stresses that gossip outside group meetings is non-sanctioned, she facilitates gossip during group meetings. This supports my claim that gossip is a means for creating intragroup solidarity and support. Gossip functions as a supportive interactional activity in this self-help group setting. Within the support group setting gossip is both a way to establish social norms as well as a way to establish relationships between members. Although gossip may be viewed as idle talk, in the support group it is productive talk.

Problems at the Center

In this final example SOWN group members gossip about other Center employees who do not belong to the group. Eva describes an unpleasant incident that occurred between a Center employee and another self-help group member, Jossie. Group members who contribute to this interaction are Eva, Andra, Jossie, and this researcher.

Example 4—Problems at the Center

Eva:	Do you know what one of the fellas in the dining room	
	told her today?	1
	She was complaining about the food or something	2
	He said, "Look when you reach your age,	3

	it's all down hill."	4
Andra:	No	5
Jossie:	To me?	6
Andra:	No	7
Jossie:	He didn't say it to me.	8
Eva:	Yes he did,	9
	you didn't hear him.	10
	He said, when you get to [your age]	11
Researcher:	[Crazy]	12
Eva:	It's all down hill=	13
Andra:	=Do we have something to talk about or what?	14
	do we have something to talk about,	15
	that bum	16
Eva:	I thought that was insulting.	17

In example 4, overlap and questions show that gossip is a multiparty interaction. On line 12, this researcher overlaps with cooperative assessment of Eva's story. This overlap is a supportive evaluation of Eva's description of the facts. In addition on lines 14–15, Andra asks a question that validates Eva's gossip narrative as an important topic for group discussion. This question is less a request than an expression of enthusiasm. Her question is a cooperative move that validates Eva's gossip narrative. This researcher's interjection on line 12 and Andra's questions support this gossip narrative as a multiparty interaction.

This is an example of gossip because a self-help group member is evaluating the behavior of an absent non-group member. One function of this gossip example is to relay information about another group member. This information enables the group to rally together to support Jossie. This gossip also serves another function that is to emphasize the status between group members and non-group members. By describing the unacceptable actions of a non-group member towards a group member, this gossip activity creates cohesiveness and reaffirms friendships within the group.

It is important to recognize other interpretations of Andra's role as group facilitator given that she is also activities director at the Center. Andra is in a position to take this kind of gossip and alert the administration regarding residents' complaints. By encouraging this kind of gossip, Andra may be collecting information about the residents' quality of life at the Center. She may use this information to aid her in her job as activities director.

Also inherent in this example is the ageist content of the employee's comments to Jossie on lines 3–4. Andra may be trying to encourage discussion about the issue of ageism within the support group. As group facilitator of an older women's support group and activities director of a geriatric facility, Andra's job description includes promotion of an anti-ageist message.

CONCLUSION

This chapter discusses gossip within the social context of a self-help group. These gossip interactions serve two main functions: the transfer of information and the reinforcement of social norms. First, gossip serves as the transfer of information between group members. As seen in Example 4 about problems at the Center, the group leader and the group members exchange information about other members in the form of gossip narratives. The transfer of information within the group about group members keeps members informed of each others' activities, allowing them to stay connected. This exchange also helps them to provide support for one another during group meetings as well as to provide a basis for support outside group meetings. This transfer of information creates cohesion between individuals and within the group.

Second, as seen in Example 2, gossip about sexual practices of other residents in the Center enforces social norms about sex and dating among older people. Gossip accomplishes this by identifying and explicating certain values held by the group members. The communication of these values helps the group to understand and embrace them as individuals and as a group. Thus the process of gossiping serves first, as a means to identify, and second, as a means to affirm social norms within the local speech communities.

Gossip doesn't have to be about people in the local community for it to carry normative significance. Gossip can be about celebrities as well as familiars. While on one level, gossip about political figures and celebrities is focused on concerns outside the local speech community, on another level, celebrity gossip constructs and affirms social norms within the SOWN group. Such that Barbara Bush and Nancy Reagan are celebrities depicted by the media for their fashions and deportment, it is these images that are translated into representations of femininity. These representations are evaluated and perhaps incorporated into the value system of the SOWN group members. Thus gossip about what Barabara Bush wears and how she acts (e.g., like a lady) also impacts the lives of these older women by establishing value judgments about social issues.

At the level of micro-analysis, this chapter looks specifically at how overlap and questions function in gossip activity. Using gossip as the frame for the speech activity, these examples illustrate how overlaps and questions are means through which speakers construct gossip as multiparty interaction. By using an overlap, a speaker can show agreement or interest in what another speaker is saying. Similarly, a question allows a speaker to expand or clarify another speaker's claim thus supporting the gossip interaction. Discursive devices such as overlaps and questions help speakers to create intragroup solidarity which leads to the establishment and maintenance of friendships.

This study suggests that gossip is not merely idle talk, but a productive way for older women to create friendships. From my conversations with older female residents of the Geriatric Center, I have observed the meaning of friendship to be different for older women. These SOWN group women don't always consider their co-inhabitants to be friends. They are hesitant to make friends with other old people who might die soon. Rather their definition of friendship encompasses lifetime relationships. One resident told me that friends are people with whom she shared common experiences such as strolling with their baby carriages. They don't expect to find friends at a retirement facility in this stage of life. And yet, despite this hesitation, these women did indeed construct friendships—not of the kind formed around strolling with their baby carriages but ones facilitated by gossip.

This study expands on previous work on gossip by integrating both social and linguistic approaches. I have illustrated in this chapter that gossip is not just idle talk, but a productive means for establishing friendships among older women. This study is just one of many that need to be conducted on the discursive practices of older women and men. The study of language and aging is gaining momentum in social psychology, communication studies, sociolinguistics, and gerontology. Further research needs to be conducted in order to understand the linguistic as well as the social implications of language and identity in late life.

NOTES

1. This chapter grew out of data collected during my dissertation fieldwork at the Philadelphia Geriatric Center. A preliminary version of this chapter was

also given at Berkeley Women and Language Conference, April 1994. Special thanks go to Philip A. Saunders, Daniel S. Lefkowitz, Heidi E. Hamilton, and Anis Bawarshi for commenting on various drafts. The data for this chapter were collected with the support of pre-doctoral research grants from American Association of University Women and Sigma Xi Scientific Research Society. The preparation of this chapter was completed with the support of post-doctoral traineeships from the Training Program in Sociocultural Gerontology, University of California, San Francisco, Division of Medical Anthropology and Institute for Health and Aging (NIA Grant # T32 AG 00045) and NIA grant #AG00226, Research Training Program in Communication and Aging.

2. Gerontology Center, 4089 Dole, KU, Lawrence, KS 66045-2160. Most of the work for this chapter was conducted during a post-doctoral fellowship at UCSF.

3. As a project manager of a research project at the Philadelphia Geriatric Center, I had access to many of the activities that went on at the Center. In addition to conducting in-depth interviews with residents, I had the opportunity to participate in the SOWN group as part of my fieldwork on language and aging. I introduced myself to the SOWN group as a student doing a research project. The members knew I was observing and tape recording the meetings. In acting as a group member and as a group leader, I got to know the women in the group very well.

4. Group members' status as gossip participants is most clear when gossip about other residents or Center staff occurs. My observation is that active gossip participants behave differently from passive gossip participants. The active participants initiate gossip about Center residents or staff; however, while passive and non-gossipers may not object to gossip about famous people, they do object to gossip about people they all know at the Center. This reveals that SOWN members are aware of the popular notions of gossip as idle talk and frame gossip about different people in different ways. I do not fully pursue this theme of active and passive gossipers in this chapter.

5. Transcription conventions are adapted from Tannen (1984) and Schiffrin (1987).

( )	extralinguistic commentary
,	rising intonation, signaling more to come
.	falling intonation, signaling conclusion
[ ]	overlapping talk
=	contiguous talk
CAPS	emphasis, stress

REFERENCES

Almirol, E. B. 1981. Chasing the elusive butterfly: gossip and the pursuit of reputation. *Ethnicity* 8: 293–304.

Besnier, N. 1989. Information withholding as a manipulative and collusive strategy in Nukulaelae gossip. *Language in Society* 18(3): 315–341.

Campbell, J.K. 1964. *Honour, Family, and Patronage: A Study of Institutions and Moral Values in a Greek Mountain Community*. Oxford: Clarendon Press.

Clark, N.M, and Rakowski, W. 1983. Family care givers of older adults: Improving helping skills. *The Gerontologist* 23: 597–604.

Colson, E. 1953. *The Makah Indians*. Manchester: Manchester University Press; Minneapolis: University of Minnesota Press.

Cox, B. 1970. What is Hopi gossip about? Information management and Hopi factions. *Man* 5: 88–98.

Edelsky, C. 1981. "Who's got the floor?" *Language in Society* 10:383–421.

Epstein, A. L. 1969. Gossip, norms, and social network. In J. Clyde Mitchell, ed., *Social Networks in Urban Situations*. Manchester: Manchester University Press, 117–127.

Ervin-Tripp, S. 1976. Is Sybil there? The structure of American English directives. *Language in Society* 5: 25–66.

Fine, G.A. 1977. Social components of children's gossip. *Journal of Communication* 27(4):181–185.

Fine, G.A. 1985. Rumors and gossiping. In Tean A. van Dijk, ed. *Handbook of Discourse Analysis*, vol. 3. New York: Academic Press. 223–237.

Fishman, P. M. 1978. What do couples talk about when they're alone? In Douglas Buttruff, ed., *Women's Language and Style*. Akron, Ohio: University of Akron, 11–22.

Frankenberg, R. 1957. *Village on the Border*. London: Cohen and West.

Gilmore, D. 1978. Varieties of gossip in a Spanish rural community. *Ethnology* 17:89–99.

Gluckman, M. 1963. Gossip and scandal. *Current Anthropology* 4(3): 307–316.

Gluckman, M. 1968. Psychological, sociological and anthropological explanations of witchcraft and gossip: a clarification. *Man* 3: 20–34.

Goffman, E. 1959. *The Presentation of Self in Everyday Life*. New York: Doubleday Anchor.

Goodwin, M. H. 1990. Tactical uses of stories: participation frameworks within girls' and boys' disputes. *Discourse Processes* 13(1).

Greenwood, A. 1989. *Discourse Variation and Social Comfort: A Study of Topic Initiation and Interruption Patterns in the Dinner Conversation of Preadolescent Children.* Ph.D. dissertation, City University of New York.

Greenwood, A., & A.F. Freed. 1992. Women talking to women: questions in conversation. In K. Hall, M. Bucholtz, and B. Moonwoman, eds., *Locating Power.* Berkeley, California: Berkeley Women and Language Group, 1: 197–206.

Halliday, M.A.K. 1973. *Explorations in the Functions of Language.* London: Edward Arnold.

Hamilton, H. 1994. *Conversations with an Alzheimer's Patient: An Interactional Examination of Questions and Responses.* New York: Cambridge.

Hannerz, U. 1967. Gossip networks and culture in a Black American ghetto. *Ethnos* 32: 35–60.

Harris, C. 1974. Hennage: a social system in miniature. New York: Holt, Rinehart and Winston.

Haviland, J.B. 1977. *Gossip, Reputation, and Knowledge in Zinacantan.* Chicago: University of Chicago Press.

Hotchkiss, J.C. 1967. Children and conduct in a Ladino community of Chiapas, Mexico. *American Anthropologist* 69: 711–718.

Hymes, D. 1961. Functions of speech: the evolutionary approach. In F. Gruber, ed., *Anthropology and Education.* Philadelphia: University of Pennsylvania Press, 55–83.

Jacobson, R. 1960. Closing statement: linguistics and poetics. In T. Sebeok, ed., *Style in Language.* Cambridge, MA: MIT Press, 350–77.

Kaye, L. W. 1995. Assessing the efficacy of a self-help support group program for older women. *Journal of Women & Aging* 7(4).

Kalcik, S. 1975. ' . . . Like Anne's gynecologist or the time I was almost raped': personal narratives in women's rap groups." *Journal of American Folklore* 88: 3–11.

Klapp, O. E. 1968. *Currents of Unrest: An Introduction of Collective Behavior.* New York: Bantam Books.

Leech, G., and Svartvik, J. 1975. *A Communicative Grammar of English.* Essex: Longman.

Levin, J., and Arluke, A. 1987. *Gossip: The Inside Scoop.* New York: Plenum Press.

Lieberman, M.A., Yalom, I.D., and Miles, M.B. 1973. *Encounter Groups: First Facts.* New York: Basic Books.

Maltz, D. N., and Borker, R. A. 1982. A cultural approach to male-female miscommunication. In J. J. Gumperz, ed., *Language and Social Identity.* Cambridge: Cambridge University Press, 196–216.

Murray, S. O. 1985. Toward a model of members' methods for recognizing interruptions. *Language in Society* 13: 31–40.

Paine, R. 1968. Gossip and Transaction. *Man* 3: 275–278.

Paine, R. 1967. What is gossip about? An alternative hypothesis. *Man* 2: 79–285.

Quirk, R., Greenbaum, S., Leech, G., and Svartvik, J. 1972. *A Grammar of Contemporary English.* London: Longman.

Rosnow, R. L. 1974. On rumor. *Journal of Communication* 24(3): 26–38.

Rysman, A.. 1977. How the "gossip" became a woman. *Journal of Communication* 27: 176–180.

Schiffrin, D. 1987. *Discourse Markers.* Cambridge: Cambridge University Press.

Schiffrin, D. 1994. *Approaches to Discourse.* Oxford: Blackwell.

Searle, J. 1975. Indirect speech acts. In P. Cole and J. Morgan, eds., *Syntax and Semantics. Volume 3: Speech Acts.* New York: Academic Press, 59–82.

Szwed, J. 1969. Gossip, drinking, and social control: consensus and communication in a Newfoundland parish. *Ethnology* 5: 434–441.

Tannen, D. 1984. *Conversational Style.* Norwood, New Jersey: Ablex.

Tannen, D. 1990. *You Just Don't Understand! Women and Men in Conversation.* New York: William Morrow.

Ting-Toomey, S. 1979. Gossip as a communication construct. Paper presented at the Annual convention of the Western Speech Communication Association, Los Angeles, California, Feb. 17–21, 1979.

West, C., and Zimmerman, D. 1983. Small insults: a study of interruptions in cross-sex conversations between unacquainted persons. In B. Thorne, C. Kramarae, and N. Henley, eds., *Language, Gender and Society*, Rowley, Massachusetts: Newbury House, 102–117.

Yalom, I. D. 1995. *The Theory and Practice of Group Psychotherapy* (4th ed). New York: Basic Books.

Yerkovich, S. 1977. Gossiping as a way of speaking. *Journal of Communication* 27: 192–196.

Zarit, S., Anthony, C., and Boutselis, M. 1987. Interventions with care givers of dementia patients: comparison of two approaches. *Psychology and Aging* 2(3): 225–232.

CHAPTER 12

Elders' Complaints

Discourses on Old Age and Social Change in Rural Kenya and Urban Philadelphia

Maria G. Cattell

Two workmen were chatting during their lunchbreak.
John (shaking his head): You know, my wife, she just complains
all the time. That's all she does: complain, complain, complain.
Dave: Yeah? What does she complain about?
John: I dunno. She don't say.
—A favorite joke of my father, Munsey Gleaton

INTRODUCTION

To borrow from my father's oft-told joke, when people complain they do not always say what it is they are complaining about. Or to put it another way, people do not always mean what they say. Even when complaints are about "facts" or observable realities, the complainers may be expressing hidden meanings and/or negotiating status or other advantages.

This paper examines the language of complaint in two very different cultural settings, among rural Samia in western Kenya and among white ethnics in an urban American neighborhood known as Olney in Philadelphia, Pennsylvania.

In rural Kenya, Samia elders complain in order to get young people to do the right thing toward the elderly. People of all ages complain about shameful behavior toward the elderly as a way of debating and reinforcing cultural ideals of family care and respect for old people. This discourse is occurring in a situation of rapid social change, stresses on families, and shifts in intergenerational relations.

In Olney the research focus was on the neighborhood rather than on the family, so these examples focus on old people's complaints about their community. Older Olneyites make their complaints in private conversations, formal interviews, and the public discourse of meetings such as civic, special interest, and senior groups. As in Kenya, Olney is in a state of flux or rapid change. Thus when people complain about graffiti or neighbors who never sweep their steps or sidewalk, their words reflect on the meanings of neighborliness, express fears for personal safety, and reveal perceptions of the community as in disorder or under attack by alien forces.

In both places, oldtimers' complaints often include explicit comparison with the "old days" or "the way it used to be." While the past is probably more or less idealized, nevertheless such comparisons give elders' language the dimensions of historical experience and moral or evaluative assessment.

The research was done as anthropological fieldwork involving participant observation, formal and informal interviews, and survey questionnaires. I lived in Samia, I commuted to Philadelphia. Initially, I was a total stranger to Kenyan culture, whereas in Philadelphia, my cultural identity and background were very similar to those of the people I encountered during my research. In short, I was more or less a native in Philadelphia.

In Kenya older women most often spoke only their local language (Lusamia); many older men also spoke Swahili; most younger people knew both of these and at least some English. In Philadelphia the research language was English (or American), though many informants spoke some European language as well. My competence in the various languages varies from being a native speaker to having modest capability (especially conversational) and working from translations. In addition, my knowledge of linguistics is slim. So this is not a fine-tuned linguistic analysis but a broad anthropological approach to cultural and personal meanings expressed in complaints viewed as cultural discourses on old age and social change.

COMPLAINTS AND SOCIAL CHANGE

In both Samia and Olney, socioeconomic and cultural changes have been going on at a rapid pace in recent decades, within the lifetimes of those now elderly. The changes have created environments very different from the elders' earlier experiences of the same places.

Such broad-scale changes are sometimes labeled by social scientists as "social change" or, in developing countries, "modernization." There are problems with these concepts, including lack of specificity, historicity, and comparability (Fischer, 1978; Foner, 1984). Nevertheless, in aging studies in particular, modernization theory (Cowgill, 1974; Cowgill and Holmes, 1972)—in spite of its shortcomings—stimulated a body of research on the impacts of change on the status and wellbeing of elders in developing countries. My own researches in Kenya, Philadelphia, and more recently, South Africa, all fall under this rubric.

In this paper I look at elders' perceptions of their lives in their changing worlds as revealed by their complaint discourse.

COMPLAINT DISCOURSE

Complaints are expressions of dissatisfaction and resentment, uneasiness, pain, and anguish. They are protest and lament, accusation and blaming. They can result from rational assessments but often are tied to feelings. Anyone can make them, probably almost everyone does.

The idea of "complaint discourse" came from Harriet Rosenberg's (1990) article on the !Kung San of Botswana.[1] In this article Rosenberg analyzes !Kung elders' complaints as a form of discourse in their negotiation of caregiving for themselves in a society which has experienced rapid and radical change in the last three decades of the 20th century.

Rosenberg and others (Lee, 1969; Marshall, 1961; Shostak, 1981) have described !Kung discourse style as characterized by a high level of verbal aggression in the form of complaints and insults ranging from mere exaggeration to total untruth. !Kung complain, joke, and make fun of others all the time to reduce status differences, keep everyone humble, and impose a measure of social control in a society which has no formal system of governance. They complain consciously, competitively, and unremittingly, sparing no one, not even visiting anthropologists. For example, !Kung repeatedly called Lee's (1969) huge fat ox "a bag of bones" and complained that they would all leave the feast hungry if that skinny ox was the meal—though they knew very well that the ox was extraordinarily large and they would feast extremely well. Their put-downs were their way of dealing with what they perceived as Lee's "boasting." They helped to reduce status differences between themselves and a powerful outsider.

Another effect of this discourse style is the relief of social tensions among people who spend most of their time in the same small group (Marshall, 1961). In this sense complaints have expressive value as they allow individuals to "let off steam" without exposing them to much danger from physical retaliation and fights.

Rosenberg found that the needs of frail elderly !Kung are generally met by caregiving networks within their small communities. "Yet the discourse used by elders to describe their situation is often one of unrelenting complaint and blaming" (p.23). Asked who looks after them, these elders often say that no one does—although it is usually patently not true. The readily observable reality is that elderly !Kung receive a high level of care. But elders' talk about their care takes the form of complaints about the high level of neglect they experience.

By the time they reach old age, !Kung have perfected complaint discourse. And they give complaints a special twist. They use complaints to reinforce the intergenerational caregiving contract—even if it means telling a monstrous and readily disproved lie about being totally abandoned in a crisis as one old man did. Such a "big story" is a way of saying the unthinkable, projecting what *might* happen if old people were neglected. Thus it is a story to remind the young of their duty rather than a genuine accusation of neglect, a verbal form of norm reinforcement (cf. Nugent 1990).[2]

While the !Kung have polished complaint discourse to high art, elders in many cultures complain; indeed, complaining may be a nearly universal characteristic of the elderly as they experience social, physical, and mental losses and find that complaining can be a strategy for maximizing or insuring support (Foner, 1984, 1985). For example, among the Black Carib (Garifuna) of Belize, support from children is considered the right of older people (Kerns, 1980). Garifuna culture idealizes both filial and parental responsibility and lifelong intergenerational reciprocity. Black Carib women in particular make themselves centers of redistributive support, hounding negligent sons on payday and publicly criticizing their children's neglect. They praise their children's generosity, too, while also reminding the children how much is done for them by their mothers—just as crazy Mary "reminded" me how much she had done for me, her daughter-in-law (see below).

Perhaps complaining by old people is even expected in many cultures, as with the !Kung and Black Carib. Kenyan young people have said to me, "Oh, old people always complain." Makoni (1996:13) suggests that in South Africa the elderly are "socialized into mastering the art of complaint," like the old Xhosa woman who said, "Every mother of my age complains."

Myerhoff (1978:146) describes the transformation of the Jewish tradition of the *kvetch*, the complainer, into competitive public performance among elderly Jews in a California senior center. These elders are not trying to encourage supportive behavior from younger people. Rather, they use complaints to gain attention and honor or "visibility" within their own center community.

While the literature on complaints, with the exception of Rosenberg's article, consists of bits and snippets, it does suggest a complexity of motivations for old people's complaints and the multivocal, multidimensional nature of complaints which can simultaneously hold several meanings, fulfill several needs, and/or have one or more intended results. Complaints can have instrumental value for the complainers in helping them fulfill perceived needs. They can also have expressive value by venting feelings about the social, physical, and mental losses of old age and disquieting environmental changes.

In particular, and relevant to the case studies presented here, complaints can be expressions of person-environment dissonance. This is the sense of unease that follows from being in an environment which has changed so much that one feels like a stranger. It involves threats to the self, to one's sense of identity, social roles, and personal safety, which arise from perceived qualities of the physical, social, and cultural environment.

I will return to these themes in the conclusion, following the presentation of two case studies on elders' complaints based on my own research.

RESEARCH METHODS: KENYA

My anthropological fieldwork among the Samia of rural western Kenya has focused on aging and old age and the lives of elderly Samia under circumstances of rapid socioeconomic and cultural change. The research extended over two years from November 1983 through November 1985, with visits of four to six weeks in 1982, 1987, 1990,

1992, and 1993. It was done in western Kenya among two Abaluyia subgroups, primarily the Samia, and among families of my rural informants in the cities of Kisumu and Nairobi. Since initially I knew nothing of the local language, Lusamia (which is unwritten), and never became proficient enough to engage in complex discussions, I had research assistants. They were secondary school graduates who were fluent in Swahili and English in addition to their mother tongue.

While I have used field-designed formal instruments (including a survey of 416 women and men age fifty years and up, dubbed the "Old People of Samia" survey), the major data sources are participant observation including informal and in-depth interviews. I have lived among the Samia and been incorporated as a member into two Samia families (plus another family in Bunyala); as a family member, I am expected to behave appropriately and to participate in family reciprocity. I have observed and interacted with numerous people in many homes, on roads and footpaths, and in other public places such as markets, churches and schools. I have shared daily activities, serious illness, theft, house fires, the struggle to educate children, marriages, births, and deaths. My contacts include females and males of all ages with a range of social and economic characteristics.

The result is a wide-ranging knowledge of Samia society and culture, recorded in extensive and varied fieldnotes and what Ottenberg (1990) calls "headnotes" or data recorded only in one's memory. In addition to the survey questionnaires (reproduced in Cattell, 1989a:604–693), the written fieldnotes include a narrative field journal and topical notes which describe events and conversations. In addition, there are biographical interviews (tapes and transcriptions), a household census in one village, focused interviews (mini-surveys on a particular topic), essays by 7th and 8th grade schoolgirls, funeral speeches (tapes and transcriptions), maps ranging from a map of Samia (see Cattell, 1994) to sketches of family compounds and house interiors, photographs and videos, cultural materials (folktales, proverbs, riddles, songs), language materials, genealogies, archival materials from Nangina Hospital, and others. Not all these materials relate directly to the topic at hand, though many do; but all taken together (along with others' publications) constitute the sources of my knowledge of Samia culture and the lives of Samia people.

Perhaps the best validation of this knowledge has come from literate Samia who have read my dissertation and articles. While not uncritical, invariably they tell me: "You really know our culture."

SAMIA OF KENYA: A DISCOURSE OF NEGLECT

Samia in the 1990s is decidedly rural. Most Samia are peasant farmers, smallholders growing both subsistence and cash crops by labor-intensive hoe agriculture; girls and women carry water and firewood from external sources to their homes and cook over open fires; most transportation is by foot.

However, despite its continuing agrarian orientation, the physical and social world of the Samia has undergone enormous changes in the 20th century. Only one hundred years ago the Samia lived in small walled villages; they had a self-sufficient agropastoral economy, no machines, and a social system and culture virtually untouched by European influences. Now they live on small farms scattered over the Samia hills. Colonialism and incorporation into the world political economy brought money, cash cropping, labor migration, Christianity, literacy, medicine and clinics, a small hospital, a centralized bureaucratic political system, trading centers and markets, public transportation, schools, churches, telephones, postal service, electric lines. All these new things and institutions, and more, in one lifetime!—roughly 60 to 80 years.

Along with these changes—and like millions throughout subsaharan Africa—the Samia have become materially impoverished. Families, though still tied to rural homelands, are geographically dispersed by schooling, employment, and the attractions of urban living. Young people have sources of knowledge, money, status, and power which are external to the family system and have weakened the social and economic control of elders. Ideals about intergenerational relationships have perhaps changed more slowly. People of all ages agree that younger family members owe elders respect and service, that elderly parents must be cared for by their children, especially sons and daughters-in-law. Many sons and other family members in fact try to live up to the ideals, but the factors mentioned make it more difficult. So the old people complain. Maybe elders complained a century ago. But probably they have more to complain about today in a setting which is conducive to feelings of unease or person-environment dissonance.

During my two years in Samia I rented a hospital staff house. Many people passed my house every day. One who went by often was Mary, an old woman who came to take vegetables from the hospital gardens. She was stealing, but no one tried to stop her. What was the use? Everyone knew that she was *omulalu*, a crazy person who could not be reasoned with. But Mary gave me a vivid lesson in the power of complaint.

One day as Mary passed my house she spotted the cat's plate on the porch and took the plate with her. The protests of my research assistant, JB, did not deter her, and a request to return the plate brought Mary to my window to harangue me: "I have given you everything," she said, "this house, a free house, these people to work for you. I have given you everything. How can you deny me such a small thing as a plate?" JB commented to me that Mary was behaving like a mother-in-law who takes some little thing from her son's wife. When the daughter-in-law asks for its return, the mother-in-law will say: "I suffered to give birth to my son, I struggled to bring him up, yet you object if I take something little. How can you deny me such a small thing?"

This was a good object lesson in the value of complaining. Had I indeed been Mary's daughter-in-law, I suppose I would have been ashamed not to just give her the thing. And in this case Mary's complaint about my lack of appreciation for her suffering achieved her goal: she got to keep her "something little."

I heard many other complaints directly in conversations, during interviews, and in my "Old People of Samia" survey ($n = 416$). In the survey, most elders agreed with statements that young people nowadays do not respect the old people as they used to, and that there is a gap between young and old. Often they added spontaneous comments in responding to these questions: "The young don't want to walk with us," "They don't want to sit and eat with us," said many old people. "They prefer talking among themselves. Young people just want to speak English," they complained. "When they want to know something, they go to books for advice."

At the conclusion of the lengthy questionnaire, a number of elderly said they were glad to have answered the questions, or they invited the interviewer to come back any time and ask more questions. Several said, "I thought I would just die with my knowledge"—a poignant commentary on how they saw the value of their own knowledge in the modern world and the diminution of their roles as advisers and teachers of the young.

There is a large measure of objective reality in such complaints. Young people today do spend much less time with elders. The generations are separate physically by spending their days in school and intellectually by formal education with instruction in two foreign languages (English and Swahili) which conveys knowledge most older people lack. This separation continues into adulthood with urban residence and employment. So the complaints, even those made under survey conditions which encourage normative responses, nevertheless reflect the world of everyday behavior.

My research assistants confirmed the generation gap from their side of it. They said that they had never really sat down with old people as they did while doing the interviews and were grateful for having met so many interesting people and learned so much about their own customs.

In conversations I heard from people of all ages complaints about neglect, particularly about children who neglected their old parents, sometimes coupled with remarks about how "the family is falling apart." From social workers at Nangina Hospital I sometimes heard about actual cases of serious neglect of older persons, but most elders I knew personally were getting at least some support from their families, primarily from children, daughters-in-law, grandchildren, and wives (Cattell, 1990). Even in the survey of 416 elderly, most people admitted to getting some help from family members. I say "admitted" because their preference in ordinary conversation was to complain about how they were suffering, not getting things they needed, and so on.

A good example of that is Mzee Oyioma, a man then in his late sixties whose home I visited a number of times. Mzee Oyioma was probably a bit more prosperous than many, but he lived the same rural lifestyle as others and was certainly not wealthy. He lived in a compound with several large, well-constructed houses and five granaries (an unusually large number). He had several educated children with good jobs, with one married schoolteacher son living at home. Another son was a medical technician working in an urban hospital.

Mzee Oyioma was thin but vigorous and seemingly healthy. From time to time I would meet him in places several miles from his home (walking anywhere took vigor since Samia is hill country). On such occasions he wore ordinary, even torn or patched, shirts and trousers and the usual rubber sandals. He looked like any other *mzee* (old man, an honorific). But when I paid a formal visit to his home he always dressed in a white shirt, sometimes even with a tie, trousers, and formal jacket, everything clean with no patches or rips. I was always given a fine meal, and his grandchildren who lived in the homestead looked well fed and strong. Not only that, all were in school, which is an expensive proposition for most families.

However, Mzee Oyioma, in spite of his obvious prosperity, had what sounded like a serious complaint: "If I could have had more educated children [to care for me], then I couldn't be suffering now. When I was younger, I had strength and money from my fishing business. It was a life of happiness. Now all that I had, I don't have that now."

Mzee's complaints were similar to complaints I heard in conversations with others who, like him, appeared reasonably healthy and well cared for. Eventually I realized that such complaints had several meanings. One was that, indeed, life was not as good as it used to be. It was not good to lose strength, be unable to work and care for your family, be deprived of food, help and companionship. In short, it was not good to become old. I heard such evaluations of old age in many conversations and interviews and from hundreds of old people in the survey, for example, in two questions which asked "What is the goodness of being an old person?" and "What is the badness of being an old person?"

Since the often-expressed Samia cultural ideal is that old age is a time of high prestige and respect, leadership and authority, one would expect many answers reflecting the ideal. In fact, both questions— separately and together—overwhelmingly amounted to a general opinion among old people that there is not much about old age that is good and plenty that is bad.[3] An unusually high number of elders had non-responses or uninterpretable responses to the "goodness" question; 63% said unequivocally that there is "no goodness in being an old person." They should know! In contrast, nearly everyone (n = 406) answered clearly the "badness" question. While many could not find the goodness in old age, nearly everyone was explicit about the badness. Only 18 said there is "no badness"; the other 388 had nearly three times as many separately coded comments (in multiple responses, or what one might call multiple complaints about old age) to the badness question as they did to the goodness question. In fact, some even complained about the bad behavior of old people who are demanding, complaining, and never satisfied!

Back to Mzee Oyioma, well fed, well clothed, surrounded by healthy grandchildren, still making oars to sell to fishermen on Lake Victoria. Why did he say he was "suffering"? Surely in part because old age was not so great, as hundreds of his compatriots said. He used to be a fisherman, now he only carves oars. He is not as strong and able as he was. But he was more fortunate than many, that was obvious. And even though his own abilities were declining, his family was taking care of him. Why was he complaining?

I puzzled over such complaints of Mzee Oyioma and other elders until I realized that there was a reason for them, not in his life circumstances, but in the need to uphold cultural ideals and remind the younger generation of their duty. Conversations and interviews are seldom private in Samia, so almost everything is heard by others who are not immediate to the discussion. Mzee Oyioma was doing his duty as an elder to remind anyone within hearing that children should care for aged parents. He was right in line with crazy Mary when it came to complaints—and both were right in line with elders in many societies, as Foner (1985) reports from her cross-cultural comparisons. Nydegger (1983) has also pointed out that old people throughout history and in differrent cultures have complained of younger generations and contrasted the present unfavorably with an earlier golden age.[4]

However, it is likely that Samia elders' complaints are particularly intense today. Today's elderly grew up in a fairly inward-looking, localized community which was just beginning to be transformed by British colonialism. Their past was lived in communities in which useful, valuable knowledge was local knowledge, and high status came with age. Most elderly men in the survey said that when they were boys, they used to sit every evening around a certain fire (*esiosio*, the "men's fire"), listening to the men talking and being advised by their elders. Women, older girls, and young children similarly sat together in the kitchen around the cooking fire. Many of these older people (both men and women) said they had slept in *esibinje*, the "grandmother's house" and had learned many things from their grandmothers. The oldest (in the survey and in in-depth interviews) recalled a world without money, without books, schools, hospitals, or churches, without cities, motor vehicles, or radios. If those old days were not entirely golden, they were surely much more under the control of Samia elders, both women and men, than is the case today with a national government which reaches into every rural village, no matter how remote, and a local economy which reverberates to changes in the world economy.

Samia old people contrast their memories of childhood, youth, and young adulthood with the situation today. Today children and grandchildren go off to school for much of the day and even for months at a time if they go to secondary school, most of which are boarding schools. The young people go to books for advice because much of the old people's knowledge has been devalued in the modern situation (Cattell, 1989b). As one active woman in her sixties said, quite reasonably, "Nowadays it is not easy to advise the young." She meant that she lacked the proper knowledge for giving advice to the young, who were going to school, books, their (usually young) schoolteachers for advice. Her complaint, and similar complaints of many other Samia elders concerning intergenerational relationships which contrasted present and past, reflected person-environment dissonance, the sense of no longer feeling at home in their environment, particularly the sociocultural environment.

Thus in Samia today elders' complaints appear to do double duty. They have instrumental value in terms of reinforcing ideals of filial obligation. They have expressive value in allowing old people to bring out their disappointments about changes over which they have had little control and disappointments about their culturally and experientially derived expectations for a good old age. They may also serve to let off steam about feeling weak and more or less useless (which no one wants to be). They may even have another purpose, that of concealing possessions. All Samia try to conceal what they have in order to protect themselves from the jealousy of others and from dunning requests to share what they have. Here one has to walk a fine line of understanding, however. One old man I knew well had his share of complaints like Mzee Oyioma's, but he gave up a night watchman job because he thought he was too old to be working and his neighbors and kin might think his children were not taking care of him. He did not want to shame his children nor reduce his own status as an elder by working at a paid job when he should be relaxing and letting his children provide for him.

In Kenya, complaint discourse is not confined to local situations such as the one I have described in Samia. Kenyan government officials (including the president and members of parliament), social workers, social scientists, and the print media are also engaged in complaints, which are part of a national discourse of norm reinforcement. Common complaints are that "the family" or "the extended family" is disintegrating, dying, or even that it is completely dead, that old people are neglected, that "no one" takes care of the elderly any more. Such complaints have the flavor of the "big story" of the !Kung man about having been abandoned in a crisis, that is, they appear rather to be commentary on the way things could go wrong if cultural ideals of elder care are forsaken.[5]

I have written about this debate on the intergenerational contract elsewhere (Cattell, 1997) and will say here only that the complaint discourse on intergenerational relationships and obligations, and on the role of the extended family in the lives of modern Kenyans, is carried on everywhere, from the most public arenas at the national level to the footpaths and homesteads of rural Samia—and no doubt will continue, given the intense pressures on the resources of most Kenyan families.

RESEARCH METHODS: PHILADELPHIA

The Kenyan discourse of norm reinforcement should reverberate with Americans, who are currently debating intergenerational equity in the allocation of healthcare resources and elder entitlements. However, let us come down to the local level again, this time to Philadelphia, specifically, to the neighborhood of Olney.[6]

This research was an 18-month community study carried out from September 1989 through February 1991 with intermittent return visits up to the present. The aim was to explore the relationship between older persons' residential continuity (aging-in-place), subjectively defined resources, and social change in Olney. The research used the multimethod approach of anthropological fieldwork, including participant observation and in-depth interviews.

I began by reading about Olney and touring the community on foot and in my car, city map and notebook to hand. I hung out at the McDonald's on 5th Street, known as the "old people's breakfast club," read the *Olney Times*, shopped. I became a member of the Greater Olney Community Council and, for a few years, the chair of its Senior Citizens Committee. I even wrote two articles for the *Olney Times* and gave a talk to one senior group on my research in Kenya!

Through attending community meetings I met several people who became key informants, including Olney's unofficial historian who provided information on the development of Olney during this century (it was farmland until the 1920s). My seven key informant relationships involved home visits, observation of daily routines, informal and focused interviews, collection of life history materials, and participation in activities outside the home such as shopping and going to meetings. In addition, another 25 persons were interviewed on several occasions, and a further 11 persons were interviewed once.

Except for occasional overnight visits with one woman, I did not live in Olney but commuted there from my home in the Greater Philadelphia area. Nevertheless, when my report on this research (Cattell 1991) was read by Community Council members, they told me that "it sounds like us."

PHILADELPHIA: COMPLAINTS AND COMMUNITY

Olney is both big city and small town. It is a blue collar rowhouse neighborhood in lower northeast Philadelphia. It suffers the usual problems of big cities. At the time of my research, the city was on the brink of bankruptcy (this is no longer the case). Everyone of every age complains about things like dirt, crime, reduced city services, inadequate police protection, do-nothing politicians. Such complaints have some obvious justification, as a walk around the streets and attention to daily media news will make immediately clear.

Olney residents have a distinct sense of their community which is reinforced by various eponymous institutions including a newspaper, several civic organizations, Olney High School, Olney Symphony Orchestra, even a community-minded citizen who is known as "Mr. Olney." In fact, when you get to know Olney and its people, it has many aspects of a small town, such as my own hometown of Lancaster, Pennsylvania. Olney's population in the 1990 census was close to 60,000—about the same as Lancaster's population. Many aspects of Olney's physical environment (Lancaster is also a rowhouse city) and community life reminded me of Lancaster, and, unexpectedly (because I was thinking "big city"), I felt at home from the beginning of my research. The feeling of at-homeness grew as I got to know Olney and some of its residents (who of course call themselves Olneyites).

Less than a year after I ended my research I drove up 5th Street and thought it looked dingier and dirtier than it had, with many new and vacant stores. Worse yet, the senior "breakfast club," a McDonald's restaurant, was boarded up! I found myself muttering about how could "they" do this to Olney and realized I was probably feeling that same person-environment dissonance older Olneyites had so often expressed to me. One woman had summed it up keenly: "I feel like an immigrant in my own community."

While my research in Kenya focused on older persons within their families, the Philadelphia research focused on older persons within their community. Specifically, the research concerned older white ethnics who have lived in Olney for decades and have seen Olney shift from being 92% white in 1980 to being a multi-ethnic community only 59% white in 1990. These new people include immigrants from many different Asian countries, Latinos, and African Americans. They are widely distributed throughout Olney's residential areas (most of Olney on either side of 5th Street); Olney is one of the most highly integrated neighborhoods in the city.

I heard many complaints from older Olneyites about their community. However, there were different patterns of complaints about their own block and the wider community. This distinction seemed to reflect a sense that if you live in a good neighborhood (block), you can tolerate more threats to self-identity and personal safety in the wider community.[7]

Complaints about One's Own Neighborhood

Several people said, with pride, that "my block is a League of Nations." Many insisted that "in my block everyone gets along." This insistence on "getting along" did not seem to be mere euphemistic gloss. In general, immediate neighbors did get along, though they certainly recognized, discussed, and complained about the physical appearance of their block and neighbors' observable imperfections.

People expressed many feelings of loss of control of their neighborhood in complaints about abandoned cars, vacant houses, and vandalism, crackhouses and other dangers to themselves and neighborhood children. People can do something about some problems, and some do: they pick up trash, paint over graffiti, take the parking space illegally "reserved" by a plastic crate and/or complain to the neighbor who put out the crate. But to do anything about a vacant house or abandoned car[8] requires dealing with Philadelphia's bureaucracy, which moves slowly at best. So complaints about these very real threats to neighborhood security seemed to have primarily expressive value to help relieve fears by sharing common concerns and anxieties.

There were also numerous specific complaints about specific neighbors—as no doubt has always been true. Many negative comments focused on behavior that impinged on physical space and privacy, for example, "reserving" a parking space or being noisy. Since people are concerned about the appearance of their block, they readily remark on the neighbor whose house is poorly maintained or who never sweeps outside. Other problems such as trash thrown on the street, graffiti, and abandoned cars tended to be blamed on outsiders, the anonymous and ubiquitous "they."

One of the most frequent complaints about neighbors was: "We don't speak the same language. We can't even talk to each other." Elders recalled "when my block was mostly German" and complained about the "different" people who live here now. "I'd rather be with my own kind of people," they said. People brought up pleasant memories of neighborhood sociability when they sat on their proches or in their backyards on summer evenings and their children played together. "But now I can't even talk to my neighbor, who is Cambodian" (or whatever: specific labels were usually used). Such complaints certainly arose from unease about the people who lived close by. They also invoked a sense of loss of neighborliness, a diminution of neighborly behavior including small exchanges (such as bringing in the mail for an absent neighbor) and neighborly trust, made impossible by so many newcomers, especially newcomers with whom the oldtimers could not communicate.

There were also multitudinous complaints about "dirt," which both describes easily seen reality and is a favorite code word for the undesirable changes in Olney. Elderly Olneyites complained about neighbors who never swept their steps or raked their leaves. They complained that the city no longer swept the streets. But they reserved their severest complaints about dirt for the wider community.

They complained about the untidiness of newcomers' gardens, especially Asians' gardens, which did not fit their European-derived concept of a tidy, rather formal flower garden (or "mini-Versailles" gardens). One seventy-year-old woman, speaking of the garden next to hers, said that her former neighbor had won prizes in the city-wide garden contest. "If she could come back and see what her garden is like today, she'd be shocked. They grow those yardlong peas or whatever they are, and hang things from strings," she said, with a verbal shiver of disgust. Ethnic slurs were rarely used, but if a Thai neighbor's squash or cucumber vine wound through a backyard fence, there would be complaints about "those vines that grow everywhere," with the vines clearly symbolic of the forces of disorder and alien invasion.

However, such breaches of neighborly behavior did not divert people from insistence on neighborhood harmony as the way life should be nor from perceiving their own neighborhood as actually being harmonious. Complaints about these minor problems were probably nothing new and did not make one's immediate living environment unacceptable in personal, esthetic or moral terms. Vacant houses, grafitti and abandoned vehicles in one's own block were more threatening, however, and brought forth stronger condemnations.

Complaints about the Wider Community

The verbal restraint often used in complaints about one's own neighborhood did not apply to comments about the wider community, especially the main shopping district along 5th Street. It is likely that unrestrained complaints about 5th street served as at least partial release for frustrations about one's own block. Complaints about 5th Street often were angry or bitter, sometimes included ethnic slurs, and had no redeeming disclaimer to compare with "we all get along in my block." Indeed, the wider community of Olney, and 5th Street in particular, was perceived as a place of strangers, interethnic conflict, crime—and DIRT.

The landscape of 5th Street has changed dramatically in recent years. In the past 10 or 15 years the 5th Street business district has shifted from European ethnic owners to predominantly Korean ownership. Many store signs are in Korean (and some other Asian language) characters, sometimes with nothing in English, which in general means "keep out: Koreans only wanted" to elderly Olneyites. Asked what how 5th Street used to be, people reminisced fondly about specific stores: the hardware store where you could get exactly what you needed, even just two nails, or the drugstore with a German-speaking pharmacist; the cleanliness of the streets; being able to get "everything you needed" on 5th Street. People complained at length about the disappearance of old family-run businesses, clerks who do not know their stock, rapid changes of store ownership, and "all those signs I can't even read."

Today 5th Street is seen as a place of strangers: "I never see anyone I know on 5th Street any more." This complaint was sometimes made in the same conversation in which the speaker mentioned meeting so-and-so on 5th Street that morning. They were neither lying nor forgetful. Rather, their hyperbole reflected the perception that the sidewalks and stores of 5th Street today throng with strangers, people of different ethnicities and cultural backgrounds (obvious to anyone walking the area).

Of course older Olneyites saw 5th Street as "soooo dirty!"—but to my eyes as well it seemed dirtier than most of the residential blocks.

The City of Philadelphia no longer does streetcleaning, so the only cleaning is done by the occasional broom-wielding merchant. In residential areas many people sweep their sidewalks, even the gutters, and pick up stray trash. The result is an obvious difference between 5th Street and the residential blocks.

Oldtimers long for Olney's former cleanliness. In their vocabulary of complaint, dirt has become a key metaphor for discomfort about the changes in Olney. "We can't say those ethnic words any more," one woman said, almost choking in her effort to keep them unsaid. But one can talk about dirt, and in Olney's complaint discourse, dirt is the highly visible antithesis of community.

Sometimes the older people were reluctant to recognize that there still is a community Olney. But for the older white ethnics who have chosen to stay in Olney ("I love Olney; I'm staying right here"), their community was to a considerable extent themselves as they met in public along 5th Street, in stores, at meetings, and in the privacy of their homes. When they got together they exchanged information and complaints, reinforcing ideals of neighborhood and community and their sense of self through shared memories of the past and common experiences (negative and positive) in the present. While they did not seem to be engaging in the "competitive complaining" of the Center Jews (Myerhoff, 1978:146), older Olneyites' complaints did contribute in their own way to their "visibility" or sense of identity and self-worth derived from recognition by their peers. Older Olneyites achieved their visibility through a well developed sense of "us" (oldtimers) against "them" (alien newcomers). Through their complaints they provided each other with comfort and sympathy, a sense of shared memory and identity, and some defense against perceived attacks on their community, neighborhoods, and themselves.

TOWARD A THEORY OF COMPLAINTS

These case studies suggest the value of listening to the words, and to the meanings behind the words, when old people complain. Not to be dismissed as "just what all old people do," their complaints are strategies for assuring their physical security and reassuring themselves as persons in settings of rapid social and cultural change which induced feelings of person-environment dissonance.

As Makoni (1996:10) points out, person-environment dissonance may itself may create an environment "conducive to complaints." This suggests a topsy-turvy take on the idea of what constitutes an environment. "One can not enter the same river twice"—because one changes, the river changes. It may be that for many who live long lives, even in relatively stable settings, person-environment dissonance grows as individuals' capacities diminish. That is, they no longer feel themselves to be the same person they were if physical or mental impairments make it difficult or impossible for them to do things they are accustomed to doing. Or the self feels trapped in a stranger's body. The person rather than the environment has changed, producing feelings of alienation and unease.

It is possible that an oppositional, complaining interpersonal style allows elders to demonstrate that they are still in control, like the old Xhosa woman who complained that young people no longer obey their elders—except in her own house where she ruled with an iron hand and things were different (Makoni, 1996). Similarly, complaining may enable impaired elders to exert competencies they still have and to maintain power over others while also keeping distant from impaired peers (Albert and Cattell, 1994:246). Here again, just as changed external environments may be conducive to complaints, so the changed internal environment of the self, or frailty, may be conducive to complaints.

Finally, there are elders who do not engage in complaints and arguments. Instead, they live lives characterized by silence and stigma, by the "silent anguish" of dementia and the stigma of silence as deviant behavior (Savishinsky, 1991:133,137). Savishinsky and also Shield (1988) found this to be the case among elders with dementia in nursing homes in the United States who come from a cultural background ("American") in which people are uncomfortable with silence. However, as Savishinsky points out, in some cultures (for example, Native American), silence is not an absence of speech, a failure, disability, or deviance. Rather, it is part of speech.

The meanings of becoming "old" vary cross-culturally, but within each culture there are cultural guidelines for old age, what Cohen (1984) calls "indigenous social policy." While cultural details differ, becoming and being old entail transformations of the self in terms of personal identity and social roles in all cultures. Thus old age, frailty, the imminence of death combine with cultural beliefs to make old age an experience of individual exploration into the unknown—an experience intensified in changing social environments. Is it any wonder that old people, everywhere, complain? Not because there is nothing else they can do, but because their complaints are a multi-vocal, multi-dimensional discourse strategy for defending social norms, negotiating care, and affirming the self.

ACKNOWLEDGMENTS

An earlier version of this article was presented in the Language and Aging pre-session at the Georgetown University Round Table on Languages and Linguistics in April 1992 with the title, "Old People and the Language of Complaint: Examples from Kenya and Philadelphia."

As always I am grateful to those who have made my Kenyan research possible over the years, especially my late husband Bob Moss; John Barasa Owiti, my Samia co-researcher since 1984, and his family; Frankline Teresa Mahaga and her family; the Medical Mission Sisters and Holy Family Hospital at Nangina, Kenya. Above all, *mutio muno* to the many people of Samia and Bunyala who have allowed me to share their lives—and tell others about them. The research in Kenya was partially funded by the National Science Foundation (grant BNS8306802), the Wenner-Gren Foundation for Anthropological Research (grant 4506), and Bryn Mawr College (Frederica de Laguna Fund grant).

I am most grateful to the people of Olney who welcomed me to their community, especially the many "senior citizens" who allowed me to visit in their homes and to attend, as a junior citizen, their senior group meetings. I thank especially Erna Rath, who adopted me as her daughter; Alfie, Bea, Elsie, and Jack; Amy Zoniriw and her family; and the Greater Olney Community Council. The research in Olney was funded by The Retirement Research Foundation in a grant made to the Philadelphia Geriatric Center (Robert L. Rubinstein and Mark R. Luborsky, Principal Investigators).

NOTES

1. The !Kung have been known by various names; their own self-chosen name is Ju/'hoansi but much of the literature refers to them as !Kung or !Kung San. I use !Kung here to accord with Rosenberg.

2. Nugent describes more stern types of norm reinforcement such as the bequeathal of property and threats of disinheritance.

3. Interestingly, in a survey of school children, most of them saw old age along the lines of the ideal, as a good time, a time to relax and enjoy life.

4. Of course young people also complain: about old people and other matters. Is complaining a cultural universal?

5. Kenyans know very well the power of the extended family in their lives. In 1992 I attended a conference on the family in Kakamega, Kenya. When I challenged the assembled Kenyan social scientists to tell me the Kenyan family is disappearing, when they know very well that tomorrow or at least by next week some family member will be asking them for help of some sort, everyone laughed, and the honsho seated next to me leaned over and said in a loud whisper, "The family is *there!*"

6. Philadelphia is a city of many "neighborhoods," named local areas which are used by everyone including the media and city officials. They are not officially delimited, however, so boundaries are a bit fuzzy. Nor are they locally administered: City Hall for all such neighborhoods is in Center City Philadelphia.

7. "Neighborhood" is used by residents to refer to the block in which they live as well as to the larger neighborhood subdivisions of Philadelphia.

8. There are vacant houses in many blocks, especially in southern Olney, and hundreds of abandoned cars.

REFERENCES

Albert, Steven M., and Cattell, Maria G. 1994. *Old Age in Global Perspective: Cross-Cultural and Cross-National Views.* Social Issues in Global Perspective Series. New York: G.K. Hall/Macmillan.

Cattell, Maria G. 1989a. Old age in rural Kenya: gender, the life course and social change. Bryn Mawr College: Ph.D. dissertation.

Cattell, Maria G. 1989b. Knowledge and social change in Samia, Kenya. *Journal of Cross-Cultural Gerontology* 5:225–244.

Cattell, Maria G. 1990. Models of old age among the Samia of Kenya: family support of the elderly. *Journal of Cross-Cultural Gerontology* 5:375–394.

Cattell, Maria G. 1991. Aging-in-place: older persons' assessment of urban neighborhood resources. Final report to The Retirement Research Foundation (unpublished).

Cattell, Maria G. 1994. "Nowadays it isn't easy to advise the young": grandmothers and granddaughters among Abaluyia of Kenya. *Journal of Cross-Cultural Gerontology* 9:157–178.

Cattell, Maria G. 1997. The discourse of neglect: family support for elderly in Samia. In *African Families and the Crisis of Social Change.* Thomas S. Weisner, Candice Bradley, Philip L. Kilbride, eds. Westport, Connecticut: Greenwood Press. 253–300.

Cohen, Ronald. 1984. Age and culture as theory. In *Age and Anthropological Theory*. David Kertzer and Jennie Keith, eds. Ithaca: Cornell University Press. 234–249.

Cowgill, Donald O. 1974. Aging and modernization: a revision of the theory. In *Late Life: Communities and Environmental Policy*. Jaber F. Gubrium, ed. Springfield, Illinois: Thomas. 123–146.

Cowgill, Donald O. and Lowell D. Holmes, eds. 1972. *Aging and Modernization*. New York: Appleton-Century-Crofts.

Fischer, David Hackett. 1978. *Growing Old in America*. Expanded ed. New York: Oxford University Press.

Foner, Nancy. 1984. *Ages in Conflict: A Cross-Cultural Perspective on Inequality between Old and Young*. New York: Columbia University Press.

Foner, Nancy. 1985. Caring for the elderly: a cross-cultural view. In *Growing Old in America: New Perspectives on Old Age*. 3d ed. Beth B. Hess and Elizabeth W. Markson, eds. New Brunswick, New Jersey: Transaction. 387–400.

Kerns, Virginia. 1980. Aging and mutual support relations among the Black Carib. In *Aging in Culture and Society: Comparative Viewpoints and Strategies*. Christine L. Fry, ed. Brooklyn: J. F. Bergin. 112–125.

Lee, Richard. 1969. Eating Christmas in the Kalahari. *Natural History* (December):14–22, 60–63.

Makoni, Sinfree B. 1996. "They talk to us like children": language and intergenerational relations in first-time encounters in an African township. *Southern African Journal of Gerontology* 5(1):9–14.

Marshall, Lorna. 1961. Sharing, talking and giving: relief of social tensions among !Kung Bushmen. *Africa* 31:231–249.

Myerhoff, Barbara. 1978. *Number Our Days*. New York: Simon and Schuster/Touchstone.

Nugent, Jeffrey B. 1990. Old age security and the defense of social norms. *Journal of Cross-Cultural Gerontology* 5:243–254.

Nydegger, Corinne N. 1983. Family ties of the aged in cross-cultural perspective. *The Gerontologist* 23:26–32.

Ottenberg, Simon. 1990. Thirty years of fieldnotes: changing relationships to the text. In *Fieldnotes: The Makings of Anthropology*. Roger Sanjek, ed. Ithaca & London: Cornell University Press. 139–160.

Rosenberg, Harriet. 1990. Complaint discourse, aging and caregiving among the !Kung San of Botswana. In *The Cultural Context of Aging: Worldwide Perspectives*. Jay Sokolovsky, ed. New York: Bergin & Garvey. 19–41.

Savishinsky, Joel S. 1991. *The Ends of Time: Life and Work in a Nursing Home.* New York/Westport/London: Bergin & Garvey.

Shield, Renee Rose. 1988. *Uneasy Endings: Daily Life in an American Nursing Home.* Ithaca: Cornell University Press.

Shostak, Marjorie. 1981. *Nisa: The Life and Words of a !Kung Woman.* New York: Vintage.

CHAPTER 13

Elderly Women Speak about Their Interactions with Health Care Providers

Joyce Allman
Sandra L. Ragan
Chevelle Newsome
Lucretia Scoufos
Jon Nussbaum

INTRODUCTION

Women's unique health communication issues traditionally have been underrepresented in the health care literature. In fact, until very recently neither medical research nor national policy has recognized the critical importance of investigating women's health issues (Office of Research, 1992). As a result, we have a dearth of information about how being female affects one's health; only recently have any measures been taken to correct the virtual absence of women subjects in major medical research programs and trials.

Likewise, women's health issues have not received adequate attention in the health care communication literature. Although women are the largest consumers of health care in the United States, we know little about the intersection between women's health and their communication with physicians, nurses, and other health care providers. Given the aging of the "Baby Boom" generation in combination with the fact that women live longer than men, the time is at hand to identify the outcomes and consequences of communication between elderly women and their physicians in an effort to enlighten scholars, caregivers, and the medical community as to the needs and concerns of this population.

To explore the world of elderly women's perceptions of their physicians' communicative behaviors and the perceived importance of these behaviors to their overall health care, 20 middle-class women over the age of sixty-five were interviewed about their medical experiences. These women represented a cross-section of elderly females that included four ethnic groups (African American, Asian, Caucasian, and Hispanic). Marital statuses included married, divorced, and widowed; all considered themselves to be in good health. The sample was purposive, as most of the women were acquainted with the interviewers and were willing to openly discuss their experiences. The open-ended interviews, which were audiotaped, revealed that physicians' communication skills can decidedly affect the degree of medical success achieved with their sixty-five and older female patients. A review of literature combined with the voice of the women themselves highlights the importance of exploring the perceptions of this population.

LITERATURE REVIEW

Gerontological Issues

The elderly are the fastest-growing segment of the United States population. In fact, according to Dychtwald and Flower (1990), "In July of 1983, the number of Americans over the age of 65 surpassed the number of teenagers" (p. 8). Whereas the eighty-five and older group now comprise 1.2% of the population, that percentage will increase to 1.8% or 4.9 million by the year 2000 (Cetron and Davies, 1989), and by 2050, the number will increase to 16 million ("The Coming Crisis," 1990). Even if the aging Baby Boomers are healthier, the fact that they will live longer means that greater numbers of the population ultimately will require medical care.

Specific to the female population, Mylander (1979) states that females are the fastest growing group in the United States, with the female/male ratio projected for the year 2035 at 33.4 million/22.4 million. Thus, the problems of aging are principally the problems of women. These women are more vulnerable than men to excesses, abuses, and inequities in long-term care, insurance, and services (Friedman, 1994a).

Although facts and figures confirm that ours is an aging population, studies relative to communication and aging are lagging behind other disciplines. Butler (1989) states that despite the emergence of gerontology as a field of study and the establishment of the National Institute on Aging in 1975, the study of aging still remains "the poor stepchild" (p. 687) of research support and scientific interest. Yet, with the elderly comprising a significant portion of the population and age becoming an increasing factor in society (Kreps, 1984), studies relative to communication and aging are slowly gaining momentum, and research on the elderly has moved from studies that focus simply on the physical aspects of aging to studies that include interaction patterns of the elderly. One such study by Giles, Coupland, Coupland, Williams, and Nussbaum (1992) described the elderly as a subculture, and, based on intercultural theories developed by Kim (1988), Giles et al. stated that intergenerational communication was analogous to intercultural encounters. According to Ruben (1990), this subculture phenomenon carries over into the health care arena as well, so that ". . . to the extent that physicians, nurses, volunteers, and administrators become enculturated into their own subsystem cultures, the interaction between them and patients is essentially intercultural communication" (p. 57). The Giles et al. study concluded that patterns of intergenerational interactions were counterproductive, which suggests implications for the health care of the elderly, as many of their physicians are of a younger generation. "The way older people talk and are spoken to by younger people is, of course, a central research focus . . . especially as it relates to noninstitutionalized older people" (Giles et al., 1992, p. 281). According to Adelman, Greene, and Charon (1991), age, gender, and race often are mismatched in the physician-elderly patient relationship. And because there are very few older practicing physicians, heterophilous pairing is the norm.

Relational roles between physicians and patients come into play often based on stereotypes. For example, occupational roles, gender, status, age, and physical appearance can influence physician-patient expectations (Kreps and Kunimoto, 1994), and elderly patients generate different expectations than children or adult patients (O'Hair and McNeilis, 1993). Roter and Hall (1992) specify several characteristics or stereotypes that have the potential of affecting physicians' expectations about patients including age, gender, social class, ethnicity or culture, physical appearance, and attitude. Studies have shown that each of these factors contributes in some way to the physician-patient encounter (Beisecker, 1996; Beisecker and Beisecker, 1990; Hooper, Comstock, Goodwin, and Goodwin, 1982; Koopman, Eisenthal, and Stoeckle, 1984; Roter, 1991; Waitzkin, 1985). As noted by Tamir (1979), differences in past experiences, socioeconomic status, life stage, and a variety of other factors make the sharing or cocreation of meaning more difficult. In sum, research suggests that young and old are very likely to misperceive and misunderstand one another because of these factors (Nussbaum, Thompson, and Robinson, 1989).

In a study by Greene, Adelman, Charon, and Hoffman (1986), in which they compared communication of patients younger than forty-five with communication of patients older than sixty-five, the medical encounters were tape-recorded and coded for medical topics, communication content, and emotional exchange. Although the researchers found little evidence of blatant ageism, they found that more medical topics and fewer psychosocial issues were discussed in interviews with older patients. Physicians generally were less responsive to psychosocial issues raised by older patients compared to the younger patients, and coders rated physicians higher relative to information provided and support given to younger patients compared to older patients. Adelman et al. (1991) also analyzed audiotapes of 88 physician-patient encounters and found that "physicians provided better information to younger patients than to older patients on issues that the physicians themselves raised. Physicians were more supportive of younger patients than of older patients on patient-raised issues . . . and were more condescending, abrupt and indifferent with older patients" (pp. 141–142). Finally, in a test for concordance between older and younger patients and their physicians, evidence from audiotapes, patient postvisit interviews, and physician postvisit questionnaires revealed greater concordance among younger physicians and patients relative to goals of the medical interview and topics discussed (Greene, Adelman, Charon, Friedmann, 1989).

Giles et al. (1992) also suggest that the way the elderly describe themselves may contribute to stereotypical responses. The elderly may feel that they need to "act their age," and by placing a stereotypical prototype on themselves, they may reinforce negative images. A study by Tarbox, Connors, and Faillace (1987) revealed that, indeed, negative images of the elderly are present among freshman and senior medical students, although the degree of negative attitudes has improved since the 1960s. These self-fulfilling prototypes may be a factor that contributes to faulty communication between the elderly and their physicians. Adelman, Greene, Charon, and Friedmann (1992) express concern that "older patients and their physicians may be more at risk for miscommunication, possibly because of physicians', and even patients', ageist beliefs" (p. 371). To combat such negativity, Rabinowitz (1988) suggests that geriatric medicine "should focus on the person who has a face, a name, a uniqueness, and it should encourage him or her to resist classification" (p. 530).

The necessity for increasing research related to communication and aging is self-evident. As the Baby Boom generation ages, it behooves us to ask questions of our elderly so that we may know not only how to improve the quality of life for them in their remaining years but also how to better prepare for our own aging.

Physician-Patient Issues

Health care has changed significantly in the last 30 years: costs have increased and health care has become market based, spawning a new breed of health care delivery. For example, health maintenance organizations have emerged; reimbursement methods have changed with the introduction of Medicare and Medicaid; hospitals have undergone organizational changes, with many consolidating into or being bought out by mega-hospital corporations; the government has introduced new regulations; and society has become litigious (Kotler and Clarke, 1987). Whereas physicians once practiced medicine only, they now must practice business management and public relations. Much of the responsibility for patient satisfaction today rests with physicians (DiMatteo, Hayes, and Prince, 1986), and a major portion of the literature on physician-patient communication focuses on the physician's role in the medical exchange.

Physician Training

Communication between doctors and patients can be traced to physician training. Although many students begin medical school with humanistic ideals, demands on technological competence eventually overtake the humanistic quality and there is an increase in rejecting behaviors—ignoring emotions, not listening, and avoiding eye contact—as students progress through medical school (Kramer, Ber, and Moore, 1987). Anderson, Rakowski, and Hickey (1988) state that during residency, physicians can examine personal attitudes and beliefs and develop satisfactory interpersonal interaction with patients.

However, Linn, Oye, Cope, and DiMatteo (1986) contend that physicians' levels of humanistic behavior may be well established by the first year of residency, and the physicians do not return to their early ideals about medical service as suggested by Goffman (1959).

Factors in Physician-Patient Communication

According to a 1988 Harris and Associates poll (cited in Kovner, 1990, p. 3), "Only 54% of Americans report being 'very satisfied' with their last physician encounter." A review of the literature identified three specific areas for this general dissatisfaction among patients: language, social structure, and physicians' demeanor.

Language. Communication with the elderly is a concern because it can affect the elderly's sense of life satisfaction (Nussbaum, 1983a, 1983b, 1985) and quality of life (Giles, Coupland, and Wiemann, 1990). At a fundamental level is the issue of stereotypes and ageism when communicating with the elderly, as research suggests that caregivers may address the elderly based on ageist stereotypes. Ryan, Giles, Bartolucci, and Henwood (1986) refer to this as the *communication predicament of aging*: "By this term, we refer to the situation in which undesirable discrepancies occur between the actual communicative competence of an elderly person and the negative perception of his/her competence" (p. 6). Whereas other age groups may have negative perceptions about the elderly, the elderly themselves (who once were young) may convey these internalized negative connotations to others. Thus, communication stereotypes of the elderly may not emanate strictly from others but may in fact be fostered by self-fulfilling prophecies.

In this vein, research by Ryan, See, Meneer, and Trovato (1992) found that the elderly had a more negative self-perception of language performance than did the younger subjects, which could have implications for self-fulfilling prophecies. Negative expectations by both the elderly and others could lead to a type of condescending speech known as baby talk (Caporeal, 1981; Caporeal and Culbertson, 1986; Caporeal, Lukaszewski, and Culbertson, 1983), patronizing speech (Ryan et al., 1986; Harwood, Giles, Fox, Ryan, and Williams, 1993) or elderspeak (Cohen and Faulkner, 1986). Baby talk is distinctive in its lexical simplicity, high pitch, and exaggerated intonation contour. Characteristics of patronizing speech and elderspeak include slow speaking rate, lexical simplicity, careful articulation, and loud volume. Any of these three speaking styles can perpetuate negative stereotypes of the elderly, as they convey nurturance and affection and promote dependency. Miscommunication can occur when caregivers mistakenly assume the elderly person falls into stereotypical categories (Coupland, Nussbaum, and Coupland, 1991).

Relative to language as a barrier, Shuy (1976) analyzed tape-recorded physician-patient interviews and documented evidence in which communication breakdowns occurred because the doctor's language and patient's language were not concordant. For example, the recorded interviews with mostly with African American women from inner city Washington, D. C., revealed that the doctors spoke in medical jargon and patients spoke in non-medical or near-social terms, employing short formal responses permeated with grammatical errors. "The doctor's over use of technical language tends to estrange him from the patient by setting himself on a much higher intellectual level" (Shuy, 1976, p. 381). Because doctors neither speak nor understand the language of the subculture, they cannot adapt their communication style to that of their patients. Williams and Giles (1991) in their macro perspective of literature regarding the socio-psychological meanings of older people's language and communication note that we use linguistic cues to make judgments about others and highlight perceptions of vocal qualities of the elderly, perceptions of their language, and beliefs about talk. Their literature review paints a picture of ageism among younger people.

Social structure. Social structure is the second barrier to positive physician-patient interactions. The traditional physician-patient relationship, referred to by Parson's (1951) as the Sick Role Model, renders an asymmetric physician-patient relationship: the patient assumes the role of the sick person and the physician plays a paternalistic role. Doctors traditionally have been accorded a position of all-knowing and, therefore, perceived with awe, which reinforces the social structure that elevates their status. Physicians are expected to exert authoritative control over the relationship, and patients are expected to accept control (Ragan, Beck, and White, 1995; Shuy, 1976; Smith, 1992; Street, Gold, and McDowell, 1995; von Friederichs-Fitzwater, Callahan, Flynn, and Williams, 1991). Consequently, patients are at a distinct disadvantage because the power in the interaction resides with the physician. Furthermore, the patient's social class can influence physician-patient interaction. For example, doctors talk more with patients who are higher in social class and give more time and explanations to higher-class patients. In addition, college-educated patients receive more information. However, patients of different classes do not differ in the amount of information they say they want (O'Hair, Behnke, and King, 1983; Roter and Hall, 1992; Waitzkin, 1984). "It has long been known that poorer and less educated patients have trouble finding health care and get less of it. Now it appears that the problems of these groups are not entirely structural. They suffer poorer treatment even after they gain access to the health care system" (Roter and Hall, 1992, p. 48).

Physician's demeanor. The third cause for dissatisfaction among patients is the physician's demeanor. Some of the characteristics that patients look for in physicians include warmth, friendliness, and awareness of the patient's psychosocial and medical concerns (O'Hair, 1986); rapport (Stein, 1985), empathy (Matthews, Suchman, and Branch, 1993; O'Hair, 1986); attention and interest (Turner, Deyo, Loeser, Von Korff, and Fordyce, 1994); and concern (O'Hair, 1986; Turner et al., 1994). However, in Shuy's (1976) study, the doctor's attitude was assessed negatively approximately 50% of the time, with 39% indicating that the doctor's attitude was sometimes unfriendly. Specific to the elderly, Adelman et al. (1991) state that the literature is "replete with anecdotal examples of health providers' ageist behavior, but there have been few studies to document the magnitude or exact nature of the phenomenon" (p. 132). A study by Greene et al. (1986) provided evidence that physicians were less friendly, patient, engaged, and respectful with older patients than with younger patients.

So why would a physician's demeanor be anything less than warm and friendly? According to Roter (1977), reasons include patients' incompetence to understand medical implications, informed patients posing a threat to the status and control of the doctor, and the physician's perceived need to protect the patient from emotional upset or worry. Dr. Michael DeBakey (cited in Shuy, 1976, p. 369) stated, "Most doctors don't want their patients to understand them! They prefer to keep their work a mystery. If patients don't understand what a doctor is talking about, they won't ask him questions. Then the doctor won't have to be bothered answering them." Also, physicians' time constraints and the need to stay on task may leave an impression of negative affect with the patient. Because medicine is a market-based commodity (Starr, 1982), physicians can afford to spend only a given amount of time with each patient. Therefore, physicians expect patients to make the visit as succinct as possible and not turn it into a social foray (O'Hair, Allman, and Moore, 1996). Waitzkin (1984) refers to this as the "voice of medicine" in the medical encounter: the doctor maintains control and keeps the patient on track through repetitive questioning and elicits a medical history that meets the technical requirements of diagnosis, treatment, and record keeping.

Other factors. Regarding specific communication behaviors of physicians, Frankel (1984) performed a microinteractional analysis of a medical encounter that revealed the following patterns of interaction between doctors and patients:

- Doctors asked questions approximately 90% of the time, while patients asked questions approximately 10% of the time.
- In simultaneous competing utterances, 94% of interruptions concluded with the doctor winning the floor.
- Third-turn options were used by doctors 61.6% of the time, although the majority of third-turns were acknowledgment (neutral) statements. Frankel concludes that third-turn options operate as a controlling device whereas overlapping talk is used to limit patient participation.

In this same vein, Beckman and Frankel (1984) found that physicians took control of the medical interview after an average of 18 seconds "by asking increasingly specific, closed-ended questions that effectively halted the spontaneous flow of information from the patient" (p. 694). In their examination of the relationship between physicians' verbal behavior and levels of patient satisfaction and understanding, Smith, Polis, and Hadac (1981) found that higher levels of information giving was associated with increased patient satisfaction, and patient understanding was associated with the amount of time spent providing information.

The importance of physician-patient communication cannot be overstated. In their book *Communication and Aging*, Nussbaum et al. (1989) provide a thorough review and summary of studies regarding physician-patient interactions. They note a discrepancy between doctors' and patients' perceptions of the doctors' friendliness, that patients complain they do not receive enough information (although often patients do not demand it), that doctors often ignore information provided by another family member, that doctors use jargon when communicating with their patients, and that patients are intimidated by their doctors. Kreps (1990) summarizes problems that can occur when both providers and consumers are dissatisfied with health communication. For example, providers experience higher rates of burnout, leading to deterioration of professional performance, and consumers are less likely to comply with medical advice or to avoid needed treatment. A considerable body of research exists that correlates communication with patient understanding, satisfaction, compliance, and health benefits. In sum, when patients have a basic understanding of their illness, its implications, and treatment and are satisfied with their health care delivery, compliance rates increase, which has the potential for improving the patient's overall health. (For summaries of studies related to compliance and satisfaction, see Kreps and O'Hair, 1995; Kreps and Thornton, 1992; Ray and Donohew, 1990; and Stewart and Roter, 1990).

Women's Health

The women's health movement can be traced to the 1820s–1830s and a health movement that opposed interventionist techniques and heroic medicine. Although women willingly assumed the role of homemaker, they embraced the ideologies of the Ladies Physiological Societies and believed that women should be educated in proper health and hygiene for the benefit of their families. It was not until the late 1960's and early 1970's, however, that the civil rights and student movements helped change social structures such that women found a collective voice through which to act on their concerns regarding feminist issues that included health concerns. The fundamental assumption underlying women's health concerns was that women did not have ultimate control over their own bodies and health, as health policy, health legislation, and health care delivery were dominated by men (Zimmerman, 1994). According to Friedman (1994a), compounding issues such as birth control, abortion, natural childbirth, breast cancer, and correlations of estrogen levels with uterine cancer served as the impetus to involve women in their own health care. One of the outgrowths of this movement was that women, recognizing the asymmetrical physician-patient relationship, began deconstructing it, choosing to question physicians and recommended procedures. "Middle-class women, better educated and better paid than their mothers and older sisters, were often unwilling to tolerate longer waits in the doctors office, being called by their first names, or having their concerns dismissed. . . .Physicians resented having their judgment questioned or their recommendations challenged, sometimes becoming openly hostile" (Eagan, 1994, pp. 22–23). Furthermore, Laurence and Weinhouse (1994) report that women have complained that physicians are "insensitive, uninterested, rushed, arrogant, and uncommunicative" (p. 329). Finally, Laurence and Weinhouse state:

> Surveys show that women are more dissatisfied with their physician than men are. And the dissatisfaction is not necessarily due to the quality of the medical care women receive, but to the lack of communication and respect they perceive in the encounter. . . .One out of four women said she had been "talked down to" or treated like a child by a physician. Nearly one out of five women had been told that a reported medical condition was "all in your head." (p. 331)

Despite the dissatisfaction that many women express relative to their health care, a positive outgrowth of the women's health care movement was the creation of the new Office of Research on Women's Health at the National Institutes of Health. But even that has its down side: as Armbruster (1992) states, ". . .only 13% of the research conducted by the NIH is in women's health. . ." (p. 63). The argument also can be made that too little attention has been paid to the unique province of women's health care in the health communication literature. Whereas several studies have addressed women's health problems (e.g., Corea, 1985; Emerson, 1970; Fisher and Todd, 1986; Smith, 1992), few have looked at the role of interpersonal communication in the context of women's health care. A number of studies of gynecologic health care in the medical education literature report that the interpersonal relationship or the communication skills of the practitioner comprise an important dimension of patient satisfaction in the gynecologic exam interaction (e.g., Domar, 1985–86; Fang, Hillard, Lindsay, and Underwood, 1984; Lesserman and Luke, 1982); yet these studies have neither described physician-patient interaction nor discovered the interaction patterns that constitute desirable interpersonal or communication skills. Several recent explorations of the gynecologic health care context have yielded descriptive data about naturally occurring patient-physician interactions (Beck and Ragan, 1992; Ragan, 1990; Ragan and Glenn, 1990). Unfortunately, however, the population of elderly women has received little to no attention in the health care communication literature, whether in gynecologic or more generalized women's health care interactions.

RATIONALE AND RESEARCH FOCUS

Riley (1971) says that chronological age is important to us as an indication of personal experience that carries probabilities of behavior and attitudes. However, aging is not only an individual phenomenon but also a collective process whereby the structure of an overall population is altered. Thus, "aging individuals" and "aging population" can refer to the aging of cohorts (Myers, 1990). Macroevents— historical experiences that influence development of individuals (Martin and Smyer, 1990)—influence cohorts as a population and affect attitudes and behaviors among the individuals who experience the event.

Considering that a woman who is at least sixty-five years of age in 1997 was born not later than 1932, she was conceivably a child of the Great Depression, the sibling or wife of a World War II soldier, the mother of a Vietnam-era soldier, and the last of a generation of "traditional" females. Because these women have aged as a cohort group with the attendant influences of their era, do their medical experiences suggest a pattern in their interaction with physicians? Because the women of that era were socialized in the traditional paradigm (prior to the feminist and women's health movements) whereby they had little or no influence over medical policy, legislation, and health care delivery, is it possible that what these women say about their doctors will reflect similar attitudes?

If one adopts the feminist perspective that regards gender roles as having direct impact on the phenomenon under investigation—as considering women's experiences not only as different from men's but as appropriate and undervalued data for analysis—then an additional argument can be offered for investigating women's health care from the perspective of the women receiving that care. McBride and McBride (1981) advocate incorporating the phenomenon of "lived experience" as the beginning point and the theoretical underpinning for women's health care: "To take seriously the lived experience of women as one's starting point, is to reject, whatever the details of one's subsequent methodology may be, a long-standing alternative tradition of preferring the standpoint of the external, supposedly 'scientific' and 'objective' observer to that of the actual subjects of one's study in their real-life situations" (p. 46). One of the goals of this study was to investigate this "lived experience" of a subgroup, who by virtue of being both female and elderly, have been overlooked by most researchers. The specific focus was to capture the voice of elderly women relative to their perceptions about their physicians' communicative behaviors and the importance placed upon physicians' communication skills in their overall health care.

METHODOLOGY

Using the boundary of age sixty-five to define "elderly" (Myers, 1990; Neugarten and Hagestad, 1976; Neugarten and Neugarten, 1986), this exploratory qualitative study focused on the interpersonal communicative behaviors of physicians as described by 20 ambulatory female patients sixty-five years of age or older. The researchers participated in a three-hour training session with an experienced ethnographer to ensure that similar interviewing techniques would be employed in all of the interviews. To elicit the first-person life-voice of these women, a non-structured interview using open-ended questions was employed to explore the importance that this population places on physicians' interpersonal communication skills relative to the patients' positive or negative responses to their medical care.

The 20 women interviewed for this study represented a purposive sample, as most of the women were acquainted with the interviewers and were willing to openly discuss their medical experiences. Requirements for the women to participate in the study included that they be at least sixty-five years old, in good health, and ambulatory. The good health and ambulatory criteria were specified to counterbalance any confounding factors that may have influenced the women's physician-patient interactions, such as the necessity of a third party to accompany the patient to medical appointments (Adelman et al., 1991). The women represented a cross-section of middle-class elderly females who were married, divorced, or widowed; they currently lived in California, Texas, Oklahoma, and New Mexico; 80% were Caucasian and 20% were from minority ethnic groups (African American, Asian, and Hispanic).

Interviews were conducted either face to face or by telephone. All interviews were audio-taped, but no identifying information was included on the tape, thus guaranteeing anonymity to the subjects. Although there might have been differences in how the information was elicited because face-to-face interaction can account for nonverbal cues and prompts, acquaintance of the interviewers and interviewees possibly mitigated that factor.

At the time of the interview, each woman was told that with our population getting older, the researchers were interested in older women's experiences with their physicians. Each interview began with the question, "Please tell me about your health," which was the only scripted question of the interview. As the interview progressed, interviewers asked questions only to clarify points or elicit further information. Although the interviewees were not specifically asked about interactional communication with their doctors, their stories described such elements.

RESULTS AND DISCUSSION

Emergent Themes

The results of these interviews were analyzed thematically and results indicate that physicians' interpersonal communication skills can decidedly affect the degree of medical success achieved with their sixty-five and older female patients. As a group, the researchers discussed the interviews and identified recurring themes. Specifically, seven themes consistently reappeared in these interviews: forms of address, socioeconomic status, nonverbal communication, immediacy, the role of support staff, patients asking questions, and how the women perceived changes in physician-patient communication over time.

In evaluating medical care, this research showed that the women interviewed expressed satisfaction and/or dissatisfaction with received medical attention relative to the perceived quality of communicative behaviors. Further, the themes that emerged from these interviews indicate that in their evaluation of medical care, elderly female patients may rely more heavily on the physician's interpersonal communication skills than on the actual medical treatment given to them as patients. The fact that physicians' interpersonal communication skills can decidedly affect the degree of medical success achieved with their sixty-five and older female patients is supported with evidence as extracted from the interviews.

Forms of Address

The issue of control, power, and status is evident in medical encounters. Patients generally defer to the physician's medical expertise, thus granting him/her power in the medical encounter. However, forms of address within the encounter solidify the notion of power and status.

Tannen (1994b, p. 207) states, "Status reigns when one speaker addresses the other by first name but is addressed by title-last name. For example, a patient addresses his doctor as 'Dr. Henderson,' but the doctor calls him 'Sidney.'" To be on an equal-naming basis indicates a shared experience or equal status (Tannen, 1994b). In what she calls the "first-name syndrome," Haug (1996) notes that how physicians and patients address each other sets the tone for the relationship and symbolizes the relative power of the participants. Specific to the elderly, Stoeckle (1987, p. 45) states that sometimes physicians may use first names to appear nonauthoritarian or to "fake chumminess" (p. 45). The use of "dearie" and "honey" with older persons may in fact serve to diminish an elderly person's sense of status and self-esteem (Conant, 1983).

Each woman who was interviewed for this study commented on how the physician addressed her. As might be expected, doctors called some of the women by their first names and some by their last names. Short (1993) notes that the current trend in medical practice is towards calling patients by their first name, although some (e.g., older patients and higher social classes) object to this practice. The women interviewed for this study had mixed reactions relative to the first-name practice. Although some of the women said being called by their first name was fine, others objected to the first-name basis. One interviewee, an African American, stated:

> Once my doctor tried to call me by my first name, and I set him straight. You see, I call him "Doctor" to show respect, so he can pay me the same courtesy. He said, "Ah, ah, excuse me." I just told him, "No excuses are necessary. This is a business deal and you are providing me with a service."

Another woman stated, "We're not friends, and my visit should be kept on a professional basis." The mother of a doctor of national prominence noted that she is addressed as "Mrs." when in the offices of doctors; however, on social occasions these same doctors address her by her first name. She also noted that when any examination or treatment involves pain, the doctors will address her by her nickname. She could not recall any other occasions in which this was the case. Tannen (1994a) explains that diminutive names are markers of closeness. Therefore, in this woman's instance, when physicians found themselves in social settings with the patient or when attempting comfort, the protocol of power via address was subordinate to the shared experience or equal status.

Another physician, however, must have wanted to promote the perception of shared experience or equal status. One of the interviewees related that the physician insisted she (the physician) be called by her first name:

> I think she really wanted me to feel comfortable and at ease. . . . You see, I wasn't brought up like that. That young lady had spent her time earning a degree; she deserved to be called doctor. But she put that straight-laced authority stuff up. She wanted to be a friend, and I needed that.

There were several women who could not recall ever being addressed by any name. One interviewee said that in the two years she has gone to this doctor, "she has never called me by any name at all."

Socioeconomic Status

As noted in the literature review regarding social structure as a factor in physician-patient communication, the patient's social class can influence the medical interaction. Friedman (1994b) states, "Women represent 60 percent of Medicare beneficiaries and the vast majority of adults who receive Medicaid benefits" (p. 13). Furthermore, according to Dimond (1995), "Very few older women have private pensions, in part because of their interrupted work careers and because mandatory laws addressing work-related private pensions were not in effect during the years that the current cohort of older women were employed" (p. 106). Consequently, Medicare and Medicaid become both a class and gender issue because more older women than men are likely to be poor (Muller, 1988). However, because medicine has become a market-driven commodity (Kotler and Clarke, 1987), physicians must take into account the additional time and resources necessary to adequately care for elderly persons, which has the potential of resulting in less-than-optimal communication between the physician and patient. Medicare pays only 80% of the reasonable charges for physicians' services (Kotler and Clarke, 1987); therefore, the financial incentive for spending optimal time and delivering optimal care—employing optimal communication—to this class of patients is lacking.

Although all of the women interviewed were Medicare eligible, the cross-sectional differences were evident. Some of the women selected their physician simply because s/he accepted Medicare payments, while others who had supplemental insurance gave no thought to that selection criterion. To the women with only Medicare coverage, their perception was that the physicians did not really care about them personally. One woman, who was seeing a doctor for neck treatments, related that the doctor had a "hurry-hurry attitude and kept telling me to come back for one more treatment." Then when she had the final treatment, that was it: "No caring or compassion. He seemed to run a patient mill strictly for the money that Medicare would pay." Another interviewee stated,

> . . . sometimes you don't have a choice, like me. I mean, only so many doctors want an old lady like me. I just have to watch out for myself as best I can. It's difficult because they see you only have Medicare and you get bounced around. It's like, "Oh, you're poor; I can treat you any ole way." It's just hard to get what you need.

Finally, one woman, when asked about her physician, said she did not like him, but that all the "old" women in town go to him because he takes Medicare.

Nonverbal Communication

Nonverbal communication encompasses not only "body language" (e.g., gestures and body movement) but also facial expressions, gaze, dress, touch, use of the voice (paralanguage), use of time (chronemics), use of space (proxemics), and so forth. Because approximately 79 percent of meaning can be accounted for by nonverbal cues or the interaction with verbal cues (Burgoon, 1994), this component of physician-patient communication cannot be overemphasized. The fact that nonverbal communication emerged as one of the themes of this study indicates the importance that these elderly women placed on nonverbal cues as part of their medical experience.

Nonverbal communication cut across all socio-economic and cultural lines. As might be expected, however, the levels of nonverbal skills were as varied as the interviewees themselves. All of the women commented in some way about whether the doctor touched her in a caring manner—a handshake upon entering the examination room, a friendly pat on the shoulder—beyond the cursory professional touch. Some appreciated that extra touch; others insisted they wanted no part of it. As one woman said, "I don't want him touching me, patting me on the shoulder, telling me I'm going to be ok. He even came around his desk to help me up. I'm not an invalid!" They also commented about whether the doctor stood or sat during the medical interview or follow-up explanations; about whether s/he looked at them or focused somewhere else, e.g., a clipboard or dictaphone.

> It really bothers me when a doctor comes in for an examination and he doesn't even look at my face. I feel like I'm in an animal shelter or something. If they just looked at me, they would make me feel like a person and not the next specimen for inspection.

A Hispanic woman commented that the doctor never really made eye contact with her. She said, "My gynecologist always looks at me. She's a real nice lady, but my GP hardly even talks to me. He just does the exam and writes on his note pad."

Personal appearance is a nonverbal cue of impression management. Older patients seem to prefer a doctor's professional attire as a symbol of professionalism, authority, and therapeutic efficacy (Stoeckle, 1987). Short (1993) states that the way a physician dresses conveys a message to the patient, "particularly with regard to the confidence he places in his doctor. Most patients expect a doctor to look like a doctor" (p. 217). One woman in this study commented on the physician's appearance, inferring a question relative to the physician's credibility:

> She didn't have a professional image; she was unkempt. For instance, her hair was greasy and didn't look like it had been combed; she didn't have on any makeup; and she was pregnant with her tenth child. I know she was tired, but to convey competence, you have to *look* as if you know something about it.

Another woman commented on the doctor's office itself, stating, "It is cheap looking, with indoor-outdoor carpeting and cheap furniture. If she would take calls and express concern, I could put up with inadequate office surroundings." The physician probably had not considered how the presentation of the office directly affects the patient's perception of the physician (Short, 1993).

Another area of nonverbal communication that was evident in how physicians treated these women relates to chronemics, which includes such elements as punctuality and waiting time (Burgoon, 1994). Specifically, more than one woman complained of not being able to get through to the doctor on the telephone because of the "fortress" nature of the front office staff or of having to talk to the doctor "through" the nurse. Thus, by having the patient go through another person, the physician controls the element of time. "If I don't pay $36 I can't talk to the doctor." One woman questioned the doctor at her next appointment about why he had not returned her telephone call and was told he had been busy. "I have to make an appointment and pay money for him not to be too busy to talk to me." A health maintenance organization patient expressed her frustration at the doctor's not returning calls promptly:

> It is very frustrating to call in for a simple question and not have the doctor call you back for several days. Hell, I could have died by the time he called me back, but I guess he figures if I'm dying I would go to the emergency room. But it does make me nervous to think that if he doesn't return my call when I'm well, he's probably not going to call me back if I ever get down.

Finally, cultural differences between physicians and patients surfaced in the area of nonverbal communication. A Caucasian woman visiting a Pakistani doctor said he could not pick up on her not wanting him to touch her. Although she said she considered herself a "touchy-feely" person, she did not want him to touch her and freely admitted that it was a cultural thing.

Immediacy

Immediacy is defined as stylistic differences in expression from which like-dislike is inferred (Mehrabian, 1981)—in other words, whether or not someone is personal or caring. In a medical context, this would relate to whether a patient perceives his/her physician as being personally caring and how that caring is conveyed. This issue of immediacy was another theme that emerged from the interviews with these elderly women.

Although three of the women had relatives who were physicians, each expressed differing opinions as to how this connection might/might not affect her treatment. For example, the mother of the nationally prominent doctor related that she most assuredly believes that she gets preferential treatment, as she does not ever have to wait to see the doctor, nor does she have to wait to get appointments (also a nonverbal issue of chronemics). She reiterated that this preferential treatment was the result of her being the mother of a doctor whom "they respect" and that she does not believe "for one minute" that all patients receive the care and attention that she does—it is simply "out of love and respect for [my son]."

In contrast, another woman has a nephew who is a professional colleague of the patient's cardiologist. This woman stated that she is not certain that her cardiologist is aware of the family relationship, and she usually must wait 30 to 45 minutes to see the doctor, who "always hurries in." She did volunteer, however, that her doctor gives her "all the time I need and is good to explain anything I need to know." Her perception of his immediacy mitigates any nonverbal chronemic cues.

Finally, the third woman (whose son-in-law is a physician) stated that she did not believe that this relationship has had any bearing on how she is treated by other physicians. She believes that the amount of time the doctors spend with her as well as the detail they provide are normal procedures. Nor does she believe the special and/or courteous considerations they display toward her is exceptional but is based rather on their "just being nice."

One woman with no familial ties to physicians related that her doctor was "awfully nice. He's pretty young and tells me I remind him of his mother. I might be getting special treatment." Another woman says that when the doctor finishes the exam, he "always says to my husband to take [me] home and go fishing. I really love Dr. F." Finally, a widow who visited a minor emergency center told of a young male doctor who said to her, "You're a real kick. If I weren't married, I could go for you in a big way." Rather than being offended, the patient considered this to be a compliment. The immediacy exhibited by these physicians is reflected in their patients' satisfaction with the interpersonal communication.

Support Staff

The role of the support staff was illustrated in several interviews. A general consensus was that the front office staff had a bearing on how the patient would be treated, which corresponds with Short's (1993) observation that the support staff is generally a reflection of the physician. Several of the women specifically mentioned the role of the nurse. For instance, the mother of the nationally prominent physician says she was immensely happy with the attention and treatment she received from the support staff, "including the nurses who give me emotional support by holding my hand." A subject whose family doctor of 40 years retired was left to find another physician

> . . . at this age when no one wants to take care of you; so I was lucky to find a doctor at all. I'm just grateful to Dr. J. He's not cranky, but he doesn't talk too much. He lets the nurse do everything. He never answers questions directly. The nurse answers most of the questions. But he could get me into the hospital if I had to go.

A Japanese American stated that she felt uncomfortable with the nurse in the room. "I know they are there to protect me, supposedly, but I really do not like it. I feel real uncomfortable with someone standing there watching me get the exam." Another woman elaborated on the general demeanor of the nurse:

> When I go to the doctor, his nurses are always friendly, and that's okay with me, but some of them are just too prissy. I don't mean flirtatious; just looks like to me they're trying too hard to impress me. They don't have to do all that. I just want them to be pleasant. I guess more than anything, when I get a bubbly one, I just feel she's being oh fake or I know, it's as if I'm incompetent. My doctor does not do that.

Patients Asking Questions

Some of the women talked about asking the doctor questions and following through with medications. One woman stated,

> I always go in with questions for the doctor. This makes my current doctor angry. I don't know why, but he gets on the defensive. It's not that I'm challenging his knowledge, but he's not an authority on my body. I have lived with this body 72 years, and I know it well.

Another interviewee commented that rather than "tormenting" the doctor for specific information, she uses other sources:

> See, at [the local hospital] they have pamphlets on the medicines and
> I read those. I also have a book on medicines and I check in there.
> You just look in there and see the side effects. I have always read
> about the medicines that I take.

Still another woman stated, "I do make sure that he knows I'm
checking with other people about what he prescribes. I refuse to let him
think I'm an idiot." And one woman related her concern about the
medicine samples provided by the doctor, stating that she prefers to get
her medicine from the pharmacist. "See, my local drugstore knows me,
and when I take in a prescription from a doctor, he checks it out for
me. . . .I have a friend who just takes whatever the doctor gives her. She
says those samples he gives her saves her money. I told her it just might
cost her her health if she keeps it up."

A cultural difference in language surfaced in this category. One
woman commented that she visited a doctor from another culture and,
although she had nothing against him personally, she could not
understand him. "That's important when medications are involved. I
want to be sure I understand what I am taking and how I am supposed
to take it. I don't want to end up dead because I couldn't understand
what he said." Perhaps patients believe it is futile to ask questions in
such circumstances.

Changes over Time

Regarding doctors in general and any differences the women may have
noticed in the physician-patient interactions through the years, one
woman said, "I had one doctor when I was young and he was very
friendly. . . .You know, it is a real change today. I guess it's my age or
maybe it's just the times, but I don't feel the warmth and friendliness
with my doctors now." An African American woman remarked, "I
guess I got better treatment by black doctors when we were segregated,
but it could have been that I was younger, too."

Finally an eighty-year-old woman, when asked what she thought
makes a good doctor, replied, "Being concerned about his practice and
patients [which he shows] by subscribing [sic] the right
medicine. . . .Today's doctors are more caring because their knowledge
is better." Asked about their bedside manner, she said, "Well, doctors
don't come to your house any more." This woman evidently equated a
good doctor with someone who is concerned about his/her patients and

wants them to have the right medicine. She also correlates caring with knowledge, and because medical knowledge is more extensive today than in the past, today's physicians must be more caring than their predecessors. However, for this woman, the bottom line is that "doctors don't come to your house any more," which to her is what bedside manner is all about.

SUMMARY AND CONCLUSION

As can be seen from the comments of these elderly women, they all have definite opinions about their health care and their physicians. Some like their doctors; some are just happy that a doctor will see them at all. All are interested in how the doctor treats them personally. These women were socialized in an era marked by "traditional" values wherein women were not encouraged to question authority, particularly medical authority. Yet these same women witnessed and experienced the women's movement. Some of these women learned that questioning authority is legitimate—particularly when it involves their own female anatomy; others still hold to the old medical model and passively comply with whatever is diagnosed or prescribed.

The stories from these 20 women appear to echo the literature relative to physician-elderly patient communication. Recommendations for improving these dyadic encounters, which also emanate from the literature, include an "other" orientation by physicians (Spitzberg and Hecht, 1984), whereby physicians allow patients to talk more, provide more statements of direct support, and focus on topics that seem most salient to patients (von Friederichs-Fitzwater et al., 1991). Ryan et al. (1986) focus on *how* a caregiver communicates with the patient, with particular attention to avoiding over-accommodating a patient's communication abilities through baby talk or patronizing speech. Giving attention to the patient's psychosocial domain is suggested by Greene and Adelman (1996), as psychosocial problems that accompany old age my influence the elderly person's health. From the fundamental problem of stereotyping the elderly, Gray (1983) suggests becoming familiar with beliefs and attitudes of both the elderly and physicians. Finally, McCormick, Inui, and Roter (1996) state, "The existing body of research information on improving clinician-elderly patient interactions has emphasized gaps, gulfs, and other glaring problems" (p. 130). Consequently, researchers now need to move on to studying methods of intervention and "'experimentation' that entails the development, fielding, and evaluation of experiences designed to enhance the capacity of clinicians for meaningful relationships with their elderly patients" (McCormick et al., 1996, p. 131).

Although the purpose of this study was to explore elderly females' perceptions of their health care relative to the interpersonal communication skills of their physicians, the researchers quickly realized this was only a thread in a tapestry rich with color and texture. The study invites additional interviews that include more minorities. It also raises a question about the other side of the dyad: How do physicians perceive elderly female patients and their interpersonal communication skills? Are there differences in how male and female physicians perceive their elderly female patients, and are these differences perceived by the patients? Finally, a third research possibility would be to conduct a similar study with elderly men to test for gender differences in their perceptions of their health care.

Given the dramatic shift in the social climate during this generation's lifetime, it behooves us to inquire how the medical experiences of these women, particularly during their later years, have shaped their perception of the health care system. Knowing the communication preferences when interacting with the physician, knowing what they deem important in their health care, determining their criteria for physician competency, and discerning whether there are differences in their perceptions of medical care based on method of payment can enlighten scholars, caregivers, and the medical community as to the needs and concerns of this population.

REFERENCES

Adelman, R. D., Greene, M G., and Charon, R. 1991. Issues in physician-elderly patient interaction. *Ageing and Society 11*, 127–148.

Adelman, R. D., Greene, M. G., Charon, R., and Friedmann, E. 1992. The content of physician and elderly patient interaction in the medical primary care encounter. *Communication Research 19*(3), 370–380.

Anderson, L. A., Rakowski, W., and Hickey, T. 1988. Satisfaction with clinical encounters among residents and geriatric patients. *Journal of Medical Education 63*, 447–455.

Armbruster, A. 1992, September. Closing the medical gender gap. *Working Woman* 63.

Beck, C.S., and Ragan, S.L. 1992. Negotiating interpersonal and medical talk: Frame shifts in the gynecologic exam. *Journal of Language and Social Psychology 2*, 47–61.

Beckman, H. B., and Frankel, R. M. 1984. The effect of physician behavior on the collection of data. *Annals of Internal Medicine 101*, 692–696.

Beisecker, A. E. 1996. Older persons' medical encounters and their outcomes. *Research on Aging 18*(1), 9–31.

Beisecker, A. E., and Beisecker, T. D. 1990. Patient information-seeking behaviors when communicating with doctors. *Medical Care 28*, 19–28.

Burgoon, J. 1994. Nonverbal signals. In M. R. Knapp and G. L. Miller, eds., *Handbook of Interpersonal Communication* (2nd ed.). Thousand Oaks, California: Sage. 229–285.

Butler, R. N. 1989. Biological markers of overall aging. *American Journal of Public Health 79*(6), 687.

Caporeal, L. R. 1981. The paralanguage of caregiving: Baby talk to the institutionalized aged. *Journal of Personality and Social Psychology 40*(5), 876–884.

Caporeal, L. R., and Culbertson, G. H. 1986. Verbal response modes of baby talk and other speech at institutions for the aged. *Language & Communication 6*(1/2), 99–112.

Caporeal, L. R., Lukaszewski, M. P., and Culbertson, G. H. 1983. Secondary baby talk: judgments by institutionalized elderly and their caregivers. *Journal of Personality and Social Psychology 44*, 746–754.

Cetron, M., and Davies, O. 1989. *American Renaissance: Our Life at the Turn of the 21st Century*. New York: St. Martin's.

Cohen, G., and Faulkner, D. 1986. Does "elderspeak" work? The effect of intonation and stress on comprehension and recall of spoken discourse in old age. *Language & Communication 6*(1/2), 91–98.

Conant, E. S. 1983. Addressing patients by their first names. *New England Journal of Medicine 308*, 266.

Corea, G. 1985. *The Hidden Malpractice: How American Medicine Mistreats Women*. New York: Harper & Row.

Coupland, J., Nussbaum, J. F., and Coupland, N. 1991. The reproduction of aging and agism in intergenerational talk. In N. Coupland, H. Giles, and J. M. Wiemann, eds., *"Miscommunication" and Problematic Talk*. Newbury Park, California: Sage. 85–102.

DiMatteo, M. R., Hayes, R. D., and Prince, L. M. 1986. Relationship of physicians' nonverbal communication skill to patient satisfaction, appointment noncompliance, and physician workload. *Health Psychology 5*, 581–594.

Dimond, M. 1995. Older women's health. In C. I. Fogel and N F. Woods, eds., *Women's Health Care: A Comprehensive Handbook.* Thousand Oaks, California: Sage.

Domar, A.D. 1985–86. Psychological aspects of the pelvic exam: Individual needs and physician involvement. *Women and Health 10*(4), 75–90.

Dychtwald, K. and Flower, J. 1990. *Age Wave.* New York: Bantam.

Eagan, A. B. 1994. The women's health movement and its lasting impact. In E. Friedman, ed., *An Unfinished Revolution: Women and Health Care in America.* New York: United Hospital Fund. 15–27.

Emerson, J. 1970. Behavior in private places: Sustaining definitions of reality in gynecological examinations. In H.P. Dreitzel, eds., *Recent Sociology, No. 2: Patterns of Communicative Behavior.* New York: Macmillan. 73–79.

Fang, W.L., Hillard, P.J., Lindsay, R.L., and Underwood, P.B. 1984. Evaluation of students' clinical and communication skills in performing a gynecologic examination. *Journal of Medical Education 59*, 758–760.

Fisher, S. and Todd, A.D., eds. 1986. *Discourse and Institutional Authority: Medicine, Education, and the Law.* Norwood, New Jersey: Ablex.

Frankel, R. M. 1984. From sentence to sequence: Understanding the medical encounter through microinteractional analysis. *Discourse Processes 7*, 135–170.

Friedman, E. 1994a. Women and health care: The bramble and the rose. In E. Friedman, ed., *An Unfinished Revolution: Women and Health Care in America.* New York: United Hospital Fund. 1–12.

Friedman, E. 1994b. Women as users of health services. In E. Friedman, ed., *An Unfinished Revolution: Women and Health Care in America.* New York: United Hospital Fund. 13.

Giles, H., Coupland, N., Coupland, J., Williams, A., and Nussbaum, J. 1992. Intergenerational talk and communication with older people. The influences of cognitive resources on adaptation and old age. *International Journal of Aging and Human Development 34*, 271–297.

Giles, H., Coupland, N., and Wiemann, J. M., eds. 1990. *Communication, Health and the Elderly.* Manchester: Manchester University Press.

Goffman, E. 1959. *The Presentation of Self in Everyday Life.* New York: Doubleday.

Gray, M. 1983. Communicating with elderly people. In D. Pendleton and J. Hasler, eds., *Doctor-Patient Communication.* New York: Academic Press. 193–203.

Greene, M. G., and Adelman, R. 1996. Psychosocial factors in older patients' medical encounters. *Research on Aging 18*(1), 84–102.

Greene, M. G., Adelman, R. D., Charon, R., and Friedmann, E. (1989). Concordance between physicians and their older and younger patients in the primary care medical encounter. *The Gerontologist 29*(6), 808–813.

Greene, M. G., Adelman, R., Charon, R., and Hoffman, S. 1986. Ageism in the medical encounter: An exploratory study of the doctor-elderly patient relationship. *Language & Communication 6*(1/2), 113–124.

Harwood, J., Giles, H., Fox, S., Ryan, E. B., and Williams, A. 1993, August. Patronizing young and elderly adults: Response strategies in a community setting. *Journal of Applied Communication Research* 211–226.

Haug, M. R. 1996. Elements in physician/patient interactions in late life. *Research on Aging 18*(1), 32–51.

Hooper, E. M., Comstock, L. M., Goodwin, J. M., and Goodwin, J. S. 1982. Patient characteristics that influence physician behavior. *Medical Care 20*, 630–638.

Kim, Y.Y. 1988. *Communication and Cross-Cultural Adaptation: An Integrative Theory.* Clevedon, England: Multilingual Matters Ltd.

Koopman, C. S., Eisenthal, S., and Stoeckle, J. 1984. Ethnicity in the reported pain, emotional distress and requests of medical outpatients. *Social Science & Medicine 6*, 487–490.

Kotler, P., and Clarke, R. N. 1987. *Marketing for Health Care Organizations.* Englewood Cliffs, New Jersey: Prentice Hall.

Kovner, A. R. 1990. Introduction. In A. R. Kovner, ed., *Health Care Delivery in the United States.* New York: Springer. 1–7.

Kramer, D., Ber, R., and Moore, M. 1987. Impact of workshop on students' and physicians' rejecting behaviors in patient interviews. *Journal of Medical Education 62*, 904–910.

Kreps, G. L. 1984. Communication and gerontology: Health communication training for providers of health services to the elderly. In G. L. Kreps and B. C. Thornton, eds., *Health Communication.* New York: Longman. 210–217.

Kreps, G. L. 1990. Communication and health education. In E. B. Ray and L. Donohew, eds., *Communication and Health.* Hillsdale, New Jersey: Lawrence Erlbaum.

Kreps, G. L., and Kunimoto, E. N. 1994. *Communicating Effectively in Health Care Contexts.* Thousand Oaks, California: Sage.

Kreps, G. L., and O'Hair, D. 1995. *Communication and Health Outcomes.* Cresskill, New Jersey: Hampton.

Kreps, G. L., and Thornton, B. C. 1992. *Health Communication Theory & Practice.* Prospect Heights, Illinois: Waveland.

Laurence, L., and Weinhouse, B. 1994. *Outrageous Practices.* New York: Fawcett Columbine.

Lesserman, L., and Luke, C.S. 1982. An evaluation of an innovative approach to teaching the pelvic examination to medical students. *Women and Health* 7(2), 31–42.

Linn, L. S., Oye, R. K., Cope, D. W., and DiMatteo, M. R. 1986. Use of nonphysician staff to evaluate humanistic behavior of internal medicine residents and faculty members. *Journal of Medical Education 61*, 918–920.

Martin, P., and Smyer, M. A. 1990. The experience of micro- and macroevents: A life span analysis. *Research on Aging 12*(3), 294–310.

Matthews, D. A., Suchman, A. L., and Branch, W. T. 1993. *Annals of Internal Medicine 118*, 973–977.

McBride, G.B. and McBride, W.L. 1981. Theoretical underpinnings for women's health. *Women and Health 6*(1/2), 37–55.

McCormick, W. C., Inui, T. S., and Roter, D. L. 1996. Interventions in physician-elderly patient interactions. *Research on Aging 18*(1), 103–136.

Mehrabian, A. 1981. *Silent Messages: Implication of Emotions and Attitudes.* Belmont, California: Wadsworth.

Muller, C. 1988. Medicaid: The lower tier of healthcare for women. *Women and Health 14*(2), 81–102.

Myers, G. C. 1990. Demography of aging. In R. H. Binstock and L. K. George, eds., *Handbook of Aging and the Social Sciences* (3rd ed.). San Diego: Academic Press. 19–44.

Mylander, M. 1979. Summary of conference on the older woman: continuities and discontinuities, September 14–16, 1978. *Women and Health 4* (3), 315–322.

Neugarten, B. L., and Hagestad, G. O. 1976. Age and the life course. In R. H. Binstock and L. K. George, eds., *Handbook of Aging and the Social Sciences.* New York: Van Nostrand Reinhold. 35–55.

Neugarten, B. L., and Neugarten, D. A. 1986. Age in the aging society. *Daedalus 115*, 31–49.

Nussbaum, J. F. 1983a. Perceptions of communication content and life satisfaction among the elderly. *Communication Quarterly 31*, 313–319.

Nussbaum, J. F. 1983b. Relational closeness of elderly interaction: Implications for life satisfaction. *Western Journal of Speech Communication 47*, 229–243.

Nussbaum, J. F. 1985. Successful aging: A communicative model. *Communication Quarterly 33*, 262–269.

Nussbaum, J. F., Thompson, T., and Robinson, J. D. 1989. *Communication and Aging.* New York: Harper & Row.

Office of Research on Women's Health. 1992. *Report of the National Institutes of Health: Opportunities for Research on Women's Health* (NIH publication No. 92–3457). Bethesda, Maryland.

O'Hair, D. 1986. Patient preferences for physician persuasion strategies. *Theoretical Medicine 7*, 147–164.

O'Hair, D., Allman, J., and Moore, S. 1996. A cognitive-affective model of relational expectations in the provider-patient context. *Journal of Health Psychology 1*(3), 307–322.

O'Hair, D., Behnke, R., and King, P. 1983. Age-related patient preferences for physician communication behavior. *Educational Gerontology 9*, 147–158.

O'Hair, D., and McNeilis, K. 1993. Advocates for the elderly patient: A case of mutual influence. In E. B. Ray, ed., *Case Studies in Health Communication.* Hillsdale, New Jersey: Lawrence Erlbaum. 61–73.

Parsons, T. 1951. *The Social System.* New York: The Free Press.

Rabinowitz, M. 1988. The challenge of combining clinical approaches with function in treating the elderly. *Public Health Reports 103*(5), 528–530.

Ragan, S. L. 1990. Verbal play and multiple goals in the gynecological exam interaction. In K. Tracy and N. Coupland, eds., *Multiple Goals in Discourse.* Clevedon, England: Multilingual Matters. 67–84.

Ragan, S. L., Beck, C. S., and White, M. D. 1995. Educating the patient: Interactive learning in an OB-GYN context. In G. H. Morris, and R. L. Chenail, eds., *The Talk of the Clinic.* Hillsdale, New Jersey: Lawrence Erlbaum. 185–208.

Ragan, S.L., and Glenn, L.D. 1990. Communication and gynecologic health care. In D. O'Hair and G. Kreps, eds., *Applied Communication Theory and Research.* Hillsdale, New Jersey: Lawrence Erlbaum. 313–330.

Ray, E. B., and Donohew, L., eds. 1990. *Communication and Health: Systems and Applications.* Hillsdale, New Jersey: Lawrence Erlbaum.

Riley, M. W. 1971. Social gerontology and the age stratification of society. *The Gerontologist 11*(1), 79–87.

Roter, D. L. 1977. Patient participation in patient-provider interaction: The effects of patient question-asking on the quality of interaction, satisfaction, and compliance. *Health Education Monographs 5*, 281–315.

Roter, D. L. 1991. Elderly patient-physician communication: A descriptive study of contact and affect during the medical encounter. *Advances in Health Education 3*, 15–23.

Roter, D. L., and Hall, J. A. 1992. *Doctors Talking with Patients/Patients Talking with Doctors: Improving Communication in Medical Visits.* Westport, Connecticut: Auburn House.

Ruben, B. D. 1990. The health caregiver-patient relationship: pathology, etiology, treatment. In E. B. Ray and L. Donohew, eds., *Communication and Health: Systems and Applications.* Hillsdale, New Jersey: Lawrence Erlbaum. 51–68.

Ryan, E. B., Giles, H., Bartolucci, G., and Henwood, K. 1986. Psycholinguistic and social psychological components of communication by and with the elderly. *Language & Communication 6*(1/2), 1–24.

Ryan, E. B., See, S. K., Meneer, W. B., and Trovato, D. 1992. Age-based perceptions of language performance among younger and older adults. *Communication Research 19*(4), 423–443.

Short, D. 1993. First impressions. *British Journal of Hospital Medicine 50*(5), 270–271.

Shuy, R. W. 1976. The medical interview: Problems in communication. *Primary Care 3*, 365–386.

Smith, C. K., Polis, E., and Hadac, R. R. 1981. Characteristics of the initial medical interview associated with patient satisfaction and understanding. *Journal of Family Practice 12*, 283–288.

Smith, J.M. 1992. *Women and Doctors.* New York: Atlantic Monthly Press.

Spitzberg, B. H., and Hecht, M. L. 1984. A component model of relational competence. *Human Communication Research 10*, 575–600.

Starr, P. 1982. *The Social Transformation of American Medicine.* New York: Basic Books.

Stein, H. F. 1985. What is therapeutic in clinical relationships? *Family Medicine 17*(5), 188–194.

Stewart, M., and Roter, D., eds. 1990. *Communication with Medical Patients.* Newbury Park, California: Sage.

Stoeckle, J. D. 1987. Introduction. In J. D. Stoeckle, ed., *Encounters between Patients and Doctors: An Anthology.* Cambridge, MA: MIT Press. 1–129.

Street, R. L., Gold, W. R., and McDowell, T. 1995. Discussing health-related quality of life in prenatal consultation. In G. H. Morris, and R. L. Chenail, eds., *The Talk of the Clinic.* Hillsdale, New Jersey: Lawrence Erlbaum. 209–231.

Tamir, L. 1979. *Communication and the Aging Process: Interaction Throughout the Life Cycle.* New York: Pergamon Press.

Tannen, D. 1994a. *Gender and Discourse.* New York: Oxford University Press.

Tannen, D. 1994b. *Talking from 9 to 5.* New York: William Morrow and Company.

Tarbox, A. R., Connors, G. J., and Faillace, L A. 1987. Freshman and senior medical students' attitudes toward the elderly. *Journal of Medical Education 62*, 582–591.

The coming crisis in long-term care. 1990, January-February. *Futurist*, p. 49.

Turner, J. A., Deyo, R. A., Loeser, J. D., Von Korff, M., and Fordyce, W. E. 1994. The importance of placebo effects in pain treatment and research. *JAMA 271*(20), 1609–1613.

von Friederichs-Fitzwater, M. M., Callahan, E. J., Flynn, N., and Williams, J. 1991. Relational control in physician-patient encounters. *Health Communication 3*(1), 17–36.

Waitzkin, H. 1984. Doctor-patient communication: Clinical implications of social scientific research. *Journal of the American Medical Association 252*(17), 2441–2446.

Waitzkin, H. 1985. Information giving in medical care. *Journal of Health and Social Behavior 26*, 81–101.

Williams, A., and Giles, H. 1991. Sociopsychological perspectives on older people's language and communication. *Ageing and Society 11*, 103–126.

Zimmerman, M. K. 1994. The women's health movement: A critique of medical enterprise and the position of women. In P. R. Lee, & C. L. Estes, eds., *The Nation's Health* (4th ed.). Boston: Jones and Bartlett. 383–390.

CHAPTER 14

Grandmothers and Granddaughters in African American Families

Imparting Cultural Tradition and Womanhood between Generations of Women[1]

Valerie Cryer McKay

INTRODUCTION

This chapter explores one aspect of African American family life that, to date, has received relatively little attention in the discipline of language, communication, and aging: the role of extended family in the lives of African American children. Previous research has recognized cultural differences in family interaction patterns by identifying the integral nature of kin networks in African American families; these networks are comprised, primarily, of extended family (grandparents, aunts, uncles, and siblings). Although non-kin networks are an important element in the structure of the African American community (Stack, 1974a and b), consanguineal bonds often supersede ties between non-blood relations (Sudarkasa, 1981); thus, this chapter focuses on kin networks comprised of extended family members.

Perhaps the strongest intergenerational bonds existing within African American families are those between female members: grandmother-mother-daughter (Dill, 1987; Ladner, 1987; Sawyer, 1973). This chapter proposes that the intergenerational transmission of a sense of *womanhood* is vital for achieving the wisdom, adaptability, and strength to overcome seemingly insurmountable economic and social obstacles. Intrinsic to the conceptualization of womanhood is the notion of continuity of African American culture imparted from older to younger generations of women. Given that discourse "may above all be the locus of partial and unsuccessful attempts at adaptation to age—at locating our own and others' selves within, or against the grain of, socially normative categories and roles" (Coupland, Nussbaum, and Grossman, 1993, p. xxvi), this chapter will focus on the discourse by which *womanhood, culture*, and *tradition* are both described and conveyed in intergenerational conversations with African American grandmothers and their biological granddaughters. Not surprisingly, an analysis of grandmothers' and granddaughters' discourse regarding their relationship, the nature and content of interaction about and between each other, and personal advice about life and family, reveals a concern that younger generations assimilate into contemporary culture while at the same time understanding and adhering to their heritage and ancestry.

THEORETICAL PERSPECTIVE

This chapter integrates three basic assumptions inherent in feminist inquiry, assumptions which emerge from criticisms or limitations identified in traditional scientific models of social research (Millman and Kanter, 1987; Sherif, 1987). First, in order to provide a more comprehensive view of social behavior, it is necessary to eliminate the effects of cultural ethnocentrism resulting in a biased view of human action. Second, theoretical and empirical evidence suggests that men and women inhabit different social worlds to the extent that generalizations intrinsic to traditional scientific models are limited in their applicability to alternative populations. Finally, and most importantly, the reductionist nature of traditional social scientific inquiry has resulted in the neglect of alternative (and perhaps more substantive) phenomena of social behavior and, specifically, women's experience (Sherif, 1987).

The effects of these limitations are perhaps most evident in extant research on African American families (English, 1974). A review of early research, such as that conducted by Frazier (1951) and Moynihan (1965), clearly illustrates the effects of a culturally ethnocentric research bias on both the public policy imposed and the social/economic status of the African American family. Furthermore, these researchers contend that the matriarchal structure of the African American family has resulted in a family pathology (i.e., dysfunction) that has led to the failure of African Americans to adapt to our predominantly white, Euro-American society. This view, often referred to as Deficit, implies that African American families are deficient in comparison with other, predominantly Euro-American, family forms (Dodson, 1981).

Acknowledging this, Dodson (1981) explains that to consider our society as homogeneous and, thus, impose an ethnocentric bias on our interpretation of non-white cultural and social patterns, assumes that all people conform to established norms; inability to conform results in inadequate or (in the terms of past research) pathological patterns of behavior. A more heterogeneous view (e.g., cultural relativity) acknowledges that variations in family functioning are intrinsic within the framework of the multicultural diversity characterizing our society. Furthermore, the mythical image of the dominant and emasculating African American woman fails to recognize her enduring strength and adaptability in the presence of harsh social and economic conditions (Gutman, 1976; Lewis and Looney, 1983).

In order to counter these perceptions, Dill (1987, p. 98) proposes "an empirically more adequate social science" that includes critical accounts of women's situation in every race, class, and culture, a feminist perspective which takes into account the view of all women that is both antiracist and antisexist. Moreover, research must seek to refute myths by "examining aspects of black family life that have been overlooked or distorted" (Dill, 1987, p. 98).[2] African American culture should be examined in and of itself—as emerging from economic and social oppression and functioning based upon a heritage characterized, historically, by the assimilation and implementation of strategies for survival. Likewise, African American womanhood should not be viewed as dominant, matriarchal or deviant from models of Euro-American womanhood but, alternatively, as adaptive and emerging as a consequence of the conditions in which it exists (Dill, 1987). To consider otherwise is to fail to recognize the effect of culture and gender on human behavior (Sawyer, 1973).

More recently, researchers have been examining the dynamics of African American family life apart from other family forms, rejecting the ineffectual and comparative Deficit model previously imposed (Burton, 1992; Burton and Dilworth-Anderson, 1991; Cheatham and Stewart, 1990). Many of these studies focus upon the integral role of Black grandparents, particularly grandmothers, in the lives of children of drug-addicted parents, young single parents, and working parents. Thus, the effects of social and economic status are integrated into our understanding of African American family life. What these studies reveal is the essential role of older women as "crucial to the maintenance and perpetuation of continuity and integrity in the extended kin network" as they pass on family history, encourage a family philosophy or theme, promote unity and continuity, and help with family responsibilities while encouraging others to follow in their footsteps (Burton and Dilworth-Anderson, 1992, p. 322). These results are consistent with what is revealed in the analysis of granddaughter-grandmother discourse within the present chapter.

EXTENDED FAMILY IN AFRICAN AMERICAN CULTURE

Perhaps there is no characteristic more ubiquitous in African American family life than the presence of extended family in the lives of its children (Burton and Dilworth-Anderson, 1992; Cheatham and Stewart, 1990; Martin and Martin, 1978; Stack, 1974a and b; and others). Extended family is described as "a multigenerational, interdependent kinship system which is welded together by a sense of obligation to relatives . . . extends across geographical boundaries to connect family units to an extended family network; and has a built-in mutual aid system for the welfare of its members and the maintenance of the family as a whole" (Martin and Martin, 1978, p. 1). Extended family members function in a variety of capacities including (but not limited to) childcare, socialization, and imparting cultural tradition from generation to generation. Although scholars of African American family life debate the historical origins of the role of extended family,[3] its endurance perpetuates solidarity and security in the lives of its younger members (Martin and Martin, 1978).

Stack (1974a and b) notes that the consanguineal extended family (including grandparents, aunts, uncles, and siblings) assists its members in meeting many and varied needs and is inherently dependent upon reciprocity for its continuance. Consistent with this view, Boyd-Franklin (1983) concludes that women are among the strongest sources of support and assistance—especially in providing aid in child-rearing—when mothers are unable to care for their children either because of work responsibilities or financial limitations.

Another key function of extended family is socialization. In fact, Billingsley (1968), Ladner (1971), and Sudarkasa (1981) propose that extended family is among the primary agents of socialization in Black families. Within this context, children learn strategies for survival and adaptation fundamental to "effective functioning within the social group" (Ladner, 1971, p. 49). Children also learn prosocial behaviors such as manners, respect for elders, and the role of strong religious beliefs in African American family life (Martin and Martin, 1985). Pertinent to this process is the notion that both family tradition and aspects of African American cultural tradition are considered vital aspects of continuity to be "passed on" between generations.

Customarily, a child selects a significant other from among extended family members with whom he or she forms a life-long bond. The significant other is regarded as someone who gives the child emotional support, acts as a role model for social and cultural learning, often serves as a source of self-validation and confirmation of self-worth, and teaches skills and knowledge necessary for goal achievement (Manns, 1981). African American children also achieve an awareness of their own family identity, described by Rainwater (1971, p. 258) as "a sense of continuity and social sameness," from hearing their elders' stories of family history. An integral function of this intergenerational bond, then, is to bestow family and cultural heritage.

In many cases the significant other is a grandparent, not surprising given the childkeeping role that grandparents (and especially grandmothers) often assume in the absence of the child's mother (Glick, 1981; Jackson, 1971; Manns, 1981; Stack, 1974a, 1974b). The selection of a significant other usually results in the formation of a same-sex (most often female) intergenerational bond (i.e., grandmother-granddaughter), and this is substantiated by evidence from extant research (cf., Boyd-Franklin, 1983; Jackson, 1971; Ladner, 1971; Stack, 1974a, 1974b). As Boyd-Franklin (1983, p. 92) notes, "there is a strong maternal instinct in our families . . . there is also a network and support system among our women which often provides the backbone for family survival." Essential to this notion is the fact that the eldest women accept the responsibility for imparting a strong sense of womanhood between generations—especially grandmothers to granddaughters.

THE CONCEPT OF WOMANHOOD

How is African American womanhood envisioned, and why is it an important aspect of continuity between generations in African American families? Perhaps this question can best be answered by analyzing the role of African American women from an historical perspective (Ladner, 1971). One of the few scholars to view African

American culture in terms of its historical development was Gutman (1976). Pertinent to his viewpoint was the belief that kinship bonds and knowledge of strategies for survival during the period of slavery were transmitted intergenerationally. The family became the agent for conveying family identity and cultural heritage from generation to generation. Not surprisingly, the eldest African American woman (who was often responsible for caring for her own as well as other children) often served as the primary agent of information dissemination and security; grandmothers continue to function in this capacity today (Bernard, 1966; Gutman, 1976; Jones, 1973). "[Grandmother] has socialized her children and grandchildren into values and patterns essential to their survival, growth, and development and they, in turn, have formed and maintained a black society despite social and economic obstacles" (Jones, 1973, p. 19).

With the rise of the institution of slavery in our country came significant changes in the cultural, social, and economic patterns of African American family life: Fathers were removed from their families, children were taken away from their parents, women cared for their own as well as other children. Yet, strong family bonds survived even if the conjugal family structure did not (Ladner, 1971; Willie, 1976). Many of the structural and interactional family patterns that emerged from the period of slavery have endured to present day; African American women have continued to adapt, overcome, and emerge as survivors, while their men continue to suffer from the effects of social and economic oppression (Stack, 1974a; 1974b).

The concept of womanhood—as it applies today—is perhaps best illustrated in the work of Ladner (1971) as she investigated the functional, as opposed to dominant and matriarchal, role of women in African American families. Moreover, Ladner (1971, p. 43) emphasizes the role of grandmothers in the socialization process, acting as role models for their granddaughters regarding "rules for Black womanhood." She states,

> The young Black girl growing up in this environment becomes consciously socialized into the role of womanhood when she is about seven or eight years old . . . the influence of the extended family upon the socialization of the young Black girl is often very strong . . . and [she] absorbs the influences of grandmother and grandfather as well as mother and father (Ladner, 1971, p. 50).

What constitutes the African American view of womanhood? Generally, it is conceptualized as the integration of women's roles, responsibilities, and relationships in African American culture. For example, Ladner (1971) describes womanhood in terms of both childbearing and motherhood. In a study of young African American women, she found that motherhood (married or unmarried) brought with it a degree of responsibility that was respected by peers. Womanhood is also conceived as a high degree of closeness in women's intergenerational relationships with other women. With this closeness comes the responsibility for caring for women and children of the extended family as previously mentioned. Womanhood also constitutes the nature of interpersonal, marital, and sexual relationships with men, and this is further substantiated by Martin and Martin (1978) who emphasize that womanhood is defined by how women relate to men—not how they dominate them. Also among the characteristics of womanhood are aspirations for education, work, and career goals; notions of independence and autonomy; money and resource management; appearance; and, not surprisingly, the role of women in the family (Ladner, 1971; Martin and Martin, 1978).

Clearly, the notion of womanhood places a particular emphasis on the strength, adaptability, and perseverance of African American women in our society. However,

> There is no single set of criteria for becoming a woman in the Black community; each girl is conditioned by a diversity of factors depending primarily upon her opportunities, role models, psychological disposition, and the influence of the values, customs and traditions of the Black community . . . the resources which adolescent girls have at their disposal, combined with the cultural heritage of their communities, are crucial factors in determining what kind of women they become . . . the concepts of motivation, roles and role model, identity, and socialization *as well as* family income, education, kin, and peer group relations are important to consider (Ladner, 1987, p. 80).

Ironically, the perseverance and determination characteristic of African American women, while often considered pathological by some scholars of African American culture, are basic to the intergenerational transmission of culture, tradition, and a sense of womanhood by which African American women achieve the wisdom, adaptability, and strength to overcome insurmountable economic and social obstacles. The focus of this chapter is on the language of African American grandmothers and granddaughters as they *talk* about who they are individually and in relationship to each other.

METHODS

Participants

Participants were ten African American grandmother-granddaughter biological pairs obtained by non-random, snowball sampling techniques: A small sample of participants was purposively selected (N = 3 pairs), and from those, additional names were obtained and their participation elicited (N = 7 pairs). Criteria for participation included: (1) biological pairs in which the granddaughter was at least twelve years old so she would have the ability to recognize integral aspects of her relationship with her grandmother, (2) pairs representing diverse educational, socio-economic, and age backgrounds in order to reflect the range of characteristics in grandmother-granddaughter relationships evidenced in extant literature, and (3) pairs in which both members were willing to participate in the interview process. As a result, our sample of grandmothers ranged in age from forty-five to eighty-four; granddaughters, from fourteen to forty-five. Participants were from low to moderate socio-economic status. Grandmothers' education ranged from near completion of high school to a master's degree; granddaughters' from junior high to a master's degree. Pseudonyms will be used in order to assure participant anonymity.

Interview Questions

The questions comprising the interview were designed to elicit information regarding the intergenerational transmission of womanhood and family and/or cultural traditions between grandmothers and granddaughters. The specific interview questions asked of grandmother participants were: (1) Do you consider yourself a role model for your granddaughter? If so, what do you try to teach her? (2) What personal, family, and/or cultural traditions do you share with your granddaughter? (3) Do you share stories of family (past or present)? (4) What does it mean to be an African American woman in today's society? And finally, (5) What advice do you have for your granddaughter for achieving a strong sense of African American womanhood?

The interview questions asked of granddaughter participants were: (1) Is your grandmother a role model for your life? If so, what have you learned from her? (2) What personal, family, and/or cultural traditions has your grandmother shared with you? (3) Does she share stories of family (past or present)? (4) What does it mean to be an African American woman in today's society? And finally, (5) What advice has your grandmother provided for achieving a strong sense of African American womanhood?

Interview Format

Interviews were conducted by a trained interviewer who was familiar with interviewing and research methods and had been trained specifically for the present investigation. In addition to presenting the prepared questions, the interviewer was encouraged to probe for additional information when and if possible without leading or imposing bias on the information obtained. Interviews were conducted in person with the participants and audiotaped; grandmothers and granddaughters were interviewed separately. The interview process was conducted over a six-week period. Transcripts of each interview were then prepared by the interviewer who was most familiar with the content; literal text from these transcripts is presented in the following portion of this chapter.

Qualitative Analysis of Interviews

The decision to offer a qualitative presentation of the transcripts obtained for this chapter is not at the expense of or at the exclusion of quantitative analytical techniques. Rather, it is consistent with the feminist view proposed as the framework for this chapter. Congruent with the recognition of the value of discourse is the appropriateness of "giving voice" to the groups of people we want to study; that is, who we are individually and in interaction with others is revealed through talk (Coupland, Nussbaum, and Grossman, 1993, p. xiii). This perspective is not new and emerges, for example, in Mead's (1932) work which assumes that identity emerges through social interaction; the lifespan developmental perspective of the process of self-identity is documented by Giddens (1990, 1991). Acknowledging that this form of analysis is open to interpretation based upon factors such as individuality, context, and experience, it might also provide the basis for more objective forms of analysis and the subsequent testing of empirical hypotheses. Here, it simply functions to reveal how grandmothers and granddaughters talk about the nature of their intergenerational relationship.

RESULTS OF ANALYSIS OF DISCOURSE

Following are excerpts from both grandmothers' and granddaughters' talk about themselves and their relationship to each other.

I. Do grandmothers consider themselves role models for their granddaughters? If so, what do they try to teach the younger women?

This question was advanced based on previous research which suggests that a young woman's concept of her own womanhood is largely dependent upon the role models she selects who are influential in socializing her in both cultural and family heritage (Ladner, 1987). In most cases, the grandmothers in our study conveyed that they do consider themselves to be role models for their granddaughters— especially when it comes to their granddaughters achieving a strong sense of womanhood. The kinds of experiences and examples they share with their granddaughters do seem to vary by age (their own education, religious faith, wisdom, and experience), but the lessons they hope their granddaughters learn from their examples are the same in most cases.

For example, Ellen (the youngest grandmother at age forty-five), holds a master's degree, and consequently, encourages Becca (age fourteen), her granddaughter, to do well in school. Becca stated, "she helps me academically, like reading and math . . . she helps me read like sometime with my homework. She explains how—the way I'm supposed to do it . . . I should—you know—study a little harder, get a good education when I get ready to go out into the real world and I should get ready for that."

Helen (age eighty-four) feels very strongly about her role in the life of her granddaughter, Sonya. When asked if she considered herself a role model for Sonya, she responded, without hesitation—"YES."

> Well, she and I sits down and we talk about life. And then I tell her about how she suppose to meet the public, and how she's suppose to carry herself as a young lady and what grandmother won't let her be

until she grows up. I want her to get that education, so she won't be beholdin' to nobody. I want her to be somebody, I want her to be a young lady and carry herself as such. But I want her to get that education first. Then I teaches her how to cook, clean, cause she helps me so much by cleaning—she come in here and help grandma clean up.

Sonya agreed that her grandmother has told her many times that she should "go to school and get [an] education so when I get older I can do whatever I want . . . she says if I finish my education I won't have to like be worried about money and stuff when I get older."

Moreen (grandmother to Debra and sixty-eight years old) stated, "I just try to show by example and tell the importance of faith in the Lord. [Debra] has told me that she looked up to me." Moreen also conveyed that faith in God was a family tradition as well. "Our family has always emphasized the importance of being a loving and caring person. With the Lord being accepted as part of our family, [Debra] has learned what it means to be a good person. . . to treat others with respect. She always treats others with respect from the heart . . . not very many people do that anymore."

Debra feels strongly about her grandmother as a role model in her own life: "I believe a role model suggest character, strength, a person that stands out, I believe Granny possesses these qualities. My grandmother has a solid foundation and her faith in the Lord has given her stability throughout life. As she continues to have faith she is strong. She doesn't try to get out of certain situations if things don't go her way—she's very strong."

II. What personal, family, and/or cultural traditions do grandmothers share with their granddaughters?

This question was advanced in order to explore specific traditions that grandmothers perceive as important (and granddaughters remember) regarding their personal, family, or cultural heritage. Not only is the content of the information conveyed being explored, but whether or not grandmothers consider this an important aspect of their intergenerational role (as a significant other) is also of interest. Generally, it was difficult for participants to remember specific "traditions," but they disclosed that family, respect, religion, and knowledge of both African and African American art and artifacts were integral in understanding cultural and personal heritage.

Becca noted, "She [grandmother] tells me about how beautiful black is . . . how beautiful they are." Consistent with this response, her grandmother, Ellen, noted,

> I think culturally that being an average person is not ok, you really have to be a super achiever because we're Black people. We really have to just dig in, you know it's just not laid out there we've really have to just dig in and keep struggling—making mistakes, not always being successful—maybe even feeling like a failure, but we've got to keep struggling . . . and I think that an appreciation for grandparents, appreciation for being a family. Culturally, appreciating all types of music . . . I think I read her a lot of Black literature—like works by Black people. The art work in my home . . . what it's like to be Black—being proud of yourself. I think the greatest thing—her biggest problem right now is her personal grooming. You know that's where I'm working on now, that's important—what your appearance is.

Ella, Rona's grandmother, noted that an important family tradition has been to pass on respect—"respect for those older than yourself . . . lots of young people today don't understand the importance of the older generation, and I believe that [Rona] understands the importance of her grandparents. She keeps in touch with us and cares about our well-being."

Helen disclosed, "I makes a parable as I go along and you know cause that what God and the Bible says. I teach her [Sonya] this book right here [points to the Bible in her lap]. As I go along, sometime I makes parables about someone that I knew. . . . " She continued, "Listen to your grandmother . . . always remember—I said when I'm dead and gone I want you [as if speaking to Sonya] to look back and say you know my grandmother told me this."

Emma noted that her grandmother, Mrs. Thompson, made it a point to take her and her sister "to museums that had lots of African and Black-American work." She also disclosed that, as a young girl, her grandmother would read stories "and that made [her] want to learn and read . . . and my sister and I learned to love ourselves for who we are and that there is nothing wrong with being Black."

III. Do grandmothers share stories of family (past or present)?

According to Manns (1981) and Rainwater (1971), the significant other (extended family member) in an African American child's life functions not only as a role model but as a source of information about family that assists the child in developing a strong sense of family identity and continuity; grandmothers often fulfill this role. Knowledge of family heritage serves as a source of self-validation and confirmation of self-worth integral to achieving, for example, relational, educational, and career goals.

As an illustration, Shirley was raised by her grandparents; she was very involved in their lives but knew very little about her parents. Her grandmother, Rose, had shared stories about Shirley's father (Rose's son): "She [Rose] was very close to my father. Basically how he just—in his day—how he was a real entrepreneur. He got along especially well with people."

Helen told us of one of the stories she often shares with Sonya:

Sometimes when I'm pressing her hair we talks about how hard it was for me growing up in Louisiana out in the cotton fields. That why I brought my children to California. I want her to finish her education and become someone. I tell stories so that she can learn from them . . . I came to California in 1970. I brought four children to California and I couldn't bring all of them at one time. So when I got off that bus in '70 on the third day of January, I had three dollars, nowhere to lay my head I could call my own—living with my niece. You see a lot of people down the county, I don't because I took the money like I was supposed to. So in February I saved and sent for five more of my children. In June I got five more and we lived in two bedroom apartment. I had six girls in one room and six boys in the other and I slept downstairs in the living room. My babies didn't have a change of clothes—so you see how good the Lord has been (she points around to the house she now owns). The good Lord and the county and me—we did it. And just about all I own I earned.

Moreen disclosed that she tells Debra about her life as a young girl: "How I was raised, things that I did. How my upbringing made me the person I am . . . things we had during my coming up period. What we used to do. Things like positions each family member played." When asked what she meant by "positions," she replied, "Well, my father had to made a living for the family so we all took positions—like cleaning the yard, the house, cooking dinner for him, and things like that; we have so many of them, I can't remember."

IV. What does it mean to be an African American woman in today's society?

Integral to this investigation is the concept of womanhood and the role it plays in terms of both individual and relational goals in the lives of African American women (Ladner, 1971, 1987; Martin & Martin, 1978; Stack, 1974a, 1974b). Responses to this question were mixed: Some participants conveyed that it was difficult, others not difficult, but in either case the conclusion was that if an African American woman works hard and takes advantage of opportunities, she can accomplish anything in life. Sources of difficulty were primarily social and economical; sources of strength were repeatedly found in family relationships and religious beliefs. In most cases, however, very little was said about these women's relationships with men, suggesting that womanhood might be individually as opposed to relationally defined and should certainly be the focus of future research.

Ellen stated, unequivocally, that "It's been very difficult." The primary source of difficulty was that she has been a single-mother since 1965; ironically, this seems to be both a source of difficulty and a valuable life experience. She contends,

> I wanted to ensure a happy valuable experience for my children, and not having a partner to do it with so that economically it would be more comfortable. And that problem solving would have be more shared and not so one-sided . . . but also, I think that economically it's been hard, I guess it's been hard in the decision making process too. What I did was use my family, my parents, my sisters would help, and my small network of friends to make it—at least try to make it balance. It's difficult being a Black women, you have to be more than just a fighter—you have to be a survivor. You have to be a survivor and an achiever—they go hand-in-hand. It's tremendously difficult being a Black woman in White America.

Rose, on the other hand, stated "it really hasn't been difficult for me. I haven't had any trouble . . . because I always worked and never had any trouble on jobs or things like that . . . in a way it has changed—

because now the younger adults they don't want to think about the older times. They'll tell you in a minute this is not the 1970s, this is the 90s." Ironically, her granddaughter Shirley replied,

> It has been hard being an Afro-American woman in today's society because it's hard to know exactly what role to play and what role is comfortable because—they did not do anything that today's women does. They—their roles for example—school teacher, nurse—it wasn't doctor or anything like that, and so it's very hard to have a role model from that generation as far as professionally. As far as socially, at home I—we probably need to get back to those roots and try to take on some of their characteristics because I do believe that Black men and Black women are very confused as to what role to play. That it's neither one of their faults because there aren't any role models.

Shirley had stated previously that she perceives her grandmother as a role model, more in terms of respecting her than following the path her grandmother has set forth. Shirley indicated more than once that her grandmother has shown her ways she could improve, but she usually fails to do so. Shirley's goals do not always match those of her grandmother—at least in terms of education and career—and this is evident in the quote above. Of particular interest was a statement by Shirley regarding her grandmother's relationship with her grandfather:

> She [her grandmother] chose to kind of be the shadow of my grandfather which I greatly respect her for that because it's something that I seem to can't do, and that takes a special person . . . I think if we could shadow our Black men a little better, but at the same time keep our own identity, the Black culture within itself would advance. It's hard to do and it's also economically hard to do because at the same time while you're trying to support the Black man and keep your own identity, you still need a dual income and I'm sure everybody wants to improve their living situation—people are just ambitious that way.

Moreen emphasized that her faith in the Lord has made her life easier: "I think I was very fortunate because I found the Lord very early in life and it is with his looking over me and my good fortune that living in America has not been hard." She believes that the same faith will help Debra in her life: "Given that she [Debra] accepted the Lord—that's one thing she had done at an early age—I would encourage her to continue on her path for the gospel. . . . She comes to me with very personal things . . . she is also very dedicated to the Lord, growing strong in the Lord at 25 years saved her from possibly going astray."

Debra disclosed that being a Black woman in today's society is not always easy: "Being a woman if you carry yourself as a lady, certain opportunities like being a doctor or lawyer, educational opportunities and basically any type of professional field is open to Black-American women. It's been hard because of the existence of racism and sexism. Me personally, looking younger than my age, I must constantly struggle for a balance to counter such discrimination . . . you must educate yourself and look above the simplicity of those who choose to discriminate. Also I think being Black has given the strength to fight and struggle for the things that I believe in."

Emma revealed that, although being Black was not difficult for her, life is a challenge primarily because she has a baby. "For me it means to prove that I can compete with the best of them. There is always the challenge to prove myself and to prove that I am somebody and will make the best of any situation. If there is one thing that I've learned from my grandmother is to always see what I start to its finish."

Like many of the other women in this study, Luella conveyed that being a Black woman is not as difficult as it used to be, but sometimes it is a struggle. "If you're Black in this country—male or female—you have to try twice as hard . . . to try twice as hard to be treated equally."

V. What advice do grandmothers have for granddaughters for achieving a strong sense of African American womanhood?

This research question was advanced in order to explore (1) grandmothers' perceptions of their role as "significant other" or socializing agent in the lives of their granddaughters, and (2) information they perceive as important to convey to their granddaughters so that they have the tools needed to survive in our society. Granddaughters' views were expected to reveal similar perspectives as an indicator of intergenerational continuity. Advice, in most cases, was given by grandmothers both directly and indirectly. Indirectly, granddaughters disclosed that their grandmothers' supportiveness ("just being there") was perhaps the most important aspect of their relationship. For example, Shirley stated that, although her grandmother [Rose] never gives advice directly, she is very supportive:

> She believes highly in education. She's just a very supportive person. She doesn't try to guide me in any particular way. She just wants me to do the right thing—that's all, just please do the right thing. And probably the one that maybe she did try to teach me is try not to make many waves . . . I will say this, you can tell she loves me unconditionally no matter what I've done wrong or what mischief I've gotten into, she's always there no matter what she loves me unconditionally and I think that's what I've learned through her was to love unconditionally.

Rona stated that her grandmother had taught her "to achieve everything that I want to accomplish in life, and if that's what you want to do—if you want to be a maid, then be the best maid—whatever you want to be—you want to be a such-and-such be a good one—be the best that you can be . . . just believe what you want to do."

Helen stated that her advice to Sonya is, "don't look at boys— don't let them fool ya, because that's what they would do. Get her education so she would not be beholding to nobody . . . I would just like all grandbabies to go on and get their education." Sonya remembers her discussions with her grandmother about education: "Well, when she do my hair she would talk to me and tell me like to go on with school and don't worry about boys—not to get involved with them and just go to school and get my education." She also disclosed, "when you try harder and do better they won't say anything but it's good. It's good to be a strong Black woman making something of herself."

As advice for coping with any adversity, Debra conveyed that her grandmother [Moreen] had a saying: "She told me when things are going bad in my life and everything is dark and bleak, to always remember that it is always darkest before dawn." She continued, "My grandmother is a believer and lover of the Lord—extremely. She love to help people all the time, mostly giving through cooking and she loves to see people enjoy themselves. If she could give more financially she would. She is surrounded by love and she is so supportive in listening. She listens when parents don't listen. She always has an open mind and ear when going into unfamiliar situations."

Acknowledging the importance of facing adversity "head-on," Mrs. Thompson recognized that many problems can be overcome with hard work and perseverance; most importantly, education was the key to success. She constantly advises Emma to "finish her education; always strive to succeed and excel at whatever path she chooses to go down in life and see through to the finish." These words convey a most powerful conviction held by grandmothers as advice for their granddaughters—in terms of achieving both a strong sense of womanhood and personal goals.

DISCUSSION AND IMPLICATIONS

This chapter began with the acceptance of three major assumptions of feminist research as the basic premises guiding this investigation; simply stated, culture and gender are critical factors in explaining or predicting patterns of behavior in our society. Consistent with this view, early research literature on African American families was acknowledged as being most illustrative of a negative interpretation of family functioning resulting from the failure to consider these factors— specifically, the myth of the dominant matriarch as the source of pathology in African American families or the Deficit view of African American family life.

In contrast, this chapter proposes that imparting a strong sense of womanhood between women is vital for achieving the wisdom, adaptability, and strength to overcome social and economic adversity; furthermore, inherent in the conceptualization of womanhood is the notion of continuity of culture imparted from older to younger generations of African American women. Pertinent to this view, then, is recognition of the vital role of extended family (and specifically a significant other such as the grandmother) in the lives of young African American women. Thus, this chapter sought to explore the means by which culture and womanhood are conveyed between African American grandmothers and granddaughters.

First, how is African American womanhood envisioned, and why is it an important aspect of continuity between generations in African American families? Not surprisingly, aspects of womanhood reported in previous research also emerged in this investigation; for example, aspirations for education, work, and career goals; notions of independence and autonomy; money and resource management; and personal appearance. However, a paucity of information was obtained (not by design) regarding the conceptualization of womanhood in terms of male-female relationships. That which was disclosed was either advice discouraging granddaughters from entering into relationships ("don't worry about boys . . . don't get involved with them . . . don't be beholdin' to anybody") or uncertainty regarding the roles of African American men and women in interpersonal relationships ("I think if we could shadow our Black men a little better, but at the same time keep our own identity, the Black culture within itself would advance . . . [but] it's hard to do"; "I do believe that Black men and Black women are very confused as to what role to play").

Although future research should endeavor to explore the nature of male-female relationships in African American culture, extant research provides some explanation for the lack of findings in this investigation. According to Glick (1981, p. 112), Black women with advanced college education are "likely to have career interests that compete with the desire to maintain a permanent marriage" and limit family size in order to be competitive in the employment market. The discourse examined in this chapter provides evidence in support of this claim. Only two of the granddaughters in this study had children (they were single parents); two were in junior high or high school; and the remaining six had either completed two- or four-year degrees, were in the process of obtaining their college education, or held master's degrees. A majority of the grandmothers were single parents themselves who had completed their education and worked hard to support their families—sometimes with the help of other family members or friends. Furthermore, in several cases, grandmothers actively encouraged their granddaughters to continue their education; likewise, granddaughters conveyed that the pursuit of education was a strong message imparted by grandmothers.

These results suggest that grandmothers and granddaughters alike perceive that (1) education is a very important part of achieving a strong sense of womanhood and independence; and (2) marriage and family come either after these have been achieved, or perhaps not at all; in either case, intergenerational continuity in attitudes toward education is apparent. Moreover, the notion of grandmothers as role models for achievement (in education and/or career) seems substantiated by these results; education is viewed as the means by which African American women overcome social and economic adversity. Less certain, however, is the role of male-female relationships in the lives of these women: How do grandmothers function as role models for male-female relationships? Do the "rules for Black womanhood" include advice regarding intimate relationships with men?

An alternative explanation can also be found in an historical perspective of African American family life. As previously mentioned, during the period of slavery, fathers were separated from their families by being sold to other estates—leaving primary childcare responsibility to mothers (Ladner, 1971). Perhaps the effects continue to the present day as African American men are, because of limited employment resources, sometimes forced to seek employment outside of the community in which they or their families reside (Stack 1974a, 1974b). The result is a significant number of single-parent families headed by women (which is not a new phenomenon in African American culture); dependence upon kin and kin networks for assistance and support; and as noted in this study, a paucity of role models for male-female relationships. Future research should endeavor to examine the viability of these explanations in interviews with both men and women.

Second, this chapter sought to explore the nature of personal, family, and cultural tradition imparted between grandmothers and granddaughters, positing that knowledge of a woman's cultural heritage enhances awareness and sense of her own identity. As previously stated, a significant other (often grandmother) selected from among extended family members is a primary source of personal, family, or cultural heritage. In this investigation, perhaps the strongest cultural message conveyed by grandmothers was for granddaughters to be proud of their African and African American heritage, to be strong and not affected negatively by those who discriminate and speak or act with racial prejudice. Some grandmothers imparted this message by exposing their granddaughters to African and African American art and literature; others simply offered advice based upon their own life experiences and wisdom. In many cases, the personal message was to rise above the effects of negative words and stereotypes and achieve your personal best. Perhaps this can best be summarized in one granddaughter's response to the question: What does it mean to be an African American woman in today's society? Her response: "To be a proud woman that happens to be Black!"

Other aspects of culture imparted by grandmothers included the importance of strong religious beliefs, family, and respect for others. More than one grandmother emphasized that her ability and determination to rise above the effects of poverty or hardship was dependent upon strong religious beliefs and faith in the Lord. Having faith was one important tradition to pass on to granddaughters so that they, too, could triumph over adversity.

One grandmother also noted that older generations have an obligation to convey information about African and African American culture to young people; she stated, "if I could do it over again, I would spend time telling her all about being Black in America—cause you don't get it in school. I didn't and maybe times have changed . . . the information is there and you need to find out what it means to be Black. We didn't come over here on a pleasure cruise or because we wanted to . . . our history has been stripped from us . . . our culture has been stripped from us . . . and so those traditions are really hard to find—we have to dig for them."

CONCLUSIONS

This chapter reveals that a key function of the relationship between generations of African American women is to bestow upon and accept a better understanding of who they are as women and the culture of which they are part. Unlike some earlier research, this chapter concludes that the determination, strength, and independence conveyed from grandmothers to granddaughters in this study is not a source of pathology or dysfunction in African American family life; rather, it is an indication of what Nobles (1981 p. 82) refers to as legitimation of beingness: "a source of connection, attachment, validation, worth, recognition, respect, and legitimacy." Not unlike their ancestors, these women adapt and prevail regardless of (and, more likely as a result of) the conditions in which they, or their families, exist.

NOTES

1. The author would like to acknowledge Reg Randles for his assistance in completing the grandmothers' and granddaughters' interviews.

2. The use of "Black," "African American," etc. is consistent with (1) each author's use in the time period during which his or her research was conducted, and (2) literal transcription of participants' interviews.

3. The Cultural Relativity school debates the African origin of extended family network or adaptation to conditions of slavery during which children were taken away from mothers; women accepted child care responsibilities even if not caring for their own children.

REFERENCES

Bernard, J. S. 1966. *Marriage and Family Among Negroes.* Englewood Cliffs, New Jersey: Prentice-Hall, Inc.

Billingsley, A. 1968. *Black Families in White America.* Englewood Cliffs, New Jersey: Prentice-Hall.

Boyd-Franklin, N. 1983. Black family life-styles: A lesson in survival (1981). In A. Swerdlow and H. Lessinger, eds., *Class, Race, and Sex: The Dynamics of Control.* New York: Barnard College Women's Center. 189–199.

Burton, L. M. 1992. Black grandparents rearing children of drug-addicted parents: Stressors, outcomes, and social service needs. *The Gerontologist 32(6),* 744–751.

Burton, L. M., and Dilworth-Anderson, P. 1991. The intergenerational family roles of aged Black Americans. *Marriage and Family Review 16(3),* 311–330.

Cheatham, H., and Stewart, J., eds. 1990. *Black Families: Interdisciplinary Perspectives.* New Brunswick, N.J.: Transaction Publications.

Coupland, N., Nussbaum, J. F., and Grossman, A. 1993. Discourse, selfhood, and the lifespan. In N. Coupland and J. F. Nussbaum, eds., *Discourse and Lifespan Identity.* Newbury Park, California: Sage Publications. x–xxviii.

Dill, B. T. 1987. The dialectics of Black womanhood. In S. Harding, ed., *Feminism and Methodology.* Bloomington: Indiana University Press. 97–108.

Dodson, J. 1981. Conceptualizations of black families. In H. P. McAdoo, ed. *Black Families.* Beverly Hills: Sage Publications. 23–36.

English, R. 1974. Beyond pathology: Research and theoretical perspectives on Black families. In L. E. Gary, ed., *Social Research and the Black Community: Selected Issues and Priorities.* Washington, DC: Institute for Urban Affairs and Research.

Frazier, E. F. 1951. *The Negro Family in the United States.* New York: The Dryden Press.

Giddens, A. 1990. *The Consequences of Modernity.* Cambridge: Polity Press.

Giddens, A. 1991. *Modernity and Self-identity: Self and Society in the Late Modern Age.* Cambridge: Polity Press.

Glick, P. C. 1981. A demographic picture of Black families. In H. P. McAdoo, ed., *Black Families.* Beverly Hills: Sage Publications. 106–126.

Gutman, H. G. 1976. *The Black Family in Slavery and Freedom, 1750–1925.* New York: Pantheon Books.

Jackson, J. J. 1971. Aged blacks: A potpourri in the direction of the reduction of inequities. *Phylon 32,* 260–280.

Jones, F. C. 1973. The lofty role of the Black grandmother. *Crisis 80(1),* 19–21.

Ladner, J. A. 1971. *Tomorrow's Tomorrow.* Garden City, New York: Doubleday & Co., Inc.

Ladner, J. A. 1987. Introduction to *Tomorrow's Tomorrow.* In S. Harding, ed., *Feminism and Methodology.* Bloomington, Indiana: Indiana University Press. 74–830.

Lewis, J. M., and Looney, J. G. 1983. *The Long Struggle: Well-Functioning Working-Class Black Families.* New York: Brunner/Mazel Publishers.

Manns, W. 1981. Support systems of significant others in black families. In H. P. McAdoo, ed., *Black Families.* Beverly Hills: Sage Publications. 238–251.

Martin, E. P., and Martin, J. M. 1978. *The Black Extended Family.* Chicago: The University of Chicago Press.

Martin, J. M., and Martin, E. P. 1985. *The Helping Tradition in the Black Family and Community.* Silver Spring, Maryland: National Association of Social Workers.

Mead, G. H. 1932. *Philosophy of the Present.* LaSalle, Illinois: Open Court Press.

Millman, M., and Kanter, R. M. 1987. Introduction to another voice: Feminist perspectives on social life and social science. In S. Harding, ed., *Feminism and Methodology.* Bloomington, Indiana: Indiana University Press. 29–38.

Moynihan, D. P. 1965. *The Negro Family: The Case for National Action.* Washington, D.C.: Government Printing Office.

Nobles, W. W. 1981. African-American family life: An instrument of culture. In H. P. McAdoo, ed., *Black Families.* Beverly Hills: Sage Publications. 77–86.

Rainwater, L. 1971. Identity processes in the family. In R. Staples, ed., *The Black Family: Essays and Studies.* Belmont, California: Wadsworth.

Sawyer, E. 1973. Methodological problems in studying socially deviant communities. In J. A. Ladner, *Death of a White Sociology.* New York: Random House. 38–54.

Sherif, C. W. 1987. Bias in psychology. In S. Harding, ed., *Feminism and Methodology.* Bloomington, Indiana: Indiana University Press. 37–56.

Stack, C. B. 1974a. Sex roles and survival strategies in an urban black community. In M. Z. Rosaldo and L. Lamphere, eds., *Women, Culture, and Society.* Stanford: Stanford University Press. 113–128.

Stack, C. B. 1974b. Personal kindreds. In *All Our Kin: Strategies for Survival in a Black Community.* New York: Harper. 45–61.

Sudarkasa. N. 1981. Interpreting the African heritage in Afro-American family organization. In H. P. McAdoo, ed., *Black Families.* Beverly Hills: Sage Publications. 37–53.

Willie, C. 1976. *A New Look at Black Families.* Bayside, New York: General Hall, Inc.

Index